# Public Health Approach to Cardiovascular Disease Prevention & Management

Cardiovascular diseases (CVDs) are the number one cause of death and disability globally, being the most important public health problem that needs to be tackled as more people die annually from CVDs than from any other cause. Over three-quarters of CVD deaths take place in low- and middle-income countries. This book on cardiovascular diseases provides an overview of the global and regional challenges associated with CVDs. Coupled with case studies and theoretical concepts, it helps the reader to contextualize CVDs in the broader public health system and the administrative aspects of practicing CVD control approaches for improved population health in their local setting.

**Key features:**

1. Covers existing and emerging issues in cardiovascular disease epidemiology and prevention.

2. Has a multidisciplinary approach in content and audience.

3. Connects with health systems and relevant sustainable development goals.

4. Provides case studies enabling readers to understand and apply evidence-based solutions to key public health issues.

5. Has inputs from globally renowned public health experts.

*The book is a master piece. There are very few books that integrate public health aspects of CVD prevention and management. The book is unique in that it addresses all the known risk factors along with introducing emerging risk factors such as air pollution while emphasizing their role across the life span. In terms of solutions it discusses a range of responses from health promotion at one end of the spectrum to universal health coverage at the other end. This book will be useful not only to clinicians but also to public health experts all over the world.*

**Dr V. Mohan**
President & Chief of Diabetes Research, Madras Diabetes Research Foundation
Chairman & Chief Diabetologist, Dr Mohan's Diabetes Specialities Centre

*Jorge Luis Borges (1899–1986) quoted "Of the various instruments invented by man, the most amazing is the book; all the others are extensions of the body of it…Only the book is an extension of the imagination and memory".*

*We celebrate the Publication of Public Health Approaches to Cardiovascular Disease Prevention & Management by Prof. Prabhakaran Dorairaj, K. Srinath Reddy, and Shuchi Anand, and invite everyone interested in cardiovascular health to the fruitful reading of it.*

*The book synthesizes the most modern concepts of the prevention and management of cardiovascular diseases, particularly from the perspective of the implementation science and Public Health.*

**Prof Daniel Pineiro**
Full Professor of Medicine, Universidad de Buenos Aires, Argentina
President-Elect, World Heart Federation, 2021–2022
Trustee, Board of Trustees, American College of Cardiology, 2018–2021

*This book provides a comprehensive overview focused on one of the most pressing public health challenges of our times. Uniquely presenting a truly global health perspective, the authors carefully dissect the complex evidence relating to the promotion of optimal cardiovascular health across the life course. For anyone engaged in the research or practice of public health relating to cardiovascular conditions, especially in low- and middle-income countries, here is an ideal "one-stop-shop" for the current state of the evidence and its practical applications.*

**Prof Anushka Patel**
Vice-Principal Director & Chief Scientist
The George Institute for Global Health
Australia

*Public Health Approach to Cardiovascular Disease Prevention and Management" fills in a needed gap in the field of cardiovascular literature by providing a more holistic approach to cardiovascular health, focusing not only on management of disease but also on promotion of cardiovascular health from a public health perspective. This very well written book will certainly be an excellent companion to all of those interested in cardiovascular health and will be another piece contributing to achieve our common goal of "cardiovascular health for everyone".*

**Prof Fausto J Pinto**
Director, Serviço de Cardiologia e Departamento Coração e
Vasos do CHULN / Head of Department
Professor Catedrático de Medicina/Cardiologia, FMUL—Full Professor
President, Centro Cardiovascular da Universidade de Lisboa (CCUL)
President, World Heart Federation (WHF) (2021–2022)
Past-President, European Society of Cardiology (ESC)

*Despite cardiovascular diseases being the leading causes of premature mortality and disability particularly in low middle income countries, policy and prevention are often neglected and this book is a timely publication to help implement evidence based recommendations to improve population level and patient outcomes.*

**Prof Kamlesh Khunti**
Professor of Primary Care Diabetes and Vascular Medicine
University of Leicester, UK

# Public Health Approach to Cardiovascular Disease Prevention & Management

**Edited By**

**Dorairaj Prabhakaran**

*Public Health Foundation of India and Centre for Chronic Disease Control*

**Shuchi Anand**

*Stanford University*

**K. Srinath Reddy**

*Public Health Foundation of India*

CRC Press

Taylor & Francis Group

Boca Raton London New York

CRC Press is an imprint of the
Taylor & Francis Group, an **informa** business

First edition published 2023
by CRC Press
6000 Broken Sound Parkway NW, Suite 300, Boca Raton, FL 33487-2742

and by CRC Press
4 Park Square, Milton Park, Abingdon, Oxon, OX14 4RN

*CRC Press is an imprint of Taylor & Francis Group, LLC*

© 2023 Taylor & Francis Group, LLC

*Library of Congress Cataloging-in-Publication Data*
Names: Prabhakaran, D., editor. | Anand, Shuchi, editor. | Srinath Reddy, K., editor.
Title: Public health approach to cardiovascular disease prevention & management / edited by Dorairaj Prabhakaran, Shuchi Anand, K. Srinath Reddy.
Description: First edition. | Boca Raton, FL : CRC Press, 2023. | Includes bibliographical references and index. | Summary: "This book provides an overview of the global and regional challenges associated with CVDs. Coupled with case studies and theoretical concepts, it helps the reader to contextualize CVDs in the broader public health system and the administrative aspects of practicing CVD control approaches for improved population health in their local setting"— Provided by publisher.
Identifiers: LCCN 2022043142 (print) | LCCN 2022043143 (ebook) | ISBN 9781032403571 (hardback) | ISBN 9781138483620 (paperback) | ISBN 9781003352686 (ebook)
Subjects: MESH: Cardiovascular Diseases | Public Health Practice | Health Policy
Classification: LCC RA645.C34 (print) | LCC RA645.C34 (ebook) | NLM WG 120 | DDC 362.1961— dc23/eng/20221103
LC record available at https://lccn.loc.gov/2022043142
LC ebook record available at https://lccn.loc.gov/2022043143

ISBN: 978-1-032-40357-1 (hbk)
ISBN: 978-1-138-48362-0 (pbk)
ISBN: 978-1-003-35268-6 (ebk)

DOI: 10.1201/b23266

Typeset in Palatino
by Apex CoVantage, LLC

Dedicated to our students, mentees, patients and the population-at-large from whom we have learnt a lot.

# Contents

# Preface

The iconic Charles Dickens novel *A Tale of Two Cities* opens with the sentence, "It was the best of times, it was the worst of times, it was the age of wisdom, it was the age of foolishness, it was the epoch of belief, it was the epoch of incredulity". While this denoted the Dickensian times, it is also applicable to the current status of cardiovascular disease (CVD) across the world. The world has witnessed tremendous advancements in prevention and management, with an amazing decline (of more than 50%) in CVD deaths and disability across most high-income countries of the world. By contrast, in most low- and middle-income countries (LMICs), where the majority of the world's population lives, deaths due to CVD have increased in the last few decades and have replaced pre-transitional conditions such as infections and nutritional diseases as the leading contributors to deaths. While this is partly explained by a demographic transition that involves population aging, a high burden of premature mortality due to CVD occurs in productive midlife years in the LMICs. The global burden of disease estimates for 2019 calculate that CVD affected 523 million people, almost double the figure of two decades earlier, with one in three CVD deaths occurring prematurely in people under 70 years of age. The majority of these premature deaths (around 90%) are in the LMICs.

There was an air of optimism in the year 2000 when Joe Flower and colleagues, on the occasion of 50 years of American College of Cardiology, wrote "Yet we can now foresee a future in which medical science might actually defeat cardiovascular disease the way it has defeated polio, smallpox, and other serious scourges of the past". They emphasized the technological advances that would bring this change in the next 50 years, where living to 100 years would be the norm. The current thinking across the world of cardiology emphasizes the individual approach, ignoring the power of prevention and public health approaches. Indeed, as a patient told one of us, "It's not until you are lying on the cold catheterization lab table that you reflect on your life choices", manifesting the crux of the problem for public health: in order to realize the true value of health and engage in preventive actions, many persons must experience a serious health event. This may be in part why the focus on health becomes one of secondary prevention. Only once a person becomes 'medicalized', in other words, only when a person becomes a patient, do they benefit from the largest share of our resources and knowledge basis. Pharmaceutical and device industries proffer lifesaving therapies, but for a small proportion of the world's population: those who are patients and those who can afford them.

While competent clinical care helps to save several lives, the cumulative risk of CVD that builds over the preceding years still snips away several years of healthy life expectancy. Many lives are lost or shortened, despite the benefit of medical care, while some die suddenly without getting to see their doctor. A public health approach to CVD has to combine prevention across the life course at both population and individual levels.

This textbook shifts the focus from the patient back to the person and the population. In the first portion, the reader will be guided through the current clinical understanding of CVDs, in parallel with key concepts and strategies that can be applied for primary and secondary prevention. We walk through the well-recognized risk factors for its development, one of which (i.e., tobacco) has been successfully addressed on the individual and sociocultural level, but many of which, including diet and physical activity, remain recalcitrant—and are ripe for creative solutions. Uniquely we acknowledge and address social determinants of cardiovascular health. The first portion of this book justifies the urgent need for a health systems approach, and the latter portion puts forward a framework for such an approach. A public health-focused health system integrates cost-effectiveness analyses with technology assessments, surveillance systems, and formal health promotion strategies.

The goal of public health is not only to add life to years but add years to life, thereby ensuring everyone has a full and fulsome life which embodies health and well-being. This requires a paradigm shift from CVD to focus on cardiovascular health. Achieving cardiovascular health for all by 2030 (the year of the Sustainable Development Goals [SDGs]) is interdependent on synergy between people adopting patterns of healthy living and the systems that enable and support them. This book attempts to emphasize the importance of public health approaches in achieving cardiovascular health through promotive, preventive, and restorative approaches. This basic tenet resonates throughout the following pages.

*Dorairaj Prabhakaran*
*Shuchi Anand*
*K. Srinath Reddy*

## Acknowledgments

We are extremely grateful to all the authors for their enriching contributions to this book and for generously sharing their expertise, experience, and time. Editing a book for a global audience and readers from diverse disciplines poses several challenges, but the authors made the task of the editors easy with their manuscripts that were simple to read, and yet comprehensive and contemporary.

The editors greatly appreciate the contribution of several individuals, colleagues, and friends who accompanied us on this journey. While we are unable to list all the names here, we are grateful to each one of you who made the editing of this book an immensely enjoyable experience.

Specifically, we would like to specially mention the contribution of Ms. Jimly Shiju, Executive Assistant to Dr Prabhakaran. Jimly is a thorough professional with excellent attention to detail. She diligently handled all communications with authors and the publisher, besides helping us organize and edit many sections. We are greatly indebted to her for the sustained efforts to ensure the highest quality.

We would like to convey our thanks and appreciation to the publishers Taylor and Francis for their abundant patience. We are thankful to Ms. Shivangi Pramanik and Himani Dwivedi for nudging us periodically with their gentle requests. Their elegant editing enhanced the readability of the final product.

We are very thankful to our students who inspired us to write this book. The book would not been conceived without the patients and communities who entrusted their health to our care, as we assisted them in promoting, protecting, or restoring their health. They taught us empathy and inspired this book.

Finally, we are very thankful to our families who never complained about the many weekends and holidays spent over the last 2 years in preparing the book. Their understanding is what the heart is all about.

*Dorairaj Prabhakaran*
*Shuchi Anand*
*K. Srinath Reddy*

## About the Editors

### Dorairaj Prabhakaran

Professor Dorairaj Prabhakaran is a cardiologist, epidemiologist and internationally renowned researcher. He is vice president of research and policy, Public Health Foundation of India; executive director of the Centre for Chronic Disease Control, New Delhi, India; and professor (epidemiology), London School of Hygiene and Tropical Medicine, UK. In addition he is an adjunct professor/scientist/fellow at Emory University, Harvard University, McMaster and Simon Fraser University, Canada. He is also a fellow of the Indian National Science Academy and the Royal College of Physicians, UK. He was recently awarded an Honorary Doctor of Science by the University of Glasgow. He has authored over 600 scholarly papers with an H index of 100. He ranks among the top 2% of researchers listed by Stanford University in 2021. He is the lead editor of *Tandon's Textbook of Cardiology*, a two volume, comprehensive book on cardiology for Indian cardiologists and fellows. His work includes mechanistic research to understand the causes for increased propensity of cardiovascular diseases among Indians and developing solutions for chronic diseases through translational research and human resource development.

### Shuchi Anand

Shuchi Anand, MD, MS, is Director of the Center for Tubulointerstitial Kidney Disease at Stanford University (http://stan.md/tikidney). She received her medical degree from Washington University School of Medicine in St. Louis and completed her internal medicine training at Brigham and Women's Hospital (Partners Healthcare, Harvard Medical School) in Boston. She completed her master's in clinical epidemiology and a nephrology fellowship at Stanford University School of Medicine.

Dr. Anand is engaged in clinical research aimed at advancing the care of patients with kidney disease living in low-resource settings using practical tools. She has active projects in collaboration with the University of Utah to promote exercise programming for underserved populations, with the Centre for Chronic Disease Control in India to study risk factors for kidney disease in South Asians, and with Kandy Hospital Sri Lanka to investigate chronic kidney disease of unknown etiology affecting agricultural communities. During the COVID-19 pandemic Dr. Anand also participated in partnership to elucidate seroepidemiology, vaccine acceptance and response to vaccination among patients on dialysis. She is part of two National Institutes of Health (NIH) consortia focused on improving the health of underserved populations.

### K. Srinath Reddy

K. Srinath Reddy is president of Public Health Foundation of India (PHFI). Trained in cardiology and epidemiology, he previously headed the Department of Cardiology at the All India Institute of Medical Sciences, Delhi. He was president of the World Heart Federation (2013–2014) and was the first Bernard Lown Visiting Professor of Global Cardiovascular Health at Harvard. He is presently an adjunct professor at Harvard, Emory, and Sydney Universities. He chaired the High-Level Expert Group on Universal Health Coverage for the Planning Commission of India and has served on many World Health Organization (WHO) expert panels. He has over 570 scientific publications. He is a member of the US National Academy of Medicine and has received the WHO Director General's Award for outstanding contributions to global tobacco control and several honorary doctorates.

# Contributors

**Yamuna Ana**
Public Health Foundation of India
Indian Institute of Public Health-Bengaluru,
    India

**Shuchi Anand**
Stanford University
Palo Alto, California, US

**Sven Andreasson**
Department of Global Public Health
Karolinska Institutet
Solna, Sweden

**Monika Arora**
Health Promotion Division
Public Health Foundation of India, Gurugram
Haryana, India

**Radhika Prakash Asrani**
Rollins School of Public Health
Emory University
Atlanta, Georgia, US

**Giridhara R. Babu**
Public Health Foundation of India
Indian Institute of Public Health-Bengaluru,
    India

**Manjusha Chatterjee**
NCD Alliance, London
United Kingdom

**Arun K. Chopra, MD, DM, FACC, FSCAI**
Fortis Escorts Hospital
Amritsar, India

**Aastha Chugh**
HRIDAY
New Delhi, India

**Thomas A. Gaziano, MD, MSc**
Department of Cardiovascular Medicine
Brigham & Women's Hospital
Boston, Massachusetts, US

**Abdul Ghaffar**
Alliance for Health Policy and Systems
    Research/WHO
Geneva, Switzerland

**Samuel S. Gidding, MD**
Genomic Medicine institute
Danville, Pennsylvania, US

**Shifalika Goenka**
Public Health Foundation of India, Gurugram,
    Haryana, India
Centre for Chronic Disease Control, New Delhi,
    India

**Tilahun Haregu**
University of Melbourne
Melbourne, Australia

**Kaitlin Harold**
Stanford University
Palo Alto, California, US

**Greg Heath**
University of Tennessee at Chattanooga
Chattanooga, Tennessee, US

**Lindsay M. Jaacks**
The University of Edinburgh
Edinburgh, Scotland, UK

**Ram Jagannathan**
Emory University
School of Medicine
Atlanta, Georgia, US

**Neha Jain**
Health Promotion Division
Public Health Foundation of India,
    Gurugram
Haryana, India

**Panniyammakal Jeemon**
Sree Chitra Tirunal Institute for Medical
    Sciences and Technology
Kerala, India

**Devraj Jindal**
Centre for Chronic Disease Control
New Delhi, India

**Arun Pulikkottil Jose**
Public Health Foundation of India, Gurugram
Haryana, India

**Prachi Kathuria**
HRIDAY
New Delhi, India

**Min Kyung Kim**
Department of Global Health and Population
Harvard T.H. Chan School of Public Health
Boston, Massachusetts, US

**Anand Krishnan**
Centre for Community Medicine
All India Institute of Medical Sciences
New Delhi, India

**Margaret E. Kruk**
Department of Global Health and Population
Harvard T.H. Chan School of Public Health
Boston, Massachusetts, US

**R. Krishna Kumar, MD, DM, FAHA**
Pediatric Cardiology
Amrita Institute of Medical Sciences and
    Research Centre, Cochin
Kerala, India

**Dorothy Lall, MD**
Institute of Public Health
Bengaluru, India

**Hannah H. Leslie**
Department of Global Health and Population
Harvard T.H. Chan School of Public Health
Boston, Massachusetts, US

**Manu Raj Mathur**
Public Health Foundation of India
Gurugram, Haryana, India

**Sailesh Mohan**
Public Health Foundation of India
Centre for Chronic Conditions and Injuries
    (CCCI), Gurugram
Haryana, India
Deakin University, Australia
Centre for Chronic Disease Control
New Delhi, India

**Prarthna Mukerjee, BDS, MPH**
Public Health Foundation of India,
    Gurugram
Haryana, India

**K.M. Venkat Narayan, MD, MSc, MBA**
Rollins School of Public Health
Emory University
Emory University School of Medicine
Atlanta, Georgia, US

**Rachel Nugent**
RTI International
Washington, USA

**Brian Oldenburg**
University of Melbourne
Melbourne, Australia

**Lorraine Oldridge**
National Cardiovascular Intelligence Network
    (NCVIN)
Health Improvement Directorate—Knowledge
    and Intelligence
Public Health England
Shrey Department of Internal Medicine
University of Texas Southwestern Medical
    Center
Dallas, Texas, US

**Rima N. Pai**
Rollins School of Public Health
Emory University
Atlanta, Georgia, US

**Rajmohan Panda**
Public Health Foundation of India (PHFI)
Gurugram, Haryana, India

**Ambarish Pandey, MD, MSCS**
Department of Internal Medicine
University of Texas Southwestern
    Medical Center
Dallas, Texas, US

**Shivani A. Patel**
Rollins School of Public Health
Emory University
Atlanta, Georgia, US

**Neil R. Poulter**
Imperial Clinical Trials Unit
Imperial College London
London, UK

**Dorairaj Prabhakaran**
Public Health Foundation of India, Gurugram,
    Haryana, India
Centre for Chronic Disease Control
New Delhi, India
London School of Hygiene and
    Tropical Medicine
London, UK

**Poornima Prabhakaran**
Public Health Foundation of India, Gurugram,
    Haryana, India

**Johanna Ralston**
World Obesity Federation
London, UK

**Shreya Rao**
University of Texas Southwestern Medical
    Center
Dallas, TX USA

**K. Srinath Reddy**
Public Health Foundation of India, Gurugram,
    Haryana, India

**Piyu Sharma**
Centre for Chronic Disease Control
New Delhi, India

**Krithiga Shridhar**
Public Health Foundation of India, Gurugram,
    Haryana, India

**Radhika Shrivastav**
HRIDAY
New Delhi, India

**Ricardo A. Peña Silva, MD, PhD**
College of Medicine
Universidad de Los Andes
Bogotá, Colombia
Lown Scholars Program
Department of Global Health and
    Population
Harvard T.H. Chan School of Public
    Health
Boston, Massachusetts, US

**Vinita Subramanya**
Rollins School of Public Health
Emory University
Atlanta, Georgia, US

**Sugitha Sureshkumar**
Institute of Global Health
University of Geneva
Geneva, Switzerland

# 1 Introduction to Cardiovascular Diseases

*Dorairaj Prabhakaran*

## CONTENTS

## INTRODUCTION

Cardiovascular diseases (CVDs) are the leading cause of death worldwide. However, there is substantial heterogeneity in the burden of CVD between high-income and low- and middle-income countries (LMICs). The United States witnessed a tremendous population-level decline in CVD mortality of 75% within a span of 50 years (1). Similar changes have been observed in many other high-income countries (HICs) (2, 3). There also has been a huge decline in the mortality of acute myocardial infarction (heart attacks) from a high of 30% in the 1960s to the current 4%. By contrast, the LMICs are witnessing an increase in CVD burden with a high burden of premature mortality due to CVD (4). Nearly 80% of CVD deaths occur in LMICs, and nearly 40% of these are premature (5). For example, the mortality due to CVD among those less than 70 years is approximately 22%. It is highly variable, and more than 50–70% in various LMICs. The reduction in CVD mortality in HICs is attributable to the advances in cardiac care as well as a decline in CVD risk factors. While the reasons for the differences between HICs and LMICs are intuitive, we need a detailed explanation of the causes for the huge differences in CVD burden across the world. This will also enable us to identify potential public health policy to combat the burgeoning CVD epidemic.

## WHAT ARE CARDIOVASCULAR DISEASES?

The World Health Organization (WHO) defines CVDs as disorders of the heart and blood vessels (6). These include:

- coronary heart disease or ischemic heart disease: disease of the blood vessels supplying the heart muscle. This includes myocardial infarction (heart attacks) and unstable and stable angina.

- cerebrovascular disease: resulting from of disease of the blood vessels supplying the brain either due to atherosclerotic occlusion, embolism or hemorrhage. These result in various forms of stroke.

- peripheral arterial disease: disease of blood vessels supplying the arms and legs, frequently manifesting as intermittent claudication (pain in the limbs on walking or while exercising) or as gangrene.

- rheumatic heart disease: damage to the heart muscle and heart valves from rheumatic fever, caused by streptococcal bacteria.

- congenital heart disease: birth defects that affect the normal development and functioning of the heart caused by malformations of the heart structure from birth.

- deep vein thrombosis and pulmonary embolism: blood clots in the leg veins, which can dislodge and move to the heart and lungs.

DOI: 10.1201/b23266-1

Heart attacks and strokes are usually acute events and are mainly caused by a blockage that prevents blood from flowing to the heart or brain. The most common reason for this is a build-up of fatty deposits on the inner walls of the blood vessels that supply the heart or brain. Strokes can be caused by bleeding from a blood vessel in the brain or from blood clots.

## WHAT ARE THE REASONS FOR THE DIFFERENCES IN CVD MORTALITY BETWEEN HICS AND LMICS?

The major reasons that can be attributed to the differences are population-level factors that include the following:

1. The epidemiological transition resulting from changes in population structure and demographic shifts

2. Globalization and urbanization resulting in adverse lifestyle changes

3. Inadequate or insufficient policy measures resulting in poor population-level prevention of CVD

4. Inadequate or rudimentary health systems not geared to address the rising burden of CVD or competing priorities such as high burden of infectious, nutritional and other diseases

5. Inherent ethnic differences

## EPIDEMIOLOGICAL TRANSITION

The Epidemiological transition is discussed in detail in Chapter 2 but a brief summary is provided here for completion. Epidemiological transition refers to a change in the pattern of disease in a country away from infectious diseases toward degenerative diseases (7). This theory was originally proposed in 1971 by Omran (8). The theory focused on the complex changes in patterns of health and disease and on the interactions between these patterns and their demographic, economic and sociological determinants and consequences. The process includes a transition from less developed to developed countries, from an agrarian economy to industrialized economy and replacement of premodern diseases such as infectious and maternal and child health diseases as the predominant disease pattern with modern diseases such as cardiovascular and other chronic diseases. In addition, healthcare undergoes a significant transformation from a primitive form of healthcare to a modern one that comprises a mix of prevention strategies as well as advanced treatments, particularly for acute care such as the management of acute myocardial infarction (AMI). For example, in India, the rapid transition has been demonstrated by the recently published State-Level Disease Burden study of the GBD study group (9). It showed that the epidemiological transition ratios (ratio of communicable diseases to noncommunicable diseases [NCDs]) for all states in India were less than 0.75 in 2016 as compared with those in the year 1990, during which only the South Indian state of Kerala and a few union territories had a predominance of NCDs and injuries. According to the study, the epidemiological transition ratios dropped to less than 1 (i.e., Disability Adjusted Life Years [DALYs] due to NCDs and injuries became greater than communicable diseases) for India as a whole in the year 2003.

## WHY DO WE NEED TO UNDERSTAND EPIDEMIOLOGICAL TRANSITION?

An understanding of epidemiological transition enables both physicians and policy makers to learn from historical patterns of transition to better anticipate the health needs of the population and intervene appropriately. Furthermore, it explains the heterogeneity in CVD patterns across nations. Many countries across the world continue to have a high burden of rheumatic heart disease, while it is virtually nonexistent in HICs with less overcrowding and high levels of development. Similarly, hemorrhagic stroke is observed frequently in early phases of transition such as in sub-Saharan Africa, while ischemic stroke is more frequent in countries with higher levels of economic development.

## CHANGING PATTERNS IN CVD

Four distinct stages of epidemiological transition have been described by Olshansky and Ault (10). A fifth stage was added later (Chapter 2), the pattern of CVDs is distinct in different stages of transition. The first stage, often called the stage of pestilence and famine with a life expectancy of 35 years, is characterized by a low prevalence of CVD (5–10% mortality). At this stage, the predominant CVD is nutritional CVD such as beriberi and rheumatic heart disease. Rheumatic heart disease is predominantly seen in upper socioeconomic classes. In the second stage (receding pandemics), the life expectancy increases to 50 years, with CVD contributing approximately to 35% of mortality. The predominant disease pattern continues to be nutritional and rheumatic heart diseases along with hemorrhagic stroke. These diseases are distributed equally among all socioeconomic classes. The predominant cardiovascular risk factors at this stage are smoking and hypertension, particularly in the upper socioeconomic classes. The third stage, described as the stage of "degenerative and man-made diseases," is characterized by a high burden of chronic midlife diseases with CVD contributing to >50% mortality. Coronary artery disease (CAD) is the predominant CVD along with both ischemic and hemorrhagic stroke. The life expectancy is around 60 years, and the poor are affected predominantly. In the final stage (delayed degenerative diseases), CVD starts declining and is responsible for less than 50% of mortality. It becomes predominantly a disease of the poor and uneducated, as is being observed in the Western populations. Life expectancy increases, and CVD mostly affects the elderly who are above 70 years of age. In addition to the earlier facts, Gaziano report a fifth stage—the age of inactivity and obesity (11). In many parts of the industrialized world, there has been a continuous decline in physical activity (PA) accompanied by an increase in total calorie intake. The slowing down in improvements of other risk factors such as smoking coupled with an increase in obesity and PA can plateau the declining trend in CVD mortality observed in HICs or, worse, may even cause it to increase in coming years.

## Ethnic Differences

Ethnic differences contribute to the occurrence and consequences of CVD in many parts of the world (5). For example, the reasons for heart failure are diverse across the world, with the predominance of heart failure related to high blood pressure and rheumatic heart disease in Africa, Chagas disease in Latin America and coronary heart disease in India. It is also unclear as to why the same disease process results in high burden of coronary heart disease among South Asians as compared to stroke in the Chinese population. The discussions on ethnic differences are beyond the scope of this book, and readers are directed to some excellent references (5).

## Why Do We Need Public Health Approaches for the Prevention of CVD?
### *History*

It has been long known that several social determinants play a major role in the causation and control of several diseases. Indeed, the German pathologist Rudolf Virchow, when asked to investigate the epidemic of typhus in upper Silesia in 1848, wrote three principles which have been the guiding principles in understanding social determinants of diseases (12–14):

> For there can now no longer be any doubt that such an epidemic of typhus had only been possible under wretched condition of life that poverty and lack of hygiene had created in Upper Silesia. If these conditions were removed I am sure this epidemic typhus would not recur.
> Do we not always find the disease of the populace traceable to defects in the society.

This reasoning for societal causes for an infection was extended to CVDs by the celebrated British epidemiologist Sir Geoffrey Rose in his seminal article "Sick Individuals and Sick Populations" (14). Therefore, the proof to this hypothesis was that if we correct or address the societal causes, we may be able to reduce the burden of several risk factors of CVD. Box 1.1 elegantly illustrates how the population prevalence of blood pressure (BP) can be reduced if we address air pollution. For example, ensuring the attainment of national ambient air quality standards (40 $\mu g/m^3$) from the

---

**BOX 1.1 HYPERTENSION 2020**

| Annual Average PM 2.5 in 2016 in the City of Delhi (in $\mu g/m^3$) | Decrease from Current Average of 125 $\mu g/m^3$ | % Decrease in Prevalent Hypertension |
| --- | --- | --- |
| 100 | 25 | 5.5 |
| 75 | 50 | 9.9 |
| 40 (national standard) | 85 | 15.1 |

*Treating sick populations: Non–personal policy interventions can have major benefits.*

*Source*: Prabhakaran et al. (15)

mean level of PM 2.5 in 2016 would potentially decrease the prevalence of hypertension by 15% in the city of Delhi, India (15). Such a change would result in major public health benefits.

Historically two major studies in the mid-20th century contributed to an understanding of the role of risk factors in the causation of CVDs. These include the Framingham Heart Study (Box 1.2) (16) which identified the most important risk factors for chronic disease, particularly the role of smoking, diet and physical activity and the British Doctors' Study (Box 1.3) which provided robust evidence for smoking and CVD (17). The success of CVD reduction in HICs is attributable to robust tobacco control policies, an enabling environment to follow healthy practices and the robust primary care that caters to CVD.

## WHAT ARE THE APPROACHES TO REDUCING CVD BURDEN?

The approaches to CVD burden can be largely classified into two groups: First, a population-based approach which attempts a modest reduction in population-level risk factors. For example, even a 2 mm reduction of diastolic BP at a population level can result in substantial gains by reducing CVD mortality and stroke. This could be done, for example, by reduction of salt consumption at a population level, alcohol control measures or reducing air pollution in communities through defined policy measures. The second example is provision of polypill or fixed-dose combinations, as proposed by Wald and Law and subsequently demonstrated in a recent individual patient meta-analysis (18, 19). Similarly, the second approach is termed a high-risk approach which attempts treatment to targets of all those with high-risk factor levels. Examples include treatment of all those with hypertension to get their BP to <140/90 or preventing a second heart attack or stroke among those who developed a myocardial infarction by secondary prevention and rehabilitation. Both of these approaches are complementary and have contributed along with advances in cardiovascular care in equal measure to the reductions observed in CVD burden across the HICs. For example, Unal et al showed between 1981 and 2000 that coronary heart disease mortality rates in England and Wales decreased by 62% in men and 45% in women 25 to 84 years old (Figure 1.1). Some 42% of this decrease was attributed to treatments in individuals and 58% to population risk factor reductions (principally smoking) (20).

## WHY DO WE NEED PUBLIC HEALTH APPROACHES?

Based on these examples, it is clear that nonpersonal population approaches have a major role to play in reducing CVD burden in several countries. Not only are they cost-effective but they can save costs to countries by preventing the need for expensive treatments of acute cardiovascular

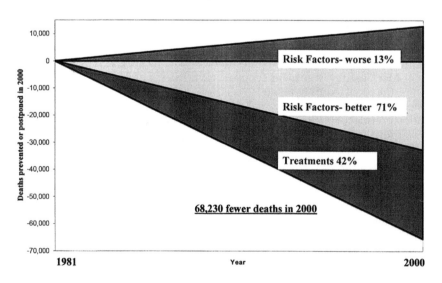

**Figure 1.1** Contributions of risk factors and treatments to the decline of CVD in the United Kingdom.

*Source*: With permission from reference (20).

illness such as myocardial infarction or stroke. Several examples of public health approaches are discussed in the subsequent chapters.

However, public health approaches have been largely ignored in many parts of the world. Thus there is a need to create awareness among public health professionals, cardiologists, physicians, policy makers and other stakeholders on the various approaches to reduce the burgeoning CVD burden in the world.

## What This Book Intends to Do

Given the rising burden of CVD in the LMICs, this book focuses on CVD prevention in LMICs. It comprehensively summarizes the role of public health approaches in preventing and managing CVD. It takes a continuum-of-care approach with importance to social determinants and upstream policy measures. It encompasses everything from early prevention to rehabilitation. Each of the chapters in the book provides simple explanations of the disease or risk factor addressed and the public health solutions to address them.

---

### BOX 1.2: FRAMINGHAM HEART STUDY (FHS)

The Framingham Heart Study is a long-term, multigenerational, ongoing cohort study that began in 1948 in the city of Framingham, Massachusetts, United States, with 5,209 participants. When US President Roosevelt died in 1945 due to a cerebral hemorrhage with a blood pressure of 300/190 mmHg, the country was presented with a grave reality—that of a CVD epidemic.

Soon after, signing of a "National Heart Act" led to an acceleration of research into the causes of CVDs that acted as a seed opportunity for CVD epidemiological studies, such as the FHS. Over the years, the FHS has led to understanding the epidemiology of heart failure; the development of "risk profiles" such as the Framingham Risk score, published in 1998 by Wilson and colleagues; and the identification and understanding of major modifiable risk factors contributing to CVDs, such as high BP, high cholesterol, smoking and diabetes.

The data from FHS has helped in understanding the immense power of a family-based approach towards the development of cohorts and understanding of various CVD risk factors. It has led to a shift from treatment of individuals with CVDs to prevention of the disease for those at risk (16).

---

### BOX 1.3: BRITISH DOCTORS' STUDY

The British Doctors' Study was a cohort study conducted from 1951 to 2001 at the University of Oxford, United Kingdom, among 33,439 male British doctors, with the overarching aim that tobacco smoking was associated with an increased risk of lung cancer and CVDs. The study was initiated by epidemiologists Richard Doll and Austin Bradford Hill, who studied the smoking habits and development of diseases among the British physicians participating in the study.

Their preliminary report indicated an association between tobacco smoking and lung cancer. Later on, they went on to track the mortality and diseases rates of the doctors and collected data on CVDs and myocardial infarction. Their preliminary findings, published in 1954 in "The Mortality of Doctors in Relation to Their Smoking Habits: A Preliminary Report" in the *British Medical Journal*, reported strong correlations between tobacco smoking and myocardial infarction and slight correlations between tobacco use and other CVDs. However, their follow-up report in 1956, "Lung Cancer and Other Causes of Death in Relation to Smoking," reported a strong correlation between smoking and CVDs (21).

The British Doctors' Study and the reports published as a result have contributed greatly to the understanding of tobacco and smoking as major risk factors for not only lung cancer but cardiovascular diseases. It has built a benchmark for further research studying smoking patterns among countries, leading to the development of effective interventions for tobacco control, higher tobacco taxations and other policies that aim at smoking cessation.

ACKNOWLEDGEMENTS

Aprajita Kaushik, Research Associate, Centre for Chronic Disease Control, New Delhi, India.

REFERENCES

1. Goff DC, Khan SS, Lloyd-Jones D, Arnett DK, Carnethon MR, Labarthe DR, et al. Bending the curve in cardiovascular disease mortality: Bethesda + 40 and beyond. Circulation [Internet]. 2021 Feb 23 [cited 2022 Apr 4];143:837–851. Available from: www.ahajournals.org/doi/abs/10.1161/CIRCULATIONAHA.120.046501

2. Mensah GA, Wei GS, Sorlie PD, Fine LJ, Rosenberg Y, Kaufmann PG, et al. Decline in cardiovascular mortality. Circulation Research [Internet]. 2017 Jan 20 [cited 2022 Apr 4];120(2):366–380. Available from: www.ahajournals.org/doi/abs/10.1161/CIRCRESAHA.116.309115

3. Moran AE, Forouzanfar MH, Roth GA, Mensah GA, Ezzati M, Murray CJL, et al. Temporal trends in ischemic heart disease mortality in 21 world regions, 1980 to 2010: the global burden of disease 2010 study. Circulation [Internet]. 2014 Apr 8 [cited 2022 Apr 4];129(14):1483–1492. Available from: www.ahajournals.org/doi/abs/10.1161/circulationaha.113.004042

4. Prabhakaran D, Anand S, Watkins D, Gaziano T, Wu Y, Mbanya JC, et al. Cardiovascular, respiratory, and related disorders: key messages from disease control priorities, 3rd edition. Lancet [Internet]. 2018 Mar 24 [cited 2022 Apr 4];391(10126):1224. Available from: /pmc/articles/PMC5996970/

5. Anand S, Bradshaw C, Prabhakaran D. Prevention and management of CVD in LMICs: why do ethnicity, culture, and context matter? BMC Medicine [Internet]. 2020 Jan 24 [cited 2022 Apr 4];18(1). Available from: /pmc/articles/PMC6979081/

6. Cardiovascular diseases (CVDs) [Internet]. [cited 2022 Mar 31]. Available from: www.who.int/news-room/fact-sheets/detail/cardiovascular-diseases-(cvds)

7. Prabhakaran D, Kumar RK, Naik N. Tandon's Textbook of Cardiology [Internet]. Wolters Kluwer; 2019. Available from: https://books.google.co.in/books?id=S3m9xgEACAAJ

8. Omran AR. The epidemiologic transition: a theory of the epidemiology of population change. The Milbank Quarterly [Internet]. 2005 [cited 2022 Apr 4];83(4):731. Available from: /pmc/articles/PMC2690264/

9. Prabhakaran D, Jeemon P, Sharma M, Roth GA, Johnson C, Harikrishnan S, et al. The changing patterns of cardiovascular diseases and their risk factors in the states of India: the global burden of disease study 1990–2016. The Lancet Global Health [Internet]. 2018 Dec 1 [cited 2022 Apr 4];6(12):e1339. Available from: /pmc/articles/PMC6227386/

10. Olshansky SJ, Ault AB. The fourth stage of the epidemiologic transition: the age of delayed degenerative diseases. The Milbank Quarterly. 1986;64(3):355.

11. Gaziano JM. Fifth phase of the epidemiologic transition: the age of obesity and inactivity. JAMA [Internet]. 2010 Jan 20 [cited 2022 Apr 4];303(3):275–276. Available from: https://jamanetwork.com/journals/jama/fullarticle/185220

12. Virchow RC. Report on the typhus epidemic in Upper Silesia. 1848. American Journal of Public Health. 2006 Dec;96(12):2102–2105. doi: 10.2105/ajph.96.12.2102. PMID: 17123938; PMCID: PMC1698167.

13. Rudolf Virchow said. "Do we not always find the diseases of . . . | by Remedy | Medium [Internet]. [cited 2022 Apr 4]. Available from: https://medium.com/@Remedy_health/rudolf-virchow-said-9b6ececb5609

14. Rose G. Sick individuals and sick populations. International Journal of Epidemiology [Internet]. 2001 Jun 1 [cited 2022 Apr 4];30(3):427–432. Available from: https://academic.oup.com/ije/article/30/3/427/736897

15. Prabhakaran D, Mandal S, Krishna B, Magsumbol M, Singh K, Tandon N, et al. Exposure to particulate matter is associated with elevated blood pressure and incident hypertension in urban India. Hypertension [Internet]. 2020 [cited 2022 Apr 4];76(4):1289. Available from: /pmc/articles/PMC7484465/

16. Mahmood SS, Levy D, Vasan RS, Wang TJ. The Framingham Heart Study and the epidemiology of cardiovascular disease: a historical perspective. Lancet. 2014 Mar 15;383(9921):999–1008. doi: 10.1016/S0140-6736(13)61752-3. Epub 2013 Sep 29. PMID: 24084292; PMCID: PMC4159698.

17. Doll R, Peto R, Boreham J, Sutherland I. Mortality in relation to smoking: 50 years' observations on male British doctors. British Medical Journal. 2004 Jun 26;328(7455):1519. doi: 10.1136/bmj.38142.554479.AE. Epub 2004 Jun 22. PMID: 15213107; PMCID: PMC437139.18.

18. Wald NJ, Law MR. A strategy to reduce cardiovascular disease by more than 80%. British Medical Journal. 2003 Jun 28;326(7404):1419. doi: 10.1136/bmj.326.7404.1419. Erratum in: British Medical Journal. 2003 Sep 13;327(7415):586. Erratum in: British Medical Journal. 2006 Sep;60(9):823. PMID: 12829553; PMCID: PMC162259.

19. Joseph P, Roshandel G, Gao P, Pais P, Lonn E, Xavier D, et al. Fixed-dose combination therapies with and without aspirin for primary prevention of cardiovascular disease: an individual participant data meta-analysis. The Lancet [Internet]. 2021 Sep 25 [cited 2022 Apr 4];398(10306):1133–1146. Available from: www.thelancet.com/article/S0140673621018274/fulltext

20. Unal B, Critchley JA, Capewell S. Explaining the decline in coronary heart disease mortality in England and Wales between 1981 and 2000. Circulation [Internet]. 2004 Mar 9 [cited 2022 Mar 31];109(9):1101–1107. Available from: www.ahajournals.org/doi/abs/10.1161/01.CIR.0000118498.35499.B2

21. Doll R, Hill AB. The mortality of doctors in relation to their smoking habits. British Medical Journal. 1954 Jun 6;1(4877):1451.

# 2 Cardiovascular Diseases Worldwide

*Thomas A. Gaziano*

## CONTENTS

## INTRODUCTION

Cardiovascular disease (CVD) is now the most common cause of death worldwide. Before 1900, infectious diseases and malnutrition were the most common causes, and CVD was responsible for <10% of all deaths. In 2019, CVD accounted for 18.6 million deaths worldwide (32.8%), with essentially the same rates now occurring in high-income countries (32.5%) as in low- and middle-income countries (LMICs) combined (32.9%) (1). CVDs include a myriad of non-infectious conditions affecting the heart (myocardial infarction, angina, valvular disease, and cardiomyopathies), major blood vessels themselves (aneurysms and peripheral vascular disease), and their blood supply to the brain, including stroke. In addition, infectious conditions still persist, including rheumatic heart disease and Chagas disease. Genetic, behavioral, socioeconomic, and environmental risk factors all have played a role to a greater or lesser extent over time contributing to both infectious and non-infectious etiologies.

This chapter will review the CVD burden over time and its changing patterns in different regions of the world. It will explore differences in risk factors and behaviors along with regional trends. There will be a review of the economic impact of these trends and a highlighting of cost-effective interventions and then the chapter will turn to diverse challenges and public health interventions and policies that decision-makers can use to influence the reduction in the current burden through screening, prevention, and treatment.

## THE EPIDEMIOLOGIC TRANSITION

The global rise in CVD is the result of an unprecedented transformation in the causes of morbidity and mortality during the twentieth century. Known as the epidemiologic transition, this shift is driven by industrialization, urbanization, and associated lifestyle and demographic changes and is taking place in every part of the world among all races, ethnic groups, and cultures (2, 3). The transition is divided into four basic stages: pestilence and famine, receding pandemics, degenerative and man-made diseases, and delayed degenerative diseases. A fifth stage, characterized by an epidemic of inactivity and obesity, is emerging in some countries (Table 2.1).

The *age of pestilence and famine* is marked by malnutrition, infectious diseases, and high infant and child mortality. Infectious diseases such as tuberculosis, dysentery, cholera, and influenza are often fatal, resulting in a mean life expectancy of about 30 years. CVD, which accounts for <10% of deaths, takes the form of rheumatic heart disease and cardiomyopathies due to infection and malnutrition. Approximately 10% of the world's population living primarily in LMICs remains in the age of pestilence and famine.

DOI: 10.1201/b23266-2

## Table 2.1 **Five Stages of the Epidemiologic Transition**

| Stage | Description | Deaths Related to CVD (%) | Predominant CVD Type |
|---|---|---|---|
| Pestilence and famine | Predominance of malnutrition and infectious diseases as causes of death; high rates of infant and child mortality; low mean life expectancy | <10 | Rheumatic heart disease, cardiomyopathies caused by infection and malnutrition |
| Receding pandemics | Improvements in nutrition and public health lead to decrease in rates of deaths related to malnutrition and infection; precipitous decline in infant and child mortality rates | 10–35 | Rheumatic valvular disease, hypertension, CHD, and stroke (predominantly hemorrhagic) |
| Degenerative and man-made diseases | Increased fat and caloric intake and decrease in physical activity lead to emergence of hypertension and atherosclerosis; with increase in life expectancy, mortality from chronic, non-communicable diseases exceeds mortality from malnutrition and infectious disease | 35–65 | CHD and stroke (ischemic and hemorrhagic) |
| Delayed degenerative diseases | CVD and cancer are the major causes of morbidity and mortality; better treatment and prevention efforts help avoid deaths among those with disease and delay primary events; age-adjusted CVD morality declines; CVD affecting older and older individuals | 40–50 | CHD, stroke, and congestive heart failure |
| Inactivity and obesity | Overweight and obesity increase at alarming rate; diabetes and hypertension increase; decline in smoking rates levels off; a minority of the population meets physical activity recommendations | 38 | CHD, stroke, congestive heart failure, peripheral vascular disease |

*Abbreviations:* CHD, coronary heart disease; CVD, cardiovascular disease.

*Source:* Data from AR Omran: The epidemiologic transition: A theory of the epidemiology of population change. Milbank Mem Fund Q 49:509, 1971; and SJ Olshansky, AB Ault: The fourth stage of the epidemiologic transition: The age of delayed degenerative diseases. Milbank Q 64:355, 1986.

Per capita income and life expectancy increase during the *age of receding pandemics* as the improvements in public health systems, water purification systems, and access to better nutrition combine to drive down deaths from infectious disease and malnutrition. Infant and childhood mortality improve, but deaths due to CVD increase to between 10% and 35% of all deaths. In addition to rheumatic valvular disease, hypertension, coronary heart disease (CHD), and stroke are the predominant forms of CVD. Almost 40% of the world's population is currently in this stage.

The *age of degenerative and man-made diseases* is distinguished by mortality from non-communicable diseases—primarily CVD—surpassing mortality from malnutrition and infectious diseases. Caloric intake, particularly from animal fat, increases. CHD and stroke are prevalent, and between 35% and 65% of all deaths can be traced to CVD. Typically, the rate of CHD deaths exceeds that of stroke by a ratio of 2:1 to 3:1. During this period, average life expectancy surpasses the age of 50. Roughly 35% of the world's population falls into this category.

In the *age of delayed degenerative diseases*, CVD and cancer remain the major causes of morbidity and mortality, with CVD accounting for 40% of all deaths. However, age-adjusted CVD mortality declines, aided by preventive strategies (for example, smoking cessation, increased leisure time and physical activity, weight loss, and effective blood pressure control), acute hospital management, and technologic advances, such as the availability of bypass surgery and new therapeutics and devices. CHD, stroke, and congestive heart failure are the primary forms of CVD. About 15% of the world's population is now in the age of delayed degenerative diseases or is exiting this age and moving into the fifth stage of the epidemiologic transition.

In high-income countries (HICs) or portions of LMIC populations with high incomes, physical activity continues to decline while total caloric intake increases. The resulting epidemic of overweight and obesity may signal the start of a fifth stage, or the *age of inactivity and obesity* (4). Rates of type 2 diabetes mellitus, hypertension, and lipid abnormalities are on the rise, trends that are particularly evident in children. If these risk factor trends continue, age-adjusted CVD mortality rates that have fallen for decades during the fourth phase could increase in the coming years, and signs are pointing in this direction.

## PATTERNS IN THE EPIDEMIOLOGIC TRANSITION

Unique regional features have modified aspects of the transition in various parts of the world in three patterns (5). A large proportion of HICs experienced declines in CVD death rates by as much as 50–60% over the last 60 years, whereas CVD death rates increased by 15% over the past 20 years in the low- and middle-income range, and the rate of change has been faster. While patterns in the last century tended to affect whole countries in general, not all populations within a country were equally affected by the changes. In HICs, wealthier populations tended to see improvements in infectious disease mortality, then worsening of some CVD risk factors (RFs) and then ultimately reductions in RFs. This pattern could be seen in some of the wealthier populations of LMICs. Later, middle- and lower-income populations of HICs developed worsening RF profiles, as there appears to be a minimal threshold of income that provides access to tobacco, processed foods, and environmental or work conditions that increase risk for CVD RFs. Thus, the pattern in many LMICs in the twenty-first century may not exactly mimic the pattern of HICs in the twentieth century, but its features are important to understand for mitigation of risk in LMIC as well as low-income regions of HICs.

The typical pattern of HICs included changes that improved mortality from infectious diseases but increased risk factors for CVD then ultimately an improvement in control of such risk factors and an age-adjusted decline in CVD mortality. This pattern in the twentieth century included a shift from an agrarian economy to an industrialized economy with improved food supplies, improvement in sanitation and public health infrastructure, introduction of antibiotics, initially worsening of lifestyle habits with mass production of tobacco and more processed foods, and reduced physical activity by the 1950s, followed by an awareness of the risk factors for CVD in the 1960s and aggressive public health and basic and clinical science research leading to advances in the prevention and treatment of CVD and its risk factors, with healthy reversals for many with poor diet, physical activity, and tobacco consumption patterns.

Currently, populations with moderate incomes in both LMICs and HICs are entering what appears to be a fifth phase. The decline in the age-adjusted CVD death rate of 3% per year through the 1970s and 1980s has tapered off in the 1990s to 2%. However, CVD death rates have declined by 3–5% per year during the first decade of the new millennium. Competing trends appear to be at play. On the one hand, an increase in the prevalence of diabetes and obesity, a slowing in the rate of decline in smoking, and a leveling off in the rate of detection and treatment for hypertension are in the negative column. On the other hand, cholesterol levels continue to decline in the face of increased statin use.

Many HICs—which together account for 15% of the population—have proceeded through four stages of the epidemiologic transition in roughly the same pattern. CHD is the dominant form of CVD in these countries, with rates that tend to be two- to fivefold higher than stroke rates. However, variations exist. Whereas North America, Australia, and central northwestern European HICs experienced significant increases than rapid declines in CVD rates, southern and central European countries experienced a more gradual rise and fall in rates. More specifically, central European countries (i.e., Austria, Belgium, and Germany) declined at slower rates compared to their northern counterparts (i.e., Finland, Sweden, Denmark, and Norway). Countries such as Portugal, Spain, and Japan never reached the high mortality rates that the United States and other countries did, with CHD mortality rates at 200 per 100,000, or less. The countries of western Europe also exhibit a clear north/south gradient in absolute rates of CVD, with rates highest in the northern countries (i.e., Finland, Ireland, and Scotland) and lowest in the Mediterranean countries (i.e., France, Spain, and Italy). Japan is unique among the HICs, most likely due to the unique dietary patterns of its population. Although stroke rates increased dramatically, CHD rates did not rise as sharply in Japan. However, Japanese dietary habits are undergoing substantial changes, reflected in an increase in cholesterol levels.

Patterns in LMICs (gross national income per capita $11,666) depend, in part, on cultural differences, secular trends, and responses at the country level with regard to both public health and treatment infrastructure. Although communicable diseases continue to be a major cause of death, CVD has emerged as a significant health concern in LMICs. With 85% of the world's population,

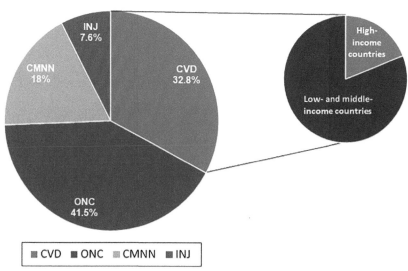

**Figure 2.1** Global deaths by cause, 2019. CMNN, communicable, maternal, neonatal, and nutritional disorders; CVD, cardiovascular diseases; INJ, injuries; ONC, other non-communicable diseases.

*Source*: Based on data from Global Burden of Disease Study 2019. Global Burden of Disease Study 2019 (GBD 2019) Results. Seattle, United States: Institute for Health Metrics and Evaluation (IHME), 2020.

LMICs are driving the rates of change in the global burden of CVD (Figure 2.1). In most LMICs, an urban/rural gradient has emerged for CHD, stroke, and hypertension, with higher rates in urban centers.

However, although CVD rates are rapidly rising globally, vast differences exist among the regions and countries, and even within the countries themselves (Figure 2.2). The East Asia and Pacific regions appear to be straddling the second and third phases of the epidemiologic transition. CVD is a major cause of death in China, but like Japan, stroke causes more deaths than CHD in a ratio of about three to one. Vietnam and Cambodia, on the other hand, are just emerging from the pestilence and famine transition. The Middle East and North Africa regions also appear to be entering the third phase of the epidemiologic transition, with increasing life expectancy and CVD death rates just below those of HICs. In general, Latin America appears to be in the third phase of the transition, although there is vast regional heterogeneity, with some areas in the second phase of the transition and some in the fourth. The Eastern Europe and Central Asia regions, however, are firmly in the peak of the third phase, with the highest death rates due to CVD (~66%) in the world. Importantly, deaths due to CHD are not limited to the elderly in this region and have a significant effect on working-age populations. South Asia—and more specifically, India, which accounts for the greatest proportion of the region's population—is experiencing an alarming increase in heart disease. The transition appears to be in the Western style, with CHD as the dominant form of CVD. Data indicate that CHD develops at least a decade earlier in the Indian population than in comparison with those of European ancestry (6, 7). However, rheumatic heart disease continues to be a major cause of morbidity and mortality. As in South Asia, rheumatic heart disease is also an important cause of CVD morbidity and mortality in sub-Saharan Africa, which largely remains in the first two phases of the epidemiologic transition, although sub-populations may be in the latter stages (1).

Many factors contribute to this heterogeneity among LMICs. First, the regions are in various stages of the epidemiologic transition. Second, vast differences in lifestyle and behavioral risk factors exist. Third, racial and ethnic differences may lead to altered susceptibilities to various forms of CVD. In addition, it should be noted that for most countries in these regions, accurate country-wide data on cause-specific mortality are not complete.

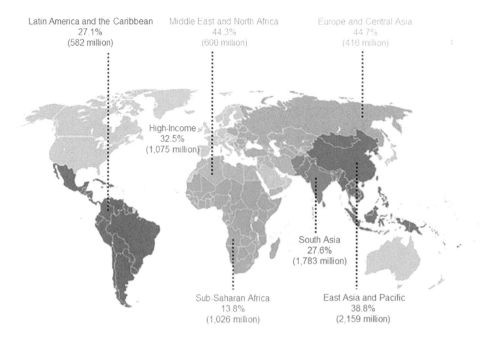

**Figure 2.2** Cardiovascular disease deaths as a percentage of total deaths and total population in seven economic regions of the world defined by the World Bank.

*Source:* Based on data from Global Burden of Disease Study 2019. Global Burden of Disease Study 2019 (GBD 2019) Results. Seattle, United States: Institute for Health Metrics and Evaluation (IHME), 2020.

## GLOBAL TRENDS IN CARDIOVASCULAR DISEASE

Over the last 5 years, there have been changes in the trends of CVD that are reflective of both trends in demographics and management of disease, but also of the way deaths and diseases have been measured and estimated. In 2017–2019, the Global Burden of Disease (GBD) Study updated its estimates, with several important changes based on newly available data, refinement in the causes of death, and the introduction of new modeling techniques. The major changes include the addition of an independent estimation of population and fertility; the addition of over 127 country-years of vital registration and verbal autopsy data; revisions of some deaths from "misclassified" to dementia, Parkinson's disease, and atrial fibrillation; and the addition of new diseases such as non-rheumatic calcific aortic and degenerative mitral valve disease. CVD accounts for 32% of deaths worldwide, a number expected to increase. In 2019, CHD accounted for 16.2% of all deaths globally, the largest portion (10.5%) of global years of life lost (YLLs), and the second largest portion (7.2%) of global disability-adjusted life-years (DALYs). In 2019, stroke remained the second largest cause of death (11.6% of all deaths globally) and the third largest contributor to global YLLs (7.5%) and DALYs (5.7%) (1).

Together, CHD and stroke accounted for more than a quarter of all deaths worldwide. The burden of stroke is of growing concern among LMICs. The impact of stroke on DALYs and mortality rates is more than three times greater in LMICs as compared to HICs.

With 85% of the world's population, LMICs largely drive global CVD rates and trends. More than 14 million (14.4) CVD deaths occurred in LMICs in 2017, compared to 3.3 million in HICs. Globally, there is evidence of significant delays in age of occurrence and/or improvements in case fatality rates; between 1990 and 2017, the number of CVD deaths increased by 49%, but age-adjusted death rates decreased by 30.4% in the same period. Age-standardized death rates, however, have declined faster in HICs than in middle-income and lower-income regions (Figure 2.3). Population growth has been greater in LMICs compared to HICs. As a result of slower rates of population growth in HICs, overall CVD deaths remained steady. However, in the LMICs, the population aging and growth outstripped gains in age-adjusted mortality reductions such that overall CVD deaths continued to climb over the last 25 years (Figure 2.4).

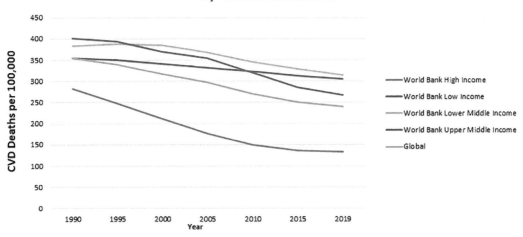

**Figure 2.3**  Age-standardized cardiovascular disease (CVD) death rate per 100,000 from 1990 to 2019, by World Bank income.

*Source*: Based on data from Global Burden of Disease Study 2019. Global Burden of Disease Study 2019 (GBD 2019) Results. Seattle, United States: Institute for Health Metrics and Evaluation (IHME), 2020.

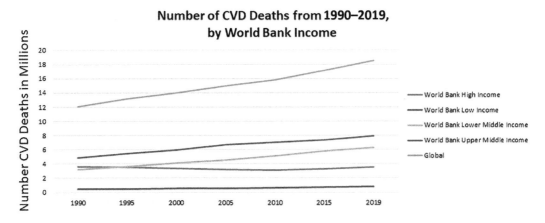

**Figure 2.4**  Number of cardiovascular disease (CVD) deaths from 1990 to 2019, by World Bank income.

*Source*: Based on data from Global Burden of Disease Study 2019. Global Burden of Disease Study 2019 (GBD 2019) Results. Seattle, United States: Institute for Health Metrics and Evaluation (IHME), 2020.

Significant portions of the population living in LMICs have entered the third phase of the epidemiologic transition, and some are entering the fourth stage. Changing demographics play a significant role in future predictions for CVD throughout the world. For example, the population growth rate in Eastern Europe and Central Asia was 1.1% between 2010 and 2017, whereas it was 11% in South Asia. CVD rates will also have an economic impact. Even assuming no increase in CVD risk factors, most countries, but especially India and South Africa, will see a large number of people between 35 and 64 die of CVD over the next 30 years, as well as an increasing level of morbidity among middle-aged people related to heart disease and stroke.

## RISK FACTORS

Global variation in CVD rates is related to temporal and regional variations in known risk factors and behaviors (8). Ecological analyses of major CVD risk factors and mortality demonstrate high correlations between expected and observed mortality rates for the three main risk factors—smoking, serum cholesterol, and hypertension—and suggest that many regional variations are based on differences in conventional risk factors.

### Behavioral Risk Factors: Tobacco

Over 1.4 billion people use tobacco worldwide. Tobacco use currently causes about 7.1 million deaths annually (12.7% of all deaths), 2.6 million of which are CVD-related (9). The population of the HIC group smokes (21.6%) at almost double the rate of the low-income countries (11.2%), while the middle-income country group's smoking rate (19.5%) approximates the global average (19.2%). From 2007 to 2017, smoking rates decreased across low-, middle-, and high-income country groups, with relative reductions of 19%, 12%, and 20%, respectively.

### Diet

Total caloric intake per capita increases as countries develop. With regard to CVD, a key element of dietary change is an increase in intake of saturated animal fats and hydrogenated vegetable fats, which contain atherogenic *trans* fatty acids, along with a decrease in intake of plant-based foods and an increase in simple carbohydrates. Fat contributes <20% of calories in rural China and India, <30% in Japan, and well above 30% in the United States. Caloric contributions from fat appear to be falling in the HICs.

### Physical Inactivity

Physical inactivity is responsible for 1.3 million global deaths annually. The global prevalence of physical inactivity has remained steady between 2001 and 2016 (28.5%–27.5%). Mortality rates attributable to inactivity are highest in North Africa and the Middle East and in Central and Eastern Europe. In urban China, for example, the proportion of adults who participate in moderate- or high-level activity has decreased significantly, whereas the proportion of those who participate in low-level activity has increased.

## METABOLIC RISK FACTORS

Examination of trends in metabolic risk factors provides insight into changes in the CVD burden globally. Here we describe four metabolic risk factors—lipid levels, hypertension, obesity, and diabetes mellitus—using data from the Global Burden of Disease, Injuries, and Risk Factors Study (GBD 2017).

### Lipid Levels

Worldwide, high cholesterol levels are estimated to play a role in 42% of ischemic heart disease deaths and 9% of stroke deaths, amounting to 4.3 million deaths annually. Although mean population plasma cholesterol levels tend to rise as countries move through the epidemiologic transition, mean serum total cholesterol levels have decreased globally between 1980 and 2008 by 0.08 mmol/L per decade in men and 0.07 mmol/L per decade in women (8). Large declines occurred in Australasia, North America, and Western Europe (0.19–0.21 mmol/L). Countries in the East Asia and Pacific region experienced increases of >0.08 mmol/L in both men and women. More recent research including Mendelian studies suggests that simple and unified biomarkers such as either lipoprotein(a) or ApoB may act as an individual predictor of CVD risk beyond traditional total or low-density lipoprotein (LDL) cholesterol through increased cellular lipid accumulation, endothelial dysfunction, and impacts on coagulation. Non-randomized data suggest higher rates among those of African descent, with twice the levels of Caucasians, with East Asians and South Asians having intermediate levels. There are limited data on clinical agents that target lipoprotein(a), although PCSK9 inhibitors lower it or specific targets, so this remains an area of intense research.

### Hypertension

Elevated blood pressure is an early indicator of the epidemiologic transition. Observational studies show increased risk of CVD beginning with those above 110–115 mmHg. Between 1990 and 2015, the global prevalence of systolic blood pressure (SBP) ≥110–115 mmHg increased from 73,119 to 81,373 per 100,000, while the prevalence of SBP ≥140 mmHg rose from 17,307 to 20,526 per 100,000 (10). In 2015, of the estimated 3.47 billion adults with SBP ≥110–115 mmHg, 874 million

(25%) had SBP $\geq$140 mmHg. While SBP $\geq$140 mmHg accounts for only 25% of those with elevated blood pressure, it accounted for 73% (7.8 million) of deaths due to elevated SBP. Worldwide, 55% of stroke deaths (3.36 of 6.17 million) and 55% of CHD deaths (4.89 of 8.93 million) are attributable to high blood pressure, accounting for 8.25 million deaths in 2017. From 1990 to 2015, the number of deaths related to SBP $\geq$140 mmHg increased in all LMIC groups but fell in HICs. Rising mean population blood pressure also occurs as populations industrialize and move from rural to urban settings. For example, the prevalence of hypertension in urban India is 33.8%, but varies between 14.5% and 31.7% in rural regions. One major concern in LMICs is the high rate of undetected, and therefore untreated, hypertension. This may explain, at least in part, the higher stroke rates in these countries in relation to CHD rates during the early stages of the transition. The high rates of hypertension throughout Asia, especially undiagnosed hypertension, likely contribute to the high prevalence of hemorrhagic stroke in the region. Globally, however, mean SBP has decreased for both sexes (0.8 mmHg per decade for men; 1.0 mmHg per decade for women).

## Obesity

Trends in obesity are concerning (11). In 2015, an estimated 603.4 million adults and 107.7 million children were obese. Global obesity prevalence was 12% among adults (5% among children) and is increasing throughout the world, particularly in developing countries, where the trajectories are steeper than those experienced by the developed countries (12). High body mass index (BMI) contributed to 4 million deaths worldwide (7.1% of deaths from any cause); CVD was the leading cause of these deaths (2.7 million) and also of associated DALYs (66.3 of 120 million), followed by diabetes (0.6 million deaths, 30.4 million DALYs). Women are more affected by obesity than are men; from 1975 to 2014, global mean age-standardized BMI increased from 22.1 to 24.4 kg/m$^2$ in females and 21.7 to 24.2 kg/m$^2$ in males, while the prevalence of obesity increased from 6.4% to 14.9% in females and 3.2% to 10.8% in males. The proportion of the world's adult women who are either overweight or obese rose from 29.8% to 38.0% between 1980 and 2013, while an increase from 28.8% to 36.9% was observed for men. Country and regional differences are observed. The highest prevalence of male obesity is in the United States, Southern and Central Latin America, Australasia, and Central and Western Europe. For females, the highest prevalence of obesity is in Southern and North Africa, the Middle East, Central and Southern Latin America, and the United States. The lowest prevalence for both males and females was observed in South and Southeast Asia and in East, Central, and West Africa. Generally, the prevalence of obesity for both sexes increased with the increase in sociodemographic index; however, the rise in adult obesity in developed countries has slowed since 2006. In many of the LMICs, obesity appears to coexist with undernutrition and malnutrition.

## Diabetes Mellitus

As a consequence of, or in addition to, increasing BMI and decreasing levels of physical activity, worldwide rates of diabetes—predominantly type 2 diabetes—are on the rise. According to the most recent data from the GBD project, the prevalence of diabetes increased 129.7% for males and 120.9% for females between 1990 and 2017 (8). An estimated 476 million people worldwide have diabetes, and the International Diabetes Foundation predicts this number will reach 693 million by 2045. Nearly 50% of people with diabetes are undiagnosed, and 80% live in LMICs. The Middle East and North Africa have the highest regional age-standardized prevalence (8.7% of the population) and incidence rates (400 per 100,000) of diabetes, compared to East Asia and the Pacific, with the lowest (5.8%; 249 per 100,000). Future growth will also largely occur in the Middle East and Africa, along with other LMICs in South Asia and sub-Saharan Africa.

### Genetic Risk Factors

A great deal of effort has recently been invested in understanding how genes impact cardiovascular health in populations. These have focused on germline genetic variants that are related to specific CVD, as well as those that are associated with cardiovascular risk factors. In either case, every year the number of associated variants has increased meaningfully to the point that it appears that hundreds or even thousands of variants are associated with these conditions, each explaining a small amount of the population variability in disease and risk factors. Collections of variants have been combined in polygenomic risk scores, but these too explain only a small amount of the variability of the disease in the population. Much more data will emerge in the coming years about these associations, mechanisms that explain these associations, relationships of variants that are specific to certain tissues such as the heart or the brain, and the interactions between genetic and lifestyle factors in causing disease. Currently, most of the data are among those with European ancestry; however, large-scale efforts are underway to understand the relationships between genes and diseases and their risk factors around the world. The early data suggest non-trivial differences among various world populations.

## Environment

Environmental pollution, especially both indoor and outdoor air pollution, has emerged as a major cause of death and disease burden (13). Exposure to particulate-matter (PM) air pollution, heavy metals (e.g., cadmium, arsenic, lead, mercury), and polyaromatic hydrocarbons is associated with increased risk of mortality and morbidity from CVD. The GBD comparative risk assessment of 2017 has shown that more than 23% of all DALYs from ischemic heart disease and about 28.9% of DALYs from ischemic strokes result from environmental risk factors, approximately the same as those attributable to tobacco smoke (8). Of these exposures, air pollution (household and ambient) is the most prominent risk factor, contributing to approximately 7 million premature deaths annually, with a majority occurring in LMICs such as India and China. In many developing countries, populations experience a continuum of exposure to ambient air pollution (from vehicles, industry, etc.) and household air pollution (from cooking, heating, and lighting), resulting in significant contributions to the health burden, as in India, where it is the second most important risk factor for poor health. More than half of all deaths associated with air pollution exposure are through cardiovascular and cerebrovascular pathways, involving ischemic heart disease, heart failure, stroke, and hypertension.

## POLICIES THAT CAN HELP CVD BURDEN AND MEET SDG GOALS

Although CVD rates are declining in the HICs, they are increasing in many other regions of the world. The consequences of this preventable epidemic will be substantial on many levels, including individual mortality and morbidity, family suffering, and staggering economic costs. As a result of these costs, the 2015 Sustainable Development Goals (SDGs) have recognized non-communicable diseases (NCDs), including CVD, as a serious obstacle to development in LMICs. With these goals includes a target to reduce premature mortality by 30% by 2030.

Fortunately, there are many cost-effective strategies recommended by the World Health Organization (WHO) (14) and the Disease Control Priorities Project (15) that LMICs can adopt to reduce the suffering and costs. In particular, three complementary strategies can be used to lessen the impact. First, the overall burden of CVD risk factors can be lowered through population-wide public health measures, such as national campaigns against cigarette smoking, unhealthy diets, and physical inactivity. Many tobacco policies have been shown to be cost-saving or highly cost-effective. Taxation has been shown to be cost-saving in Vietnam and highly cost-effective ($140/DALY averted) in Mexico. Other highly cost-effective strategies include public smoking bans (India, $2–35/DALY averted), advertising bans (Mexico, $2800/DALY averted), and mass media campaigns that are either cost-saving or up to $2800/DALY averted. Taxation on sugar-sweetened beverages has also been shown to be cost saving (16). Programs that encourage or subsidize fruit and vegetable consumption or discourage unhealthy consumption have been shown to be cost-saving and highly cost-effective as well (17). Salt reformulation by the industry appears to be more cost-effective than campaigns to reduce sodium intake. While many disease-prevention or health-promotion programs have not been assessed for cost-effectiveness in LMICs, some evidence suggests that community trails built alongside or over abandoned rail tracks, use of pedometers or step counters, and school-based health education programs are among the most promising.

Second, it is important to identify higher-risk subgroups of the population who stand to benefit the most from specific, low-cost prevention interventions. Screening by community health workers can be done simply (18), and treatment for hypertension has been shown to be cost-saving (China) and cost-effective (Argentina and South Africa, $500–7000/DALY averted). The cost-effectiveness of strategies that use lipid-lowering therapies is slightly higher than screening and pharmacological treatment of hypertension, ranging from $1200 per QALY in most large LMICs when part of a multidrug regimen to as much as $22,000 per DALY in the Philippines. As more statins come off patents this strategy is already more cost-effective. Opportunistic screening for diabetes is more cost-effective than mass screening. Screening for complications of diabetes such as for foot ulcers or for retinopathy with telemedicine (India, $1200–2400/DALY averted) are also attractive strategies.

Third, resources should be allocated to both acute and secondary prevention interventions. Use of simple diagnostic tools such as electrocardiogram (EKG) machines (India, $12/QALY gained) and prehospital thrombolysis with an established emergency transport system (Brazil) is also highly cost-effective. Use of early aspirin and beta-blockers and generic streptokinase is also highly cost-effective in acute myocardial infarction. More advanced therapies such as percutaneous coronary interventions are moderately cost-effective for middle-income countries (China, $9000–$25000/QALY gained). Management of patients with heart failure and reduced ejection fraction with generic angiotensin-converting enzyme inhibitors, beta-blockers, or aldosterone antagonists have been shown to be cost-saving or highly cost-effective. Simple, low-cost interventions, such as the "polypill"—a regimen of aspirin, a statin, and an antihypertensive agent—also need to be explored and have been shown to be cost-saving in secondary prevention and likely cost-effective in primary prevention with high-risk individuals. For countries with limited resources, a critical first step in developing a comprehensive plan is better assessment of cause-specific mortality and morbidity, as well as the prevalence, of the major preventable risk factors.

In the meantime, all countries must continue to bear the burden of research and development aimed at prevention and treatment, being mindful of the economic limitations of many LMICs. The concept of the epidemiologic transition provides insight into how to alter the course of the CVD epidemic. The efficient transfer of low-cost preventive and therapeutic strategies could alter the natural course of this epidemic and thereby reduce the excess global burden of preventable CVD.

## REFERENCES

1. Global Burden of Disease Collaborative Network. Global burden of disease study 2019 (GBD 2019) disease and injury burden 1990–2019 [Internet]. Institute for Health Metrics and Evaluation (IHME). 2020 [cited April 2021]. Available from: http://ghdx.healthdata.org/gbd-results-tool
2. Olshansky SJ, Ault AB. The fourth stage of the epidemiologic transition: the age of delayed degenerative diseases. The Milbank Memorial Fund Quarterly. 1986;64(3):355–391.
3. Omran AR. The epidemiologic transition: a theory of the epidemiology of population change. Milbank Memorial Fund Quarterly. 1971;49(4):509–538.
4. Gaziano JM. Fifth phase of the epidemiologic transition: the age of obesity and inactivity. JAMA. 2010;303(3):275–276.
5. Arroyo-Quiroz C, Barrientos-Gutierrez T, O'Flaherty M, Guzman-Castillo M, Palacio-Mejia L, Osorio-Saldarriaga E, et al. Coronary heart disease mortality is decreasing in Argentina, and Colombia, but keeps increasing in Mexico: a time trend study. BMC Public Health. 2020;20(1):162.
6. Prabhakaran D, Jeemon P, Roy A. Cardiovascular diseases in India: Current epidemiology and future directions. Circulation. 2016;133(16):1605–1620.
7. India State-Level Disease Burden Initiative CVD Collaborators. The changing patterns of cardiovascular diseases and their risk factors in the states of India: the Global Burden of Disease Study 1990–2016. The Lancet Global Health. 2018;6(12):e1339–e1351.
8. GBD 2017 Risk Factor Collaborators. Global, regional, and national comparative risk assessment of 84 behavioural, environmental and occupational, and metabolic risks or clusters of risks for 195 countries and territories, 1990–2017: a systematic analysis for the Global Burden of Disease Study 2017. Lancet. 2018;392(10159):1923–1994.
9. WHO Report on the Global Tobacco Epidemic, 2019. Geneva: World Health Organization. Licence: CC BY-NC-SA 3.0 IGO.
10. Forouzanfar MH, Liu P, Roth GA, Ng M, Biryukov S, Marczak L, et al. Global burden of hypertension and systolic blood pressure of at least 110 to 115 mm Hg, 1990–2015. JAMA. 2017;317(2):165–182.
11. Ng M, Fleming T, Robinson M, Thomson B, Graetz N, Margono C, et al. Global, regional, and national prevalence of overweight and obesity in children and adults during 1980–2013: a systematic analysis for the Global Burden of Disease Study 2013. Lancet. 2014;384(9945):766–781.
12. The GBD 2015 Obesity Collaborators. Health effects of overweight and obesity in 195 countries over 25 years. New England Journal of Medicine. 2017;377(1):13–27.
13. Landrigan PJ, Sly JL, Ruchirawat M, Silva ER, Huo X, Diaz-Barriga F, et al. Health consequences of environmental exposures: changing global patterns of exposure and disease. Ann Glob Health. 2016;82(1):10–19.
14. World Health Organization. Tackling NCDs: 'best buys' and other recommended interventions for the prevention and control of noncommunicable diseases. Geneva: World Health Organization; 2017. Contract No.: WHO/NMH/NVI/17.9.

15. Prabhakaran D, Anand S, Watkins D, Gaziano T, Wu Y, Mbanya JC, et al. Cardiovascular, respiratory, and related disorders: key messages from disease control priorities, 3rd edition. The Lancet. 2018;391(10126):1224–1236.
16. Wilde P, Huang Y, Sy S, Abrahams-Gessel S, Jardim TV, Paarlberg R, et al. Cost-effectiveness of a US National sugar-sweetened beverage tax with a multistakeholder approach: who pays and who benefits. American Journal of Public Health. 2019;109(2):276–284.
17. Lee Y, Mozaffarian D, Sy S, Huang Y, Liu J, Wilde PE, et al. Cost-effectiveness of financial incentives for improving diet and health through Medicare and Medicaid: A microsimulation study. PLoS Medicine. 2019;16(3):e1002761.
18. Gaziano TA, Abrahams-Gessel S, Denman CA, Montano CM, Khanam M, Puoane T, et al. An assessment of community health workers' ability to screen for cardiovascular disease risk with a simple, non-invasive risk assessment instrument in Bangladesh, Guatemala, Mexico, and South Africa: an observational study. Lancet Global Health. 2015;3(9):e556–e563.

# 3 Concepts of Risk and Risk Factors

*Rima N. Pai and Shivani A. Patel*

## CONTENTS

## INTRODUCTION

### Importance of Risk Factors in Public Health and Medicine

Risk factors are characteristics associated with a higher incidence of disease; they are the factors that either cause or predict the occurrence of the disease outcome. Identifying and addressing risk factors within populations is the crux of public health prevention programs for cardiovascular disease (CVD). Risk factor identification is a pillar of public health prevention efforts and plays a critical role in the disease-specific diagnosis and management of patients in clinical medicine. About 80% of CVD can be attributed to known clinical and behavioral risk factors occurring in men and women (1). Over 300 risk factors for hypertension, stroke, and coronary heart disease have been identified (1). Our efforts to reverse risks once they have developed are rarely met with success, and such risk reversal, when achieved, is also prone to rebound. Therefore, blocking the initial development of risk factors in populations and individuals through early and ongoing measures is a central priority in CVD prevention. While many of these risk factors were historically attributed to 'lifestyle choices', there is increasing interest in the environmental milieu that gives rise to individual and community-level risks (2). This chapter provides an overview of the concept of risk factors and risk in CVD epidemiology.

### History of 'Risk Factor' as a Term

The term 'risk factor' was first coined by Dr. William B. Kannel, the former director of the Framingham Heart Study (FHS), in 1961 in an article in the *Annals of Internal Medicine* (3, 4). The FHS is among the earliest and most impactful epidemiologic studies of heart disease. Before the FHS, the causes of heart disease in the population were poorly understood and poorly quantified. At the time, the pathophysiological processes underlying CVD—termed atherosclerosis—was believed to be an inevitable part of the aging process. Researchers leading the FHS study sought to understand whether it was possible to reduce the disease and death associated with cardiovascular (CV) conditions. They followed over 5,000 men residing in Framingham over decades to

DOI: 10.1201/b23266-3

identify which factors contributed to differential risk across the study participants (4). Through this systematic enumeration of characteristics of individuals who developed the disease, the FHS played a pivotal role and created a paradigm shift to identify and address 'risk factors' for CVD. Framingham investigators identified cigarette smoking, elevated cholesterol, elevated blood pressure (BP), and obesity as factors implicated in increased CVD risk (5). Conversely, exercise was identified as a factor associated with lower CVD risk in the 1960s (5). To this day, the behaviors and clinical parameters identified in FHS are the leading modifiable risk factors for CVD. This work laid the foundation of the Framingham risk scoring system and other risk assessment tools, guidelines for screening, and algorithms to determine CVDs (5). Subsequent studies have built on Framingham's lessons to explore the generalizability of findings across diverse populations and to investigate novel risk factors that contribute to an evolving landscape of risk factor classification systems for CVD.

## Risk Factors and Risk Factor Epidemiology Today

Identifying risk factors is now a cornerstone of public health for an array of health conditions, extending far beyond CVDs. There is concern that searching for 'independent effects' of single risk factors in isolation ignores disease processes' complexity. This leads to a tension between the tendency in epidemiology to focus on single, isolated risk factors and broader recognition that dynamic forces at multiple levels of influence (e.g., societal, interpersonal, individual) ultimately culminate in disease. Furthermore, not all individuals with risk factors develop the disease, and some people with no risk factors indeed develop the disease. Using risk factors to predict disease is based on average outcomes observed across individuals. It is a statistical fact that there will always be individuals who fall above and below the average. Despite these concerns and the potential simplification of disease processes through conventional risk factor epidemiology, this approach has often worked. For example, it is generally well accepted that preventing and treating CVD risk factors identified through these conventional epidemiologic methods was critical to reducing heart disease mortality in high-income countries (HICs). Furthermore, as discussed later in this chapter, many of these risk factors are collectively considered in risk assessment tools better to address an individual's risk profile totality.

## RISK CONCEPTS: DEFINITIONS AND EXAMPLES

The concept of risk factors is multifaceted. The term 'risk' can be defined in several ways, but most equate to relative frequency or percentage of probability of an unwanted event. For CVDs, it can be an occurrence of an unwanted event (e.g., myocardial infarction) or from the cause of an unwanted event (e.g., high BP). This necessitates the need for evaluating CV risk factors. These risk factors need to be understood in terms of added predictive value, practical application in day-to-day practice, and potential for therapeutic interventions.

## Absolute Risk

Absolute risk is a critical metric to understand the extent of a health problem in the population. In the technical sense, absolute risk is the probability of an event occurring over a specified time period. It is computed as the cumulative number of new disease events that occur divided by the total population at risk at baseline. The magnitude of absolute risk is contingent on the frequency of the event. For example, a stroke's absolute risk is lower than the absolute risk of myocardial infarction (MI) over one year because stroke is rarer than MI. Similarly, the magnitude of risk will depend on follow-up duration. For example, over ten years, absolute risk for an atherosclerotic CVD event is 1.6% for a 45-year-old African American woman with diabetes in the United States (6). Throughout her lifetime, however, her risk accumulates to 39%. The absolute risk of an event generally varies by person, place, and calendar year. Risks can be higher or lower based on demographic factors (e.g., risk of MI is higher in men than in women), based on setting (e.g., the risk of hemorrhagic stroke is higher in low- and middle-income countries [LMICs] than in HICs). Risks can vary over time (e.g., the secular decline in the risk of death due to heart disease in HICs).

Many epidemiologic and clinical metrics are derived from the absolute risk. In trials, treatment benefit due to the reduction of risk factor levels is estimated by the absolute risk reduction (ARR) and number needed to treat (NNT). It offers another framework through which several similar patients treated during a specific time (usually five years) are required to prevent a CVD complication for one person (7, 8). Absolute risk can be critical for a clinical decision because it measures an individual's probability of experiencing an event and benefiting from specific interventions.

Therefore, assessing absolute risk is used to differentiate high- versus low-risk patients to guide prevention and management interventions.

## Relative Risk

Risk factors either cause disease or can be used to recognize individuals at high risk for disease. We identify risk factors for a condition by estimating the relative risk of disease among individuals with and without the risk factor. As such, relative risk compares the absolute risk of disease across individuals who differ in their exposure to the putative risk factor. This comparison is expressed as a ratio, and the terms risk ratio and relative risk are routinely used synonymously. The risk ratio measures the strength of the association between a risk factor (e.g., hypertension) or intervention (e.g., receiving a statin) and an outcome (e.g., MI). If exposure is harmful, then the relative risk will be >1, and that exposure will be termed a risk factor. If the exposure is beneficial, the risk ratio is <1, and the exposure will be termed a protective factor. For example, because the relative risk of CV complications comparing people with and without hypertension is greater than 1, hypertension is deemed a risk factor for CV complications. Furthermore, there is evidence that treatment of hypertension can reverse this excess risk; antihypertensive medications decrease the risk of CV complications by 25% across men and women irrespective of age and smoking status (9). However, a single risk factor or categorical risk classification can only predict individual risk. Like absolute risks, the relative risk may also differ by personal characteristics (age, gender, race), over time, and across places.

## Population-Attributable Fraction

The population-attributable fraction (PAF) (also described as population-attributable risk) is the proportion of disease incidence in the population attributed to a particular exposure or risk factor. It is the proportion of disease that would be removed from the population if the exposure were eliminated. PAF incorporates the strength of association between the risk factor, disease outcome, and the prevalence of the risk factor and has been used to reflect the public health burden with a focus on early prevention. The INTERHEART study (10) demonstrated that approximately 60% of acute myocardial infarction (AMI) cases among South Asians were attributed to dyslipidemia, indicating that up to 60% of AMI in the community could be averted if dyslipidemia were eliminated from this population.

## ROLE OF RISK FACTORS IN THE CARDIOVASCULAR HEALTH OF POPULATIONS

Given that CVDs account for nearly one in three deaths worldwide, identifying the causes of CVD is a foremost public health priority (11). For this reason, CVD risk assessment has been developed to assist clinicians and risk-based intervention programs. For example, significant development of guidelines by the Joint National Committee on Detection, Evaluation, and Treatment of High Blood Pressure (JNC) determined risk estimates by creating cut-off levels for BP to determine when to initiate antihypertensives, which has played a crucial role in CVD (12). Adherence to those guidelines in managing hypertension has been cited as a cause for a subsequent reduction in CVD events, CVD mortality, and overall mortality (12).

## Classification of Risk Factors for Prevention and Management

Risk factors can be broadly divided into modifiable and nonmodifiable. Modifiable risk factors are amenable to intervention and are mainly lifestyle-related, such as smoking, excess alcohol, sedentary lifestyle, high cholesterol, high BP, and diabetes mellitus (1). Nonmodifiable risk factors are not amenable to intervention and include individual characteristics such as age, biological sex, genetic factors, race, and ethnicity (1). Several new and emerging potentially modifiable CVD risk factors are being researched, including coronary artery calcium score, homocysteine, thrombosis markers, carotid intima-media thickness, genotypic variations, nonalcoholic fatty liver disease, C-reactive protein, platelets, and weight at birth (13). Beyond individual-level factors, environmental determinants impact CVD outcomes and closely interact with modifiable and nonmodifiable risk factors. These environmental determinants include aspects of the physical environment (i.e., ambient particulate matter, neighborhood walkability, food environment) and the social environment (e.g., social relationships, psychosocial stressors, economic resources). The role of environmental influences in etiologies of CV health could lead to the development of new prevention strategies (14). However, their utility in clinical practice and risk scoring algorithms has only recently begun.

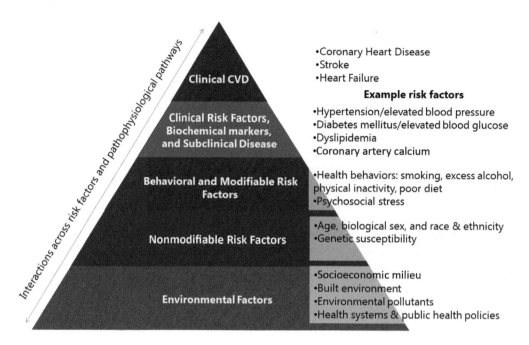

**Figure 3.1** A framework for risk factors for cardiovascular diseases.

### A Framework for Risk Factors

CVD is impacted by risks at multiple levels (e.g., at the individual level, at the societal level) and across multiple domains (e.g., social, behavioral, biological). Major atherosclerotic risk factors such as hypertension, diabetes, smoking, and high cholesterol are themselves a result of behavioral and environmental risk factors. Figure 3.1 illustrates interconnectedness of risk factors. The environments in which we live and nonmodifiable risk factors (e.g., age, genetics) are at the base of this pyramid because these factors lay the foundation for an individual's opportunities and constraints to engage in healthy behaviors and also shape physiological pathways that are related to CVDs.

### High-Risk Approach versus Population-Wide Approach

Figure 3.1 presents multiple opportunities to disrupt significant CVD risk factors and intervene in the pathway between the risk factor and CVD events (15, 16). An ideal approach would be engaging in multiple strategies with mixed interventions. Two ways of prioritizing intervention include the high risk and the population-wide approaches. The high-risk approach focuses on the identification of high-risk individuals in the population with targeted preventive services (behavior change interventions, pharmacological measures, or both). The high-risk approach strategy utilizes scoring systems to prioritize individuals with the highest risk of disease for targeted intervention. A population-wide approach focuses on shifting the distribution of risk factors in the entire population through broader population-based strategies (implementation of evidence-based policies, laws, and regulations) (17). The population-based approach seeks to change broader living conditions and social norms through public health policies for favorable shifts in risk profiles of the population at large.

### INTRODUCTION TO CVD RISK ASSESSMENT

Because of the debilitating, deadly, and costly consequences of CVDs, we are often interested in identifying individuals at high risk who may be targeted for aggressive medical monitoring and potentially treatment. We use the observed risk factor profile of an individual to estimate his or her absolute risk of CVD-related events over a specified time frame (7, 18). Both modifiable and nonmodifiable factors are incorporated into risk assessment tools. It is important to note that even individuals who do not fall into a high-risk group may go on to develop CVD. The benefit of risk stratification through CVD risk assessment is that it helps allocate preventive and clinical services to a targeted population in need and allows us to benchmark the health of populations against national guidelines and recommendations (19). However, these systems will always be imperfect because we are never able to measure all relevant factors and we are unable to measure risk factors perfectly.

## Major Risk Scoring Systems for CVD

Multiple risk scoring systems have been developed for single CVD outcomes (e.g., MI) in isolation or composite CVD events (e.g., combined MI and stroke). The most widely used cardiovascular risk prediction model is the Framingham Risk Score (FRS) and its modifications like the ten-year Framingham Risk Calculator equation. There are also many other risk scoring systems—several of which pool data across multiple cohorts—including the American Heart Association (AHA) and American College of Cardiology (ACC)–developed Atherosclerotic Cardiovascular Disease (ASCVD) calculator, QRISK2 model, and Joint British Society risk calculator 3 (JBS3) (20, 21).

The FRS is a well-characterized risk assessment tool to predict ten-year risk for MI, stroke, and cardiac death for an individual. It is useful for CV assessment by including risk factors of age, gender, total cholesterol, systolic BP, high-density lipoprotein cholesterol (HDL-C), and cigarette use (3).

The AHA/ACC ASCVD calculator predicts a ten-year risk of heart disease or stroke among individuals who have no history of MI or stroke (22). The calculator provides sex- and race-specific estimates for the first ASCVD event for black and white men and women aged 40–79. Variables included in the risk assessment equations are age, total cholesterol, HDL-C, systolic BP (including treated or untreated status), diabetes mellitus, and current smoking status.

The QRISK2 model is a multivariable risk score that is based on ethnicity and history of conditions associated with CV risk (treated hypertension, diabetes mellitus, rheumatoid arthritis, renal disease, and atrial fibrillation). Although QRISK2 has been developed for use in the UK, it is being used internationally (20).

The JBS3 calculator estimates a 'heart age' through multivariable modeling, which is referenced to someone of the same age, gender, and ethnicity with optimal risk factors (e.g., smoker, high BP). The JBS3 tool emphasizes the lifetime risk of CVD events, including competing risks like cancer. The JBS3 risk calculator helps clinicians communicate CVD risk and the benefits of either lifestyle or therapeutic interventions or both (20).

Overall, these scoring systems differ in actual estimation and integration of results in management protocols (20, 23). These and several other risk scores almost all have been developed in HICs and describe risks largely in white populations. There is a need to develop scoring systems that are contextually tailored and account for differential patterns of risk in diverse ethnic groups. For example, most existing CVD risk scores are driven by age, but the occurrence of CVD occurs in younger age groups among ethnic South Asians than in the white populations. It is therefore imperative to either develop new risk systems or calibrate existing systems to more accurately reflect risks in LMIC populations.

## Validation of Risk Scoring Systems

LMICs have historically lacked the research infrastructure to develop risk assessment tools using data from their populations, and therefore often use risk assessment tools that were created for other settings. Risk assessment tools must be validated, however, before applying them in populations outside of the one in which they were derived. Validation studies may reveal that the risk assessment tool underpredicts or overpredicts the absolute risk of an event in a new population. When this occurs, the risk assessment tool must be recalibrated to the observed risks in the population for optimal use. For example, researchers showed that the FHS risk assessment tool for CHD (developed in the United States in a homogenous population) overpredicted coronary heart disease (CHD) death among those deemed at highest risk in a Chinese cohort (24). The FHS tool could be recalibrated, however, to provide more meaningful information regarding risk in the Chinese population (24).

## CVD RISK FACTORS IN LOW- AND MIDDLE-INCOME COUNTRIES (LMICS)

The burden of CVDs in LMICs is disproportionately higher than the CVD burden in HICs (2). About three-quarters of CVD deaths occur in LMICs (2), especially among the working class between ages 30 and 69 years in sub-Saharan Africa, which is at least ten years earlier than HICs (25). The seminal work of the INTERHEART study established that major risk factors for MI are largely the same across countries (10). However, the prevalence of CVDs, their age and sex distribution, and associated fatality vary. This has led some researchers to hypothesize that the same risk factors have different effects and act at different thresholds across populations.

This chain of risk factors is intricately associated with each other and is expanded by multifold at individual and population levels in LMICs. At a population level, the dual burden of undernutrition and overnutrition among LMICs has been attributed to changes in the global diet, physical activity, environmental pollutants, chronic psychosocial stress, neuroendocrine dysregulation, and genetic/epigenetic mechanisms (26). This is also manifested in the 'double burden' of disease, or the simultaneous prevalence of infectious diseases, maternal and child disorders, and undernutrition, along with NCDs such as CVD (25).

### Global Variation in CVD and Its Risk Factors

The variation in CVD outcomes across regions, countries, and subnational localities is generally attributed to differences in modifiable risk factors like diet, activity, environmental exposures, and resulting cardiometabolic profiles. The heterogeneity in the risk factors themselves has many proposed explanations. The epidemiologic transition, in which chronic conditions such as CVDs begin to contribute to a larger share of the total disease burden than infections and undernutrition, is expected to follow broader socioeconomic development and the demographic transition. Cultural beliefs that impact behavioral norms may also be responsible for the differences across countries and variation between urban and rural settings within countries. Due to generations of marriage within countries, there may be clustering of genetic factors that predispose individuals to subclinical and clinical disorders such as lipid disorders, obesity, insulin resistance, and endothelial dysfunction. Finally, the combination of environments and genetics may interact to produce phenotypes that are at higher risk for CVD in the current environment. This may occur through prenatal and early life exposures, such as poor maternal and undernutrition, which in turn contribute to reduced insulin sensitivity (27), and overnutrition in later childhood and adulthood can lead to adipose dysfunction, dyslipidemias, and obesity (27). Similarly, migration between populations or countries affects the complex interactions of classical and novel CV risk factors in diversified environments (28).

### Unique Phenotypes in LMICs

Environmental factors can interact with biological predisposition in the development of CVD outcomes. The combinations of behavioral and environmental exposures present in a population are expected to differ in LMICs compared with HICs. The result is unique presentations of CVD, such as the high risk of CVD in nonobese individuals. A classic example of the intersection of environmental, behavioral, and biological risks is that children who have experienced undernutrition in early life may be at higher risk of CVD later in life. This phenomenon has been documented in India, where poverty and food system failures combined to result in widespread undernutrition (16, 27–29). Behaviorally, there is then a desire to compensate with nutrient-dense foods when they are available. Early exposure to undernutrition and later life exposure to caloric excess produce metabolic disturbances that have been linked to diabetes, raised blood lipids (dyslipidemia), and obesity. Together, these factors coalesce in a manner that increases the risk of heart attack and stroke.

## CHALLENGES AND OPPORTUNITIES IN CVD RISKS GLOBALLY

Many of the significant risk factors for CVD—such as hypertension, diabetes, tobacco use, high cholesterol, male sex, and older age—have remained relatively stable over time and space. Nevertheless, despite decades of research, we cannot perfectly predict—let alone effectively prevent—all CVDs. Some of the major challenges—and opportunities for future inquiry—include the dynamic nature of potential risk factors, the complexity of hitherto unidentified risk factors for CVDs, and the differential impact of risk factors across individuals and settings.

### Changing the Distribution of Risk Factors

Risk factor profiles have changed considerably in the past 50 years. Tobacco use has declined in HICs, obesity has increased globally, and with obesity, diabetes has dramatically risen. Furthermore, broader contextual and social factors have changed. Fewer people live in poverty today, and sedentary lifestyles have permeated urban metropolises and reach rural areas. Medical management of CVD risk factors such as high BP, glucose, and cholesterol are becoming more effective and possibly more widely available. Individuals with other medical morbidities—such as HIV infection and cancer—live longer with their conditions and are therefore at risk of developing CVD. The dynamic nature of risk factor distribution in response to broader environmental, social, and economic conditions and clinical discovery ensures that the study of CVD risk factors will never be final.

## Complexity of Novel Risk Factors

Much of what we have learned so far has been through careful epidemiologic studies that follow large groups of individuals over time for the differential development of the disease. Once a putative risk factor is identified through longitudinal cohort studies, they are often tested for a causal relationship through randomized trials. Several technological advancements in biomarker assessments have allowed us to evaluate such increasingly complex and dynamic exposures as risk factors for CVD. Evidence for using multiple biomarkers instead of single biomarkers is gaining more impetus to develop composite risk scores that address multiple pathophysiological pathways (30). Different biomarkers reflect unique pathophysiological pathways. For example, a combination of troponin-C elevation (myocardial damage) and C-reactive protein (inflammation) indicates acute coronary syndrome. This provides cause-specific mortality (30). However, the challenge of using multiple biomarkers is that despite achieving improved discrimination and calibration, it is more likely an exhaustive process. Also, not all factors that carry a risk for CVD are easily measured. Examples are genomics and metabolomics—or the totality of genes and metabolites, respectively. These and other -omics, such as epigenomics, have been challenging to measure at scale and analyze because they require extracting information on huge numbers of indicators, change over time, and may change in response to the environment. However, the integrative analysis of "-omics" data is not straightforward and represents several logistic and computational challenges. Even though many genes and loci are identified, the precise mechanisms by which these genes influence CVD risk are not well understood. Recent advances in the development and optimization of high-throughput technologies for the generation of -omics data have provided a deeper understanding of the processes and dynamic interactions involved in CVDs. Significant breakthroughs in novel, robust, and cost-effective multiomics (metabolomics, epigenomics, proteomics) have the potential to overcome past limitations (31, 32). Several studies have successfully applied integrative genomics approaches to investigate novel mechanisms and plasma biomarkers involved in CVDs. Furthermore, any variability source is incorporated into statistical models to identify causal genes in gene loci translation into biological processes. It has opened the possibility to mechanistically understand disease onset and progression at the molecular level, resulting in the characterization of novel pathways and targeted therapeutic interventions (31, 32).

## Heterogeneity of Risk across Individuals and Populations

As described earlier, risk scoring systems fail to predict outcomes in all individuals and perform differently across populations. Simultaneously, our ability to collect risk measures has grown phenomenally since the time of the FHS that inaugurated the era of risk prediction. These two observations have motivated the era of precision or personalized medicine (33, 34). Precision medicine involves an integrative CVD management approach through personal profiling of individuals' lifestyle, genetics, CV health, environmental exposures, and disease phenotypes. This eliminates the reductionistic approach of using average population statistics and provides unique disease risk and treatment that works best for the individual. While precision health (also known as 'precision public health') is broader, it includes approaches to disease prevention, health promotion, and precision medicine that individuals can do on their own to protect themselves and public health steps (34). However, in most LMICs, the cost of these measurements will be prohibitive and a limiting factor. Therefore, focusing on simple and common risk factors such as BP may be a better approach. Even small shifts in average BP may have huge benefits for population-level CVD mortality. As elegantly shown in Figure 3.2, an intervention that reduces average systolic BP by 3 mmHg could lead to a five percentage point reduction in CHD mortality. To provide real-world context to these numbers, a recent study from India demonstrated that a unit increase in ambient particular matter 2.5 (PM 2.5) was associated with 3–5 mmHg higher systolic BP on average, depending on whether it was short- or long-term exposure. Therefore, combating air pollution and reducing PM 2.5 may have a miniscule impact on an individual's clinical risk but has a huge bearing on population-level BP.

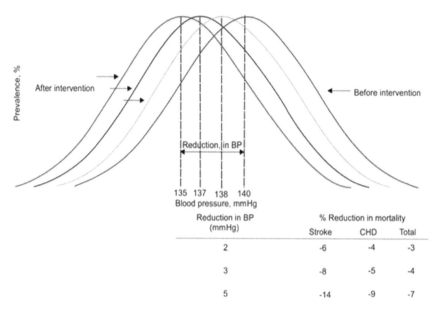

| Reduction in BP (mmHg) | % Reduction in mortality | | |
| --- | --- | --- | --- |
| | Stroke | CHD | Total |
| 2 | -6 | -4 | -3 |
| 3 | -8 | -5 | -4 |
| 5 | -14 | -9 | -7 |

**Figure 3.2**  Population impact of changes in average blood pressure (35).

## SUMMARY

Risk reduction at an individual level has multifold effects on population prevention programs. Moreover, the CVD-based public health programs will continue to rely on the more thorough implementation of existing risk tools based on putative risk factors, i.e., smoking, high BP, and high serum total cholesterol levels. Developing CVD guidelines that consider CVD's multifactorial nature is an effective strategy for lowering a patient's total CV risk. Designing and implementing a comprehensive approach towards the continuum of care requires both medical and public health approaches that are crucial in preventing the epidemic of CVD. Utilizing local applications of CV assessment models and algorithms by adding novel and emerging risk factors will help in measuring lifetime risk for CVD and tailoring our treatment approaches.

## REFERENCES

1. Payne RA. Cardiovascular risk. Br J Clin Pharmacol. 2012 Sep;74(3):396–410.
2. Ezzati M, Hoorn SV, Rodgers A, Lopez AD, Mathers CD, Murray CJL. Estimates of global and regional potential health gains from reducing multiple major risk factors. The Lancet. 2003;362:10.
3. Chen G, Levy D. Contributions of the Framingham heart study to the epidemiology of coronary heart disease. JAMA Cardiol. 2016 Oct 1;1(7):825.
4. Stampfer Meir J, Ridker Paul M, Dzau Victor J. Risk factor criteria. Circulation. 2004 Jun 29;109(25_suppl_1):IV–3.
5. Mahmood SS, Levy D, Vasan RS, Wang TJ. The Framingham heart study and the epidemiology of cardiovascular diseases: A historical perspective. Lancet. 2014 Mar 15;383(9921):999–1008.
6. ASCVD Risk Estimator [Internet]. [cited 2020 Dec 15]. Available from: https://tools.acc.org/ldl/ascvd_risk_estimator/index.html#!/calulate/estimator/
7. National Vascular Disease Prevention Alliance. Guidelines for the management of absolute cardiovascular disease risk. 2012. Available from: https://informme.org.au/guidelines/guidelines-for-the-management-of-absolute-cvd-risk-2012
8. Sedgwick JEC. Absolute, attributable, and relative risk in the management of coronary heart disease. Heart. 2001 May 1;85(5):491–492.
9. O'Donnell MJ, Xavier D, Liu L, Zhang H, Chin SL, Rao-Melacini P, et al. Risk factors for ischaemic and intracerebral haemorrhagic stroke in 22 countries (the INTERSTROKE study): a case-control study. The Lancet. 2010 Jul;376(9735):112–123.

10. Yusuf S, Hawken S, Ounpuu S, Dans T, Avezum A, Lanas F, et al. Effect of potentially modifiable risk factors associated with myocardial infarction in 52 countries (the INTERHEART study): case-control study. Lancet Lond Engl. 2004 Sep 11;364(9438):937–952.
11. Yusuf S, Reddy S, Ôunpuu S, Anand S. Global burden of cardiovascular diseases. Circulation. 2001 Nov 27;104(22):2746–2753.
12. Kotchen TA. Developing hypertension guidelines: an evolving process. Am J Hypertens. 2014 Jun 1;27(6):765–772.
13. Helfand M, Buckley DI, Freeman M, Fu R, Rogers K, Fleming C, et al. Emerging risk factors for coronary heart disease: a summary of systematic reviews conducted for the U.S. preventive services task force. Ann Intern Med. 2009 Oct 6;151(7):496.
14. Developing Countries I of M (US) C on P the GE of CDM the C in, Fuster V, Kelly BB. Framework for action [Internet]. Promoting cardiovascular health in the developing world: a critical challenge to achieve global health. National Academies Press (US); 2010 [cited 2021 Jun 13]. Available from: www.ncbi.nlm.nih.gov/books/NBK45685/
15. Schultz William M, Kelli Heval M, Lisko John C, Varghese Tina, Shen Jia, Sandesara Pratik, et al. Socioeconomic status and cardiovascular outcomes. Circulation. 2018 May 15;137(20):2166–2178.
16. Singh A, Dixit S. Socioeconomic patterning of cardiovascular disease and its risk factors among Indians: a systematic review of literature. Int J Med Public Health. 2017 Mar 1;7(1):01–17.
17. Batsis JA, Lopez-Jimenez F. Cardiovascular risk assessment—from individual risk prediction to estimation of global risk and change in risk in the population. BMC Med. 2010 May 25;8(1):29.
18. Jansen J, Bonner C, McKinn S, Irwig L, Glasziou P, Doust J, et al. General practitioners' use of absolute risk versus individual risk factors in cardiovascular disease prevention: an experimental study. BMJ Open. 2014 May 1;4(5):e004812.
19. Viera AJ, Sheridan SL. Global risk of coronary heart disease: assessment and application. Am Fam Physician. 2010 Aug 1;82(3):265–274.
20. Garg N, Muduli SK, Kapoor A, Tewari S, Kumar S, Khanna R, et al. Comparison of different cardiovascular risk score calculators for cardiovascular risk prediction and guideline recommended statin uses. Indian Heart J. 2017;6.
21. Bonner C, Fajardo MA, Hui S, Stubbs R, Trevena L. Clinical validity, understandability, and actionability of online cardiovascular disease risk calculators: systematic review. J Med Internet Res. 2018 Feb 1;20(2):e29.
22. Goff DC, Lloyd-Jones DM, Bennett G, Coady S, D'Agostino RB, Gibbons R, et al. 2013 ACC/AHA guideline on the assessment of cardiovascular risk. J Am Coll Cardiol. 2014 Jul;63(25):2935–2959.
23. Betts MB, Milev S, Hoog M, Jung H, Milenković D, Qian Y, et al. Comparison of recommendations and use of cardiovascular risk equations by health technology assessment agencies and clinical guidelines. Value Health. 2019 Feb;22(2):210–219.
24. Liu J, Hong Y, D'Agostino RB, Wu Z, Wang W, Sun J, et al. Predictive value for the Chinese population of the Framingham CHD risk assessment tool compared with the Chinese multi-provincial cohort study. JAMA. 2004 Jun 2;291(21):2591–2599.
25. Yusuf S, Reddy S, Ôunpuu S, Anand S. Global burden of cardiovascular diseases: Part I: general considerations, the epidemiologic transition, risk factors, and impact of urbanization. Circulation. 2001 Nov 27;104(22):2746–2753.
26. Ford ND, Patel SA, Narayan KMV. Obesity in low- and middle-income countries: burden, drivers, and emerging challenges. Annu Rev Public Health. 2017 Mar 20;38(1):145–164.
27. Palinski Wulf. Effect of maternal cardiovascular conditions and risk factors on offspring cardiovascular disease. Circulation. 2014 May 20;129(20):2066–2077.
28. Jeemon P, Neogi S, Bhatnagar D, Cruickshank KJ, Prabhakaran D. The impact of migration on cardiovascular disease and its risk factors among people of Indian origin. Curr Sci. 2009;97(3):378–384.
29. Yusuf S, Joseph P, Rangarajan S, Islam S, Mente A, Hystad P, et al. Modifiable risk factors, cardiovascular disease, and mortality in 155 722 individuals from 21 high-income, middle-income, and low-income countries (PURE): a prospective cohort study. The Lancet. 2020 Mar 7;395(10226):795–808.

30. Wang Thomas J. Multiple biomarkers for predicting cardiovascular events. J Am Coll Cardiol. 2010 May 11;55(19):2092–2095.
31. Lau E, Wu JC. Omics, big data, and precision medicine in cardiovascular sciences. Circ Res. 2018 Apr 27;122(9):1165–1168.
32. Leon-Mimila P, Wang J, Huertas-Vazquez A. Relevance of multi-omics studies in cardio-vascular diseases. Front Cardiovasc Med [Internet]. 2019 Jul 17 [cited 2020 Dec 15];6. Available from: www.ncbi.nlm.nih.gov/pmc/articles/PMC6656333/
33. Lacey B, Herrington WG, Preiss D, Lewington S, Armitage J. The role of emerging risk factors in cardiovascular outcomes. Curr Atheroscler Rep [Internet]. 2017 [cited 2020 Dec 11];19(6). Available from: www.ncbi.nlm.nih.gov/pmc/articles/PMC5419996/
34. Pencina MJ, Peterson ED. Moving from clinical trials to precision medicine: the role for predictive modeling. JAMA. 2016 Apr 26;315(16):1713–1714.
35. Stamler R. Implications of the INTERSALT study. Hypertens Dallas Tex 1979. 1991 Jan;17(1 Suppl):I16–I20.

# 4 Concepts in Prevention

*Radhika Prakash Asrani and Shivani A. Patel*

CONTENTS

## INTRODUCTION

In this chapter we focus on individual and population-level approaches for cardiovascular disease (CVD) prevention. As seen in previous sections, behavioral, biological, psychosocial, and health systems factors contribute to the burden of CVDs (1). The inter-relatedness of these factors provides the basis for developing a comprehensive conceptual model for disease prevention that coordinates across sectors and multiple levels of influence and intervention. In this section we discuss definitions of prevention, provide an ecological framework for CVD prevention in the developing country context, and discuss existing evidence and applications of the framework to individuals, communities, and broader society.

### Definition of Prevention

The definition of prevention has expanded over time. In 1967, prevention was defined as a means of averting the development of any pathological state broadly, irrespective of the stage of disease (2). In 1978, distinctions were made between primary, secondary, and tertiary prevention, wherein primary prevention is the prevention of overt disease (e.g., preventing coronary artery disease), secondary prevention is the prevention of worsening severity of coronary artery disease (CAD), and tertiary prevention is the prevention of clinical events. Primary prevention includes activities to reduce risk factor levels to prevent development of disease. It is targeted at individuals at risk of disease and includes activities such as risk assessment; management of risk factors such as hypertension and diabetes; and offering support for self-management such as promoting healthier diets, exercise, and other healthy behaviors. Secondary prevention dealt with early detection and diagnosis of disease based on clinical or imaging criteria with the aim of preventing acute events. Secondary prevention is targeted at individuals with pre-clinical disease and can include more aggressive management of risk factors or medical treatment. Tertiary prevention includes reversing or delaying the progression of disease such as improving adherence and compliance to treatment (2). These three types of prevention can be traditionally conceptualized to fall under the purview of formal health services with an individualistic focus.

Over time, the concept of prevention has shifted to include population health and reducing disparities in health. Population-level interventions are targeted at healthy individuals with the aim to reduce exposure and susceptibility to disease by addressing the underlying causes of exposure (e.g., social pressure to smoke). The public health approach to prevention includes public health surveillance, risk factor research, development and evaluation of programs, and the dissemination of information on what works (3). The World Health Organization (WHO) defines disease prevention as "specific, population-based and individual-based interventions for primary and secondary (early detection) prevention, aiming to minimize the burden of diseases and associated risk factors" (4). Risk factor reduction was added to prevention by the WHO in 1998 (2), and this is sometimes referred to as "primordial prevention" and is an essential component of health promotion and policy-level interventions. In the context of CVDs, this includes identification of high-risk individuals using risk scores; resetting thresholds or changes in diagnostic criteria for cholesterol, diabetes, and blood pressure; and making population-wide policy-level changes to alter risk factors such as higher taxation on alcohol and cigarettes. In a present-day context, prevention is viewed in a wider sense as a social good to include activities and improvements in the social determinants of health, reductions in health inequities, and increased access to education (3). Health education and promotion can be applied at all three levels of prevention, thereby maximizing the gains from prevention.

### Population-Based Approaches to Prevention

Prevention, when conceptualized in a broader sense, has benefits that extend beyond improvements in health measures. CVD prevention can follow a population-based approach or a high-risk approach. While each of these strategies aid in the reduction of risk factors, population-based approaches have proven to be more effective. Population-based approaches aim to reduce risk in the population as a whole, wherein a large-scale change will result in mass benefits across a wide range of risks (5). In contrast, the high-risk approach aims to identify individuals at elevated risk levels who are then targeted for interventions. For instance, a UK-based study revealed that reduction of risk factors at the population level led to a 70% decline in overall mortality and coronary mortality than improved technologies for care (30%) (6). Similarly, in the United States, population-wide changes in blood cholesterol from changes in diet and reductions in cigarette smoking led to a 54% decline in CHD mortality between 1968 and 1978, while changes in the treatment of hypertension and changes in healthcare accounted for 39.5% of the decline (7). Population-based approaches are lifestyle linked and more inexpensive than pharmacological interventions, which are more expensive. Population-based interventions in low- and middle-income countries (LMICs) have largely focused on reduction in salt intake and smoking and are found to be cost-saving or very cost-effective in CVD prevention (8). Salt reduction interventions have focused on health education via mass media campaigns, product reformulation, and relabeling. With respect to tobacco control, mass media campaigns, increasing taxes, and smoke-free laws are predominant strategies in LMICs. Other examples of population-based interventions include increasing public awareness of the importance of physical activity to prevent CVDs, promoting physical activity in workplaces and school systems, reducing consumption of refined carbohydrates such as wheat flour and white rice, population-wide advertising campaigns on healthy foods and lifestyle, and taxes on sugar and poor-quality oils.

### Framework for Prevention

A balance of population and high-risk approaches to prevention is desired, and in this chapter, we propose a framework for prevention that operates at the socio-ecological level, which postulates that individual health behaviors are shaped by their local environment and socio-cultural influences. We propose that the design of prevention strategies should consider a) intrapersonal factors, which include biologic and personal factors such as education, income, skills, and attitudes; b) interpersonal factors, which could include social networks, family, and peer networks; c) institutional factors, such as social institutions with formal or informal rules and regulations; d) community-level factors, which entail relationships among institutions and networks with well-defined boundaries; and e) public policy, which could include local, state, and national laws that govern behaviors and interventions. This framework has been adapted from Bronfenbrenner's socio-ecological model and the Institute of Medicine's approach to CVD prevention in developing countries (Figure 4.1) (9).

## TYPES OF INTERVENTIONS

Interventions may target one or more levels of the socio-ecological framework. Health research is increasingly focused on more distal levels of influence (e.g., social systems, healthcare system) as compared with proximal factors (e.g., individual health behaviors) as a target for intervention. Similarly, organizations and governments are increasingly seeking intersectoral partnerships to solve public health issues. In the context of CVDs and chronic diseases, policy and environmental changes aid in sustaining behavior changes as opposed to individually directed interventions (10).

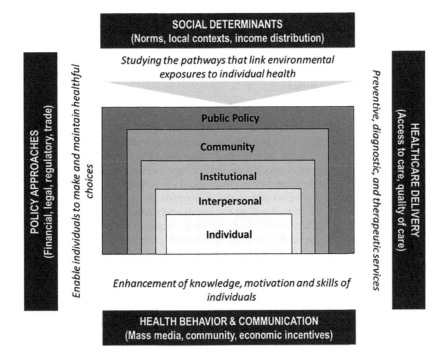

**Figure 4.1**   Socio-ecological framework for CVD prevention. (9)

## Social Determinants of Health

Inequalities in social and economic well-being lead to inequalities in health. Social determinants of health include contextual factors such as characteristics of a neighborhood (residential segregation, distribution of income) and individual factors such as availability of social support. Emphasis on social factors suggests that intervention efforts must include attention to social and economic policies, social and physical environments, and the implications of these policies and environments for health behaviors and risk of CVDs. For instance, availability of healthy foods and food subsidies influence individual dietary choices. Understanding the inter-relationships between social, economic, and clinical factors enables us to consider the implications of intervening at various points in these processes (11).

To illustrate the impact of social context, a study conducted in South India examined the prevalence of CVD risk factors in men and women in rural and urban areas and their association with measures of socio-economic status. They found that cardiovascular risk factors were higher in the urban than in the rural population. Indicators of socio-economic status (SES) were positively related to CVD risk factors, including overweight and obesity, lipid profiles, hypertension, and abnormal glucose tolerance. They found stronger associations of CVD risk factors with material wealth than with educational indicators, which likely reflects differences between lower and higher SES groups in beliefs, perceptions about body size, and dietary practices (12).

A crucial aspect for developing any policy or program is understanding the nature of the problem as it occurs in the local context where the intervention will be implemented. This requires an assessment of the needs of the population, existing and current efforts, available capacities, and infrastructure needs to address CVDs and chronic diseases and to gauge the political context. An assessment of the local needs and social determinants will inform priorities and determine choices about the implementation of evidence-based policies and programs and capacity-building efforts.

Variables for the measurement of social determinants of health include place or neighborhood of residence (rural, urban, peri-urban), house ownership, race, ethnicity, perceived discrimination, gender, partner violence, perceived role within a family, highest educational attainment, income, occupation, household wealth, ownership of land, etc. The study of ecologic-level exposures has called for innovative multilevel analysis methods. The assessment of exposures at the environmental level can lead to an understanding of the social determinants of health that is more than the sum of individual-level measures (13). Studying the pathways that link environmental exposures to individual health outcomes is a valuable research tool to epidemiologists. Additionally, models and frameworks have emerged to examine ways in which social and economic conditions influence health over the life course.

## Behavioral Interventions and Health Communication

Preventive health behavior can be defined as "any activity undertaken by an individual who believes himself (or herself) to be healthy, for the purpose of preventing or detecting illness in an asymptomatic state" (14). Health behavior change interventions have been the focus of multiple fields, including public health, health and medical specialties, psychology, health education, and social work. During the 1970s and 1980s the emphasis on an individual's behaviors as determinants of health in turn led to an increased focus on the broader social determinants of health (10). An entire body of public health research deals with incorporating the social and economic context into explanations about why some people stay healthy while others get sick. Social environments influence behavior by a) shaping norms, b) enforcing health-damaging or health-promoting patterns of social control, c) providing or not providing opportunities to engage in certain behaviors, and d) reducing or producing stress (13). More recently, we have gathered that behaviors are clustered with one another. For instance, people who drink also smoke, people who eat a healthy diet are also physically active, people who are poor also have lower levels of education and more likely to engage in risk-related behaviors. These patterned behavioral responses have led to the incorporation of the social context into behavioral interventions by targeting communities, schools, and workplaces to achieve health behavior change (13). Social context could include life experiences, social relationships, organizational structures, the physical environment, and societal influences that could act as either modifying conditions or mediating mechanisms between an intervention and an outcome (13).

Health communication and education programs are a means to alter health behaviors and are typically designed to reach a large audience. Communication programs could influence behaviors through a) directly persuading or educating individuals to change behaviors and b) changing expectations of peers in a community, which in turn could influence individual behaviors. Health education and communication efforts could occur at multiple levels, from national government to local authorities and community organizations.

## Community Interventions

Community-based interventions utilize the organization as the unit of analysis. Health behavior change theories were expanded to include community constructs that emphasize the social context. A multifactor community intervention approach can act synergistically with clinical health services and health professionals (9). For instance, adherence to a medication regimen could be easier if others in the peer network have also learned the importance of it, for example, following a certain diet or controlling blood pressure. Health education efforts at the community level could be achieved by campaigns organized by community health workers, making print materials on health available, conducting health fairs and events, and conducting educational programs at the clinical setting. The local media could also be leveraged in this regard. Special-interest groups in the community are crucial for developing and fostering capacity for CVD control by mobilizing and empowering members. Such groups may evolve and operate as neighborhood groups, self-help groups, schools, etc., and help in diffusing the effects of an intervention to the target community. A cluster randomized trial of the HRIDAY program of school-based health education in India showed that intervention students were less likely than controls to have been offered, received, experimented with, or have intentions to use tobacco (15). A worksite-based health promotion in ten sites across India and a pilot community program in southern India have also been successful in reducing risks for CVD (5).

## Mass Media

As the importance of population-based perspectives has developed, there has been an increased focus on interventions that have larger-scale impact, such that they combine the best of individually oriented interventions in a format that can be tailored to broader audiences. Media can have a strong impact on behavior of individuals, families, and society at large. Media can be used as a tool to promote community organization, accept policy changes, and achieve dietary and physical activity behaviors.

Brazil's Agita intervention aimed to increase the population's awareness of the importance of physical activity. The program organized three main types of interventions: mega-events, activities with partner institutions, and partnerships with community organizations. Nearly 21 million people were reached by means of 30 newspapers distributed in various cities, along with seven national newspapers and four broadcasts on national television. An annual survey carried out over 4 years showed increased self-reported levels of physical activity following the intervention (16). In addition to better management of information and health education, communication technologies in recent years have offered new mechanisms to deliver interventions. Telehealth and m-health approaches have been used in developing countries for better management of chronic diseases. UKIERI's Mobile Disease Management System is a joint effort by the UK and India, wherein a monitoring system using a mobile phone has been developed to collect information on physiological measures from patients, which includes information on electrocardiogram (ECG) data, blood pressure, oxygen saturation, and blood glucose level, which are then relayed to healthcare professionals (9).

### Economic Incentives

Economic and financial incentives are another means to influence a consumer's preventive health behaviors, particularly in the short term. Financial incentives for smoking cessation have been evaluated in the Philippines, wherein a program offered smokers a voluntary commitment contract to quit smoking coupled with a savings account to deposit money for 6 months without interest. Participants were given a lockbox to deposit their daily savings, with a weekly deposit collection service. Within 1 week of the 6-month maturity date, participants took a urine test for nicotine and cotinine. If they passed, their money was returned; otherwise, their money was forfeited to charity (17). The study found that smokers randomly offered commitment contract combined with savings account were three percentage points more likely to pass the 6-month test than the control group, and this effect persisted in surprise tests at 12 months, indicating that the program produced lasting smoking cessation. Conditional cash transfer programs have also been instituted to improve health, nutrition, and education in developing countries. Financial incentives can also be used to improve adherence to clinical interventions.

### Policy Approaches

Laws, treaties, policies, and regulations have played important roles in the prevention and control of disease. In a multilevel framework, a population-centric approach to CVD prevention would require "upstream" policies to make practices such as healthy eating and physical activity easier, "midstream" policies to influence population behaviors, and "downstream" policies to support health services and clinical care (18). The social determinants of health influence the extent to which communities possess the physical and personal resources to satisfy their needs. The burden of poor health, including chronic disease, is disproportionately located in economically and socially disadvantaged communities. A government's policies for chronic disease prevention would need to address the underlying determinants of health. Policy areas that influence the underlying determinants of health include finance, trade, legal systems, education, and social affairs, to name a few.

Financial policies would be those that increase the monetary costs of behaviors, such as imposing taxes on the sale of tobacco products, or reducing the cost of healthy alternatives, such as price supports for fruits and vegetables. Legal policies, under the force of law, would inhibit exposure of the population to risks with imposition of fines/penalties if found guilty of violating a law. An example would be prohibiting smoking in public spaces or increasing tobacco prices. Regulatory polices include setting standards for various determinants of risks such as air quality, trans fat content in food, requirements for communications of such risks via food labeling, etc. Not meeting the requirements could lead to fines or discontinuance of sale of products. Trade and marketing policies include those that affect production, buying, and selling of products that affect risk behaviors such as marketing regulations for tobacco products and agricultural policies to encourage fruit and vegetable production. All these policies can be viewed as "upstream" policies that influence the healthy eating and risk behavior environment. These polices alter the environment in a way such that healthier choices are the easier choices, thus indirectly influencing population behaviors. For instance, a single policy measure instituted by the government of Mauritius in 1987 changed the composition of commonly used cooking oil from being mostly palm oil (high in saturated fatty acids) to being wholly soybean oil (high in unsaturated fatty acids), which led to a reduction in the plasma cholesterol levels of its population (5).

Midstream policy approaches would aim to directly influence the population's behavior, for which they need to directly affect the settings in which people live their lives. For instance, if the aim is obesity prevention, key settings would include where people eat and can be physically active, such as early childhood settings, education settings (schools, colleges), workplaces and households, and recreational facilities. At the organizational level, schools could institute school food policies, physical activity requirements, and programs to promote healthy eating. Similarly, workplaces could offer incentives to participate in health and wellness activities and set health targets as part of performance indicators. Government policy instruments to influence individual behaviors, on the other hand, would take the form of education and campaign-based programs.

Downstream policy approaches represent actions that support health services and clinical interventions for individuals. At the primary care level, this could include subsidies for healthy lifestyle counseling, instituting a nutritionist or dietician at primary care clinics. Similarly, at the secondary and tertiary level, subsidies could be put in place for treatment by specialists.

## Healthcare Delivery

The success of any CVD prevention intervention is dependent on the quality of existing health systems at the local, state, and national levels. While we can design interventions to alter behaviors and improve awareness, the success of these interventions in reducing mortality from CVDs is dependent on its healthcare workforce and health infrastructure to deliver interventions. This includes availability of human resources at the provider level and the mechanisms and quality of healthcare delivery. An effective healthcare delivery system would need to focus on specific CVD needs as well as broader health systems needs that are relevant for chronic diseases and synergistic with integrated primary care. Incorporation of prevention messaging and education by healthcare providers would be an important step towards reducing CVD risks. The WHO defines a health system as consisting of "all organizations, people, and actions whose primary intent is to promote, restore, or maintain health". The fundamental goal of a health system is to provide effective, equitable, responsive, and efficient care.

Effective care can be described as timely, safe, improves health outcomes, and continues until a health issue is resolved such that it is responsive to the needs of the patients through technical competence and the interpersonal quality of providers. Equity in health systems ensures that health services are accessible and utilized by all members of a society and that payment for care is equitable. Efficiency refers to achieving the greatest health gains from resources that are available in a productive manner. In this section, we discuss components of healthcare delivery for successful implementation of clinical prevention and disease management of CVDs, namely patient-level interventions and provider-level interventions to improve quality and access to care. All these interventions are not intended to be used in isolation from each other, but in synergy with population and community-based approaches.

### Patient-Level Interventions

Access to CVD care entails a cost-effective primary care–centered approach with targeted screening for high-risk individuals and treatment for symptom control (9). While CVD risk scoring mechanisms exist in high-income countries, these may not be directly applicable to low- and middle-income country contexts. Screening in resource-limited areas would need to focus on simple methods such as family history, medical history, and physical measurements for body mass index (BMI) and blood pressure. As a follow-up to screening, an effective health system would need to ensure access to essential medicines, medical products, and technologies.

### Provider Interventions to Improve Quality of Care

Quality improvement strategies that impact provider behavior could focus on improving technical performance of providers (the extent to which services are performed as per standards) and interpersonal quality (meeting users' expectations to provide responsive care) (9). These can be improved by setting guidelines, disease management programs, audit and feedback on performance, public reporting, and performance incentive mechanisms (9).

With the expected increase in the burden of CVDs worldwide, shortages in healthcare workforce and leadership would be felt more acutely in low-income countries. Strategies to tackle this challenge include provision of specialized continuous training at several levels of the healthcare workforce and promoting motivation by providing satisfactory renumeration, appropriate infrastructure, and career development. Community health workers who are trusted members of the community but do not have formal health training have been used in several areas of global health and have been beneficial in community health education, ensuring increased access to basic health services, cultural sensitivity, and cost-effectiveness and improving community self-reliance. Such a task sifting policy would require determining the optimal mix of specialization and training required to meet CVD-specific needs within individual countries.

### Monitoring and Evaluation

The ultimate goal when intervention approaches are proven to be effective is scale-up, maintenance, and dissemination. This requires ongoing surveillance and evaluation of implemented strategies such that they allow policy makers to determine if programs are having the intended effect and meeting defined goals. Over time, program managers would need to reassess needs, capacities, and priorities of the community to alter policies and programs as needs change, new lessons are learned, and communities undergo transitions in economy, health, or social environments.

## CONCLUSION

Prevention seeks to avert poor health outcomes before they occur. Health behaviors are undertaken by individuals, but they can be modified by intrapersonal, familial, social, and political events that occur inside and outside of an individual. A successful prevention strategy for CVDs would be multilevel in nature and considers all levels of influence on health behaviors, wherein both individual and structural approaches are needed to improve health. The most effective approaches would arise from interdisciplinary collaborations. From the previous sections, it is evident that the prevention of CVD extends beyond the realm of the health sector. An intersectoral coordinated approach at the governmental level is required so that policies in non-health sectors (such as agriculture, urban development, education, transportation, and the private sector) can be developed synergistically to promote cardiovascular health. Furthermore, local context matters for the planning and implementation of intervention approaches, as this directly influences the effectiveness of the intervention. Implementation and translational research would be important to develop and evaluate interventions in local settings.

## REFERENCES

1. Reducing the Burden of Cardiovascular Disease: Intervention Approaches—Promoting Cardiovascular Health in the Developing World—NCBI Bookshelf [Internet]. [cited 2019 Sep 24]. Available from: www.ncbi.nlm.nih.gov/books/NBK45696/
2. Starfield B, Hyde J, Gérvas J, Heath I. The concept of prevention: a good idea gone astray? J Epidemiol Community Health. 2008 Jul;62(7):580–583.
3. Ataguba JE, Mooney G. Building on "The concept of prevention: a good idea gone astray?" J Epidemiol Community Health. 2011 Feb;65(2):116–118.
4. WHO EMRO. Health promotion and disease prevention through population-based interventions, including action to address social determinants and health inequity. Public health functions. About WHO [Internet]. [cited 2019 Oct 18]. Available from: www.emro.who.int/about-who/public-health-functions/health-promotion-disease-prevention.html
5. Goenka S, Prabhakaran D, Ajay VS, Reddy KS. Preventing cardiovascular disease in India—translating evidence to action. Curr Sci. 00113891. 2009 Aug 10;97(3):367–377.
6. Critchley JA, Capewell S, Unal B. Life-years gained from coronary heart disease mortality reduction in Scotland: prevention or treatment? J Clin Epidemiol. 2003 Jun;56(6):583–590.
7. Goldman L, Cook EF. The decline in ischemic heart disease mortality rates. An analysis of the comparative effects of medical interventions and changes in lifestyle. Ann Intern Med. 1984 Dec;101(6):825–836.
8. Aminde LN, Takah NF, Zapata-Diomedi B, Veerman JL. Primary and secondary prevention interventions for cardiovascular disease in low-income and middle-income countries: a systematic review of economic evaluations. Cost Eff Resour Alloc. 2018 Jun 14;16(1):22.
9. Fuster V, Kelly BB, editors. Promoting cardiovascular health in the developing world: a critical challenge to achieve global health. Washington DC: Institute of Medicine of the National Academies; 2010.
10. Glanz K, Rimer BK, Viswanath K. Health behavior: theory, research, and practice. John Wiley & Sons; 2015. 512 p.
11. Schulz AJ, Zenk S, Odoms-Young A, Hollis-Neely T, Nwankwo R, Lockett M, et al. Healthy eating and exercising to reduce diabetes: exploring the potential of social determinants of

health frameworks within the context of community-based participatory diabetes prevention. Am J Public Health. 2005 Apr 1;95(4):645–651.

12. Samuel P, Antonisamy B, Raghupathy P, Richard J, Fall CH. Socio-economic status and cardiovascular risk factors in rural and urban areas of Vellore, Tamilnadu, South India. Int J Epidemiol. 2012 Oct;41(5):1315.

13. Berkman LF, Kawachi I, Glymour MM. Social epidemiology. Oxford University Press; 2014. 641 p.

14. PhD SVK, Sidney Cobb MD M. Health behavior, illness behavior, and sick-role behavior. Arch Environ Health Int J. 1966 Apr 1;12(4):531–541.

15. Reddy KS, Arora M, Perry CL, Nair B, Kohli A, Lytle LA, et al. Tobacco and alcohol use outcomes of a school-based intervention in New Delhi. Am J Health Behav. 2002 Jun;26(3):173–181.

16. Matsudo SM, Matsudo VR. Coalitions and networks: facilitating global physical activity promotion. Promot Educ. 2006;13(2):133–138, 158–163.

17. Giné X, Karlan D, Zinman J. Put your money where your butt is: a commitment contract for smoking cessation. Am Econ J Appl Econ. 2010 Oct;2(4):213–235.

18. Sacks G, Swinburn B, Lawrence M. Obesity policy action framework and analysis grids for a comprehensive policy approach to reducing obesity. Obes Rev Off J Int Assoc Study Obes. 2009 Jan;10(1):76–86.

## Additional References

Aminde LN, Takah NF, Zapata-Diomedi B, Veerman JL. Primary and secondary prevention interventions for cardiovascular disease in low-income and middle-income countries: a systematic review of economic evaluations. Cost Effectiveness and Resource Allocation: C/E. 2018;16:22. https://doi.org/10.1186/s12962-018-0108-9

Correia JC, Lachat S, Lagger G, Chappuis F, Golay A, Beran D, COHESION Project. Interventions targeting hypertension and diabetes mellitus at community and primary healthcare level in low- and middle-income countries: a scoping review. BMC Public Health. 2019;19(1):1542. https://doi.org/10.1186/s12889-019-7842-6

Hills AP, Misra A, Gill JM, Byrne NM, Soares MJ, Ramachandran A, et al. Public health and health systems: implications for the prevention and management of type 2 diabetes in South Asia. Lancet Diabetes Endocrinology. 2018;6(12):992–1002. https://doi.org/10.1016/S2213-8587(18)30203-1

Krieger N. Theories for social epidemiology in the 21st century: an ecosocial perspective. Int J Epidemiol. 2001 Aug;30(4):668-677. doi: 10.1093/ije/30.4.668

Nishtar S. Prevention of coronary heart disease in south Asia. Lancet. 2002;360(9338):1015–1018. https://doi.org/10.1016/S0140-6736(02)11088-9

Pandian JD, Gall SL, Kate MP, Silva GS, Akinyemi RO, Ovbiagele BI, et al. Prevention of stroke: a global perspective. Lancet. 2018;392(10154):1269–1278. https://doi.org/10.1016/S0140-6736(18)31269-8

Schulz A, Northridge ME. Social determinants of health: implications for environmental health promotion. Health Educ Behav. 2004;31(4):455–471. https://doi.org/10.1177/1090198104265598

Schulz AJ, House JS, Israel BA, et al. Relational pathways between socioeconomic position and cardiovascular risk in a multi ethnic urban sample: complexities and their implications for improving health in economically disadvantaged populations. J Epidemiology Community Health. 2008;62:638–646. http://dx.doi.org/10.1136/jech.2007.063222

Schulz AJ, Kannan S, Dvonch JT, Israel BA, Allen III A, James SA, House JS, Lepkowski J. Social and physical environments and disparities in risk for cardiovascular disease: the healthy environments partnership conceptual model environmental health perspectives. Environ Health Perspect. 2005 Dec;113(12):1817–1825. doi: 10.1289/ehp.7913

Schulz AJ, Zenk S, Odoms-Young A, Hollis-Neely T, Nwankwo R, Lockett M, Ridella W, Kannan S. Healthy eating and exercising to reduce diabetes: exploring the potential of social determinants of health frameworks within the context of community-based participatory diabetes prevention. Am J Public Health. 2005;95:645–651. https://doi.org/10.2105/AJPH.2004.048256

# CHAPTER 5
# RISK FACTORS

# 5.1 Cardiovascular Disease Risk Factors

*Dorairaj Prabhakaran*

CONTENTS

Risk factors are defined as any attribute, characteristic, or exposure of an individual that increases the likelihood of developing a disease or injury.[1] Multiple risk factors have been identified for cardiovascular disease (CVD), and these may be classified as modifiable and nonmodifiable (Box 5.1.1). Identification and stratification of patients on the basis of number of risk factors is an important first step in the management of CVD. Knowledge of risk factors and their role in CVD is of critical importance in the initiation of preventive measures, as well as in the selection of an appropriate management strategy. In this brief introduction, we schematically summarize the various determinants of CVD and the role of risk factors (Figure 5.1.1). The reasons for the increasing burden of CVD and its risk factors are described in Chapter 1.

## ROLE OF RISK FACTORS

Several studies have been undertaken to understand the role of risk factors in CVD. However, three studies have largely contributed to our present knowledge and also stimulated further research in CVD epidemiology, namely the Framingham Heart Study (FHS), the British Doctors' Study, and the Seven Countries Study. The role of risk factors in coronary artery disease (CAD) was first identified by the seminal FHS. Over a span of 70 years, the study uncovered several CVD risk factors hitherto unknown and was cardinal in paving the path for several other studies that tried to understand the underlying mechanisms.[3] The British Doctors' Study was another landmark study that revealed the association of tobacco smoking to several diseases and, more importantly, showed conclusive evidence of its role in myocardial infarction (MI).[4] The Seven Countries Study directed by Ancel Keys was the first multicountry study that tried to understand the role of varied dietary and lifestyle patterns in CVD.[5] This study led to the much-debated and controversial diet–heart hypothesis that postulated the role of lipids in heart disease.

A large volume of evidence has been accumulated subsequently through several epidemiological studies and clinical trials. To infer the causal role of risk factors, Hill has provided a set

---

**BOX 5.1.1 MAJOR RISK FACTORS FOR CARDIOVASCULAR DISEASE**

| Modifiable | | | Nonmodifiable |
|---|---|---|---|
| **Behavioral** | **Biological** | **Environmental** | |
| Tobacco | Hypertension | Air pollution | Family history |
| Diet | Diabetes | Noise pollution | Age |
| Physical inactivity | Dyslipidemia | Light | Gender |
| Alcohol | Central obesity | Lead and other heavy metals in the water | Ethnicity |
| Stress | | | |

---

DOI: 10.1201/b23266-6

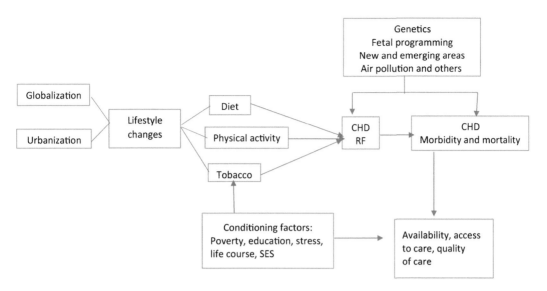

**Figure 5.1.1** Complex interplay of determinants and risk factors in the pathway of cardiovascular diseases in the population. CHD, coronary heart disease; RF, risk factor; SES, socioeconomic status.[2]

*Source*: Modified from Ref. 7.

of criteria, and based on this, the best-established risk factors for CVD are smoking, high blood pressure (BP), lipids, and diabetes.[6] Unhealthy diet and physical inactivity also confirm largely to this set of criteria. In fact, the reversal of reduction of risk factors at a population or individual level is an important feature of assessing causality. Unal, Capewell et al., Bandosz et al., and Ford et al. attribute a major role of reduction in CVD risk factors, both at a population and an individual level, for the decline in CAD.[7–10] The INTERHEART study identified nine simple risk factors that include the conventional risk factors identified by the FHS as major predictors for acute myocardial infarction (AMI) at an individual level as well as at a population level, contributing to at least 90% of attributable fraction (platelet-activating factor [PAF]).[11] Another large study that has contributed considerable evidence to our knowledge of cardiovascular risk factors is the Prospective Urban Rural Epidemiology (PURE) study.[12] The PURE study is a large, epidemiological cohort study of individuals aged 35–70 years in 18 countries that examines the impact of urbanization on the development of primordial risk factors (physical activity and nutrition changes), primary risk factors (obesity, hypertension, dysglycemia and dyslipidemia, smoking), and CVD. To this risk factor mix a recent addition is the role of air pollution and CVD. Air pollution, both indoor and outdoor, has emerged as a major risk factor for CVD, hypertension, and diabetes.

## PRINCIPLES OF PREVENTION OF CARDIOVASCULAR DISEASE

The role of a particular risk factor in CVD is often modified by the presence or absence of other coexisting risk factors. It is important to consider this coexistence and the interplay between them, rather than look at each risk factor individually. It is useful to keep the following four principles in mind while designing and constituting preventive strategies, or even while imparting health education to patients who either have or are at risk of developing CVD.

### Principle of Continuous Risk

It has been observed that risk due to a risk factor operates in a continuum and not across arbitrary thresholds. Several studies have shown how risk factors such as BP, serum cholesterol, body weight, smoking, and physical activity have a graded and continuous relationship with risk of CVD. Even within the normal range of a CVD risk factor, those with a higher level would have a higher risk for future cardiovascular events. For example, hypertension is defined as BP over 140 mmHg for systolic BP (SBP) and/or 90 mmHg for diastolic BP (DBP). Even at BP levels lower than the cutoff, there is a graded increase in risk with increasing levels of SBP.

It is important to note that the benefits of risk reduction are also continuous and operate across the range of the risk factor. An individual with an SBP level of 120 mmHg has a considerably lower risk as compared with an individual with an SBP of 130 mmHg. Clinical studies and cohort studies have shown that reduction in BP and blood lipid levels reduces the CVD events irrespective of the cutoff values of BP and cholesterol levels. Therefore, at a population level, it would be useful to shift the distribution to the left (Figure 5.1.2).

### Principle of Population-Wide Risk

The majority of coronary and stroke events arise in people who are in the midrange of a risk factor distribution curve. Although the relative risk (RR) of events is higher as we move up this distribution curve, the absolute numbers of people in the midrange of this distribution are much larger and thereby account for majority of the adverse events.

For example, evidence from Framingham Cohort shows that although RR for coronary heart disease (CHD) events is four times that among individuals with blood cholesterol levels >300 mg% than those with <200 mg%, more than twice as many CHD events arose from the <200 mg% group (who form 45% of the population) than from the >300 mg% group (who form 3–5% of the population). This principle emphasizes the importance of focusing public health interventions on individuals in this midrange group in order to attain greater impact.

### Principle of Multiplicative Risk

Evidence from large cohort studies has shown how coexistence of risk factors leads to interactive risk, which is multiplicative. In simple terms, when multiple risk factors coexist, the overall risk is multiplicative. Therefore, for maximal risk reduction, it is important to assess and manage all risk factors through nonpharmacological or pharmacological means, rather than focus on any single risk factor in isolation. Furthermore, even small elevations of multiple risk factors as compared with large elevation of a single risk factor are likely to have a higher risk of future CVD events.

To illustrate, let us compare two individuals of the same age. The first person, a male, has the following risk factor profile: serum cholesterol >245 mg/dL, SBP 118–124 mmHg, and is a non-smoker; the second person has serum cholesterol 205 mg/dL, SBP 134 mmHg, and is a smoker. If we apply the Framingham Risk Score, the risk of CHD events in the second person with multiple risk factors would be five times greater than in the first person.

A diagrammatic representation of the multiple risk factor profile attribution to the total risk is shown in Figure 5.1.2. In this figure, as the number of risk factors increases, the CVD risk increases in a linear fashion.

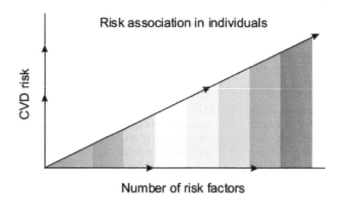

**Figure 5.1.2**  A diagrammatic representation of the multiple risk factor profile attribution to the total risk. CVD, cardiovascular disease.

*Source*: With permission from Prabhakaran D, Krishna Kumar R, Naik N, Kaul U. In: Cardiovascular Disease—Introduction to Risk Factors and Cardiovascular Disease Prevention. *Tandon's Textbook of Cardiology*, Volume 2. New Delhi: Wolters Kluwer India, 2019, Chapter 33.

## Principle of Absolute Risk

The absolute risk of a major CVD event is dependent on the overall risk profile contributed to by coexistent risk factors operating in a continuum. Essentially a combination of the aforementioned principles of continuous and multiplicative risk, this principle explains that, in most populations, the majority of CVD events arise in individuals with modest elevations of many risk factors rather than in individuals with marked elevation of a single risk factor.

## LIFE-COURSE APPROACH IN PREVENTING CARDIOVASCULAR DISEASES

In recent years, a life-course approach to the study of health and illness—which suggests that exposure to disadvantageous experiences and environments from womb to tomb accumulates throughout life and increases the risk of illness and premature death—has gained popularity. The interval between exposure, disease onset, and clinical recognition in CVDs suggests that exposures early in life are involved in initiating disease processes prior to clinical manifestations.

For example, the birth weight of babies is strongly associated with maternal nutrition, which is determined by the socioeconomic status (SES) of the family. Undernutrition of the mother during pregnancy affects the growth of the fetus inside the uterus and results in low birth weight. The fetus undergoes a state of "programming" to adapt to a low nutrient supply. "Programming" of the fetus impairs fetal development, which in turn "programs" for adult CHD, stroke, hypertension, and diabetes. The four relevant factors in fetal life are (i) intrauterine growth retardation (IUGR), (ii) premature delivery, (iii) overnutrition during gestational life, and (iv) intergenerational factors. There is considerable evidence, mostly from developed countries, that IUGR is associated with an increased risk of CHD, stroke, diabetes, and raised BP. It may rather be the pattern of growth, i.e., restricted fetal growth followed by very rapid postnatal catch-up growth, that is important in the underlying disease pathways. On the other hand, large size at birth is also associated with an increased risk of diabetes and CVD.[13]

Thus, it is clear that risk factors must be addressed throughout the life course. For interventions to have a lasting effect on the risk factor prevalence and the health of societies, it is also essential to change or modify the environment in which these diseases develop. Reversing current trends will require a multifaceted public health policy approach.

## SUMMARY

The core principles of understanding the concepts of risk factors as primary targets for population-based approaches and public health interventions for CVD prevention are presented here. The subsequent sections will discuss the individual risk factors in greater detail.

## ACKNOWLEDGMENT

This chapter is based on the manuscript originally written by the same author in the book *Tandon's Textbook of Cardiology,* Dorairaj Prabhakaran, Raman Krishna Kumar, Nitish Naik (eds). *Tandon's Textbook of Cardiology.* Wolters Kluwer, New Delhi, 2019.

Arun Pulikkottil Jose, Deputy Director, Centre for Digital Health, Public Health Foundation of India.

## REFERENCES

1. World Health Organization. *Differences between risk, risk factors, risk-behaviours, risk-conditions and at-risk.* https://apps.who.int/adolescent/second-decade/section/section_5/level5_5.php. Accessed April 22, 2022.
2. Prabhakaran D, Anand S, Watkins D, et al. Cardiovascular, respiratory, and related disorders: key messages from Disease Control Priorities, 3rd edition. *Lancet (London, England).* 2018;391(10126):1224–1236. doi:10.1016/S0140-6736(17)32471-6
3. Mahmooda SS, Levy D, Vasan RS, Wang TJ. The framingham heart study and the epidemiology of cardiovascular diseases: A historical perspective. *Lancet.* 2014;383(9921):1933–1945. doi:10.1016/S0140-6736(13)61752-3.
4. Doll R, Hill AB. Lung cancer and other causes of death in relation to smoking. *Br Med J.* 1956;2(5001):1071. doi:10.1136/BMJ.2.5001.1071
5. Keys A, Menotti A, Aravanis C, et al. The seven countries study: 2,289 deaths in 15 years. *Prev Med (Baltim).* 1984;13(2):141–154. doi:10.1016/0091-7435(84)90047-1
6. Bradford Hill SA, CBE H FRCP D. The environment and disease: Association or causation? *Proc R Soc Med.* 1965;58(5):295. doi:10.1177/003591576505800503

7. Unal B, Critchley JA, Capewell S. Explaining the decline in coronary heart disease mortality in England and Wales Between 1981 and 2000. *Circulation.* 2004;109:1101–1107. doi:10.1161/01. CIR.0000118498.35499.B2

8. Capewell S, Beaglehole R, Seddon M, McMurray J. Explanation for the decline in coronary heart disease mortality rates in Auckland, New Zealand, between 1982 and 1993. *Circulation.* 2000;26(102(13)):1511–1516. www.circulationaha.org

9. Bandosz P, O'Flaherty M, Drygas W, Rutkowski M, Koziarek J, Wyrzykowski B, Bennett K, Zdrojewski T, Capewell S. Decline in mortality from coronary heart disease in Poland after socioeconomic transformation: modelling study. *Br Med J.* 2012 Jan 25;344:d8136. doi: 10.1136/bmj.d8136

10. Ford ES, Ajani UA, Croft JB, et al. *Explaining the decrease in U.S. deaths from coronary disease.*; 1980. www.nejm.org.

11. Yusuf S, Hawken S, Ôunpuu S, et al. Effect of potentially modifiable risk factors associated with myocardial infarction in 52 countries (the INTERHEART study): case-control study. *Lancet.* 2004;364(9438):937–952. doi:10.1016/S0140-6736(04)17018-9

12. Teo K, Chow CK, Vaz M, et al. The Prospective Urban Rural Epidemiology (PURE) study: Examining the impact of societal influences on chronic noncommunicable diseases in low-, middle-, and high-income countries. *Am Heart J.* 2009;158(1):1–7.e1. doi:10.1016/J. AHJ.2009.04.019

13. Aboderin I, Kalache A, Ben-Shlomo Y, et al. *Life course perspectives on coronary heart disease, stroke and diabetes: key issues and implications for policy and research: summary report of a meeting of experts,* 2–4 May 2001.; 2002. https://apps.who.int/iris/handle/10665/67173. Accessed April 23, 2022.

## 5.2 Tobacco

*Manu Raj Mathur and Piyu Sharma*

CONTENTS

### WHY IS TOBACCO A MAJOR PUBLIC HEALTH ISSUE?

#### The Global Burden of Disease Attributable to Tobacco

Tobacco kills more than 8 million people a year worldwide, making it one of the largest public health threats faced globally today. More than 7 million of these deaths are caused by direct tobacco use, while 1.2 million are attributable to exposure to secondhand smoke (SHS).[1] Cardiovascular disease (CVD) is the world's leading cause of death, 80% of which occurs in low- and middle-income countries (LMICs.) Approximately 17% of cardiovascular deaths globally is attributable to tobacco use.[1]

Of the 10 countries with the largest numbers of smokers, China, India and Indonesia are the three leading countries. The Global Burden of Disease Study 2017 noted that the smoking-attributable disability adjusted life years (DALYs) worldwide in 2017 was 213.4 million.[2]

There are approximately 1.1 billion smokers worldwide, 80% of whom reside in LMICs; hence the burden of tobacco-related illness and death is the heaviest in these countries.[1]

The number of people consuming tobacco products has increased globally due to an increase in the population even though the prevalence of tobacco consumption has decreased from 1980 to 2012. The pattern of tobacco consumption differs between men and women across different regions. In 2012, a study established that the daily prevalence rates of smoking in men ranged from >50% (e.g. Armenia, Indonesia, Kiribati and Laos) to <10% (e.g. Ghana, Niger, Sudan and Ethiopia). For women the daily prevalence rates ranged from >30% (e.g. Kiribati and Bulgaria) to ≤1% (e.g. Azerbaijan, Algeria, Gambia, Sri Lanka, Sudan).

The prevalence of tobacco consumption has increased between 1980 and 2012 in some LMICs— in Kazakhstan, Mauritania and Serbia among men and in Tunisia, Costa Rica, Kyrgyzstan, Tonga and Bulgaria among women.[3]

Tobacco also imparts a heavy economic burden on countries, including healthcare costs for the treatment of diseases caused by exposure to tobacco and the loss of human capital because of the morbidity and mortality related to tobacco use. In 2018, the World Health Organization (WHO) reported the global economic cost of smoking to be around 1.4 trillion USD per year, which included 400 billion USD in direct costs and 1 trillion USD in indirect costs from loss of productivity due to morbidity and premature death from exposure to SHS.[4]

### TOBACCO: A BRIEF HISTORY OF ORIGIN AND SPREAD

Tobacco is mainly indigenous to the Americas, where it was cultivated by the native peoples in 6000 BCE. Christopher Columbus brought tobacco leaves and seeds back to Europe on his return in 1492. From Europe it spread to other parts of the world in the 16th century. It was introduced to

DOI: 10.1201/b23266-7

the Middle East by the Egyptians in the early 16th century and to China and Japan between 1530 and 1600. The Japanese army introduced it to Korea between 1592 and 1598. At the same time, Spanish and Portuguese traders took it to Africa. The Portuguese also traded tobacco for spices and textiles in India in the early 17th century.[5]

The Native Americans used tobacco mainly for ceremonial purposes. Thomas Harriot and Sir Walter Raleigh popularized pipe smoking in the 16th century among the British aristocracy. In India and the Middle East, hookah was popular among the noble classes in the 17th century. In the 18th century, oral and nasal forms of tobacco became popular. Cigarette smoking started during the Crimean War and became hugely popular by the end of World War II. It remains the most widely practiced form of tobacco consumption to date.[5]

The botanical name of tobacco was given by Carolus Linnaeus, a Swedish botanist, in 1753. He identified two species, namely *Nicotiana rustica* and *Nicotiana tabacum*. He named it after the French diplomat, Jean Nicot, who introduced and popularized tobacco in France.[5]

## TYPES OF TOBACCO

### Smoked Tobacco Products

The most common method of tobacco use is smoking. Of the over 1.3 billion smokers worldwide, approximate 80% live in LMICs. Apart from cigarettes, smoked tobacco products include bidis, kreteks, cheroot, pipes, cigars and waterpipes. These alternatives are often more affordable as compared to cigarettes. Some of these products have specific regional variability—for example, bidis are mainly produced and consumed in South Asia. They carry no health warning, and their sales are not subject to taxation. Another popular form of smoked tobacco in rural parts of South Asia is chillum. Kreteks are mainly produced in Indonesia, where over 90% of all smokers use them. Waterpipe tobacco consumption is popular in the Eastern Mediterranean region and some East Asian countries like Vietnam.[3]

### Smokeless Tobacco Products

All tobacco products that are not burned for consumption and used orally or nasally are included under smokeless tobacco (SLT). Their consumption is highly variable based on geography, and almost 258 million consume SLT in South Asia.[3] They can be broadly categorized as premade manufactured, premade cottage industry and custom-made vendor or individual. Premade products are commercially produced, whereas custom-made products are altered according to customer preferences and made for immediate consumption.[6]

Some popular examples are paan, gutka, zarda, khaini, toombak and dry snuff or tapkeer. These can be chewed, sucked or snuffed nasally. Chimó is popular in Venezuela and toombak in Sudan, whereas tapkeer, gutka, paan and khaini are popular in different regions of South Asia.[3] Snus (pouch) in Sweden, plug and twist tobacco in the United States, rapé in Brazil, shammah in Saudi Arabia and nasway in Uzbekistan are some other examples.[6]

The combined use of tobacco forms (both smoking and smokeless), also known as dual tobacco use, carries a higher risk for coronary heart disease when compared to either form individually.

## PATHOPHYSIOLOGY OF SMOKING ON CARDIOVASCULAR DISEASE

Smoke contains over 7000 chemicals and may be divided into the particulate and the gas phases. The particulate phase contains nicotine and total aerosol residue (tar). Nicotine is a highly addictive substance that elevates the heart rate, blood pressure and myocardial contractility. Tar and other chemicals cause inflammation, damage the endothelium, enhance clot formation and decrease formation of high-density lipoproteins (HDLs). Carbon monoxide contained in the gas phase replaces oxygen, reducing availability for heart muscle and other body tissues (Figure 5.2.1).

## TOBACCO AND CARDIOVASCULAR DISEASE

The earliest documentation of evidence of tobacco smoke and heart disease dates back to 1893 by Huchard. He documented the influence of nicotinism on arteriosclerosis. The early 1900s saw more literature published linking smoking and CVD.

The first study to depict a statistical association between smoking and coronary thrombosis was conducted by Hoffman in 1926. Evidence of higher mortality among male smokers versus nonsmokers was provided by the first US Surgeon General report in 1964. The 1971 report helped establish smoking as an independent risk factor for CVD.[5]

The pioneering study by Sir Richard Doll and Sir Austin Bradford Hill on a cohort of British doctors demonstrated that cigarette smoking in men led to a higher risk of death from coronary

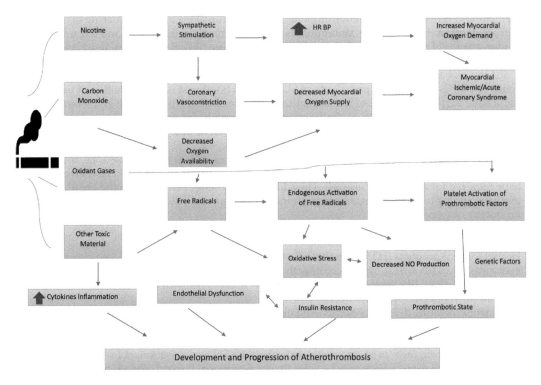

**Figure 5.2.1** Pathophysiology of cigarette smoking and nicotine on cardiovascular disease. BP—blood pressure, HR—heart rate, NO—nitrogen monoxide.

*Source*: Salahuddin S, Prabhakaran D and Roy A. Pathophysiological Mechanisms of Tobacco-Related CVD Cardiovascular disease. *Global Heart* Volume 7, Issue 2, July 2012, Pages 113–120.

thrombosis, with the odds of 2:1 in lifelong smokers under the age of 70 versus nonsmokers of the same age bracket.[5] The Framingham Heart Study, a cohort study conducted in 1960 by Boston University and the National Heart, Lung and Blood Institute, provided evidence of cigarette smoking increasing the risk of heart disease and as smoking as an important risk factor for stroke.[5]

INTERHEART, a global case-control study, assessed the modifiable risk factors for acute myocardial infarction (AMI) in 15,152 cases across 52 countries. They found nine risk factors, with more than 90% of the population-attributable risk (PAR) for AMI, with smoking as the second highest risk factor. INTERSTROKE, a global case-control study to assess modifiable risk factors for stroke, was conducted in 32 countries on 13,447 cases and found that 91% of the stroke burden was attributable to the same risk factors, with smoking ranking seventh on the list.[7]

Tobacco consumption and CVD risk exhibit a strong, albeit nonlinear, dose-response relationship. Even low levels of exposure carry significant risks, i.e. smoking 1 cigarette per day incurs half the risk of developing coronary heart disease and stroke attributed to smoking 20 cigarettes per day.[4]

SHS, also known as environmental tobacco smoke (ETS), is a combination of smoke directly exhaled by the smoker (mainstream smoke) in the environment and the smoke released by the burning cigarette (side-stream smoke). Exposure to SHS was found to increase the risk of ischemic heart disease (IHD) and myocardial infarction (MI) by 30% and the risk of congestive heart disease (CHD) by 25% by Bonita et al and He et al, respectively.[5] Around 55% of deaths caused by SHS are attributed to IHD.[8] The INTERHEART study demonstrated an elevated risk (odds ratio [OR] 1.62, 95% confidence interval [CI] 1.45–1.81) of AMI in persons exposed to SHS for more than 21 hours per week when compared to those minimally exposed—around 1–7 hours per week.[9]

Thirdhand smoke (THS) is a complex phenomenon that results from tobacco smoke pollutants that adhere to surfaces and are reemitted into the gas phase. Residual smoke on clothing, furnishings and dust in indoor environments, which remains long after the clearing of SHS, reacts with oxidants in the air to form contaminants which are mostly carcinogenic and hazardous for human health.[10] This exposure can occur long after smoking has ceased and mainly consists of unintentional intake.[11]

SLT is a global issue that impacts over 300 million people. More than 250 million adult SLT users reside in LMICs. The highest prevalence of SLT use is in Southeast Asia, where 89% of users reside. India has a higher prevalence of SLT users than cigarette smokers in both men and women. This variability provides an additional challenge in categorizing harm and introducing regulations for these products. Some, but not all, SLTs are associated with IHD and stroke.[6]

The INTERHEART study found that the odds of having AMI was 2.23 times higher (95% CI 1.41–3.52) in solely SLT users,[9] but the risk increased 4 times in dual tobacco users, i.e. those that both smoked tobacco and used smokeless tobacco products.[8] Higher cessation efforts were found to be required for these people as well. The additional challenge is that due to the broad range of products and patterns of use, it is hard to support broad generalizations of level of harm of SLT products as a category.[6]

## NOVEL TOBACCO PRODUCTS AND CARDIOVASCULAR DISEASE

Heated tobacco products (HTPs) are those that produce aerosols containing nicotine and other toxic substances upon heating tobacco or activating a device containing tobacco and may be in the form of 'heat sticks' like cigarettes or pods or plugs.[1] There is no evidence that HTPs are less harmful than conventional forms of tobacco.

Electronic nicotine delivery systems (ENDSs), also known as e-cigarettes and vape pens, are devices which heat a liquid to create an aerosol, which is then inhaled by the user. They are marketed as a safer alternative to conventional tobacco products and effective alternatives for cessation. However, there is an ongoing debate about ENDS as a cessation tool versus a gateway to smoking for adolescents.[1] They may be safer than conventional burned tobacco products, but studies show impact on cardiovascular biomarkers, including but not limited to increased oxidative stress, inflammation, platelet aggregation and poor vascular health.[12] They also contain nicotine, which can have a direct impact on cardiovascular health. Secondhand vaping may cause CVD in children and young adults.[13]

Both HTPs and ENDSs can be regulated using the MPOWER policy package outlined in the next section.[14]

## POLICIES FOR TOBACCO CONTROL

### World Health Organization Framework Convention for Tobacco Control (WHO FCTC)

This was the first treaty negotiated under the auspice of the WHO and adopted by the World Health Assembly (WHA) on 21 May 2003 and came into force on 27 February 2005. Ninety days later, it had been accepted by 40 states, and currently there are 181 parties to it, covering over 90% of the world's population.[15] It is an evidence-based treaty developed as a response to the globalization of the tobacco epidemic. In contrast to previous drug control strategies, it represents a paradigm shift to developing regulations for addictive substances and asserts the importance of demand reduction as well as supply issues.

Its demand reduction measures contain nonprice and price tax measures to decrease the demand for tobacco. The nonprice measures include protection from exposure to tobacco smoke, regulation of content of tobacco products, regulation of tobacco product disclosure, packaging and labeling tobacco products, raising public awareness through education and communication, restrictions on tobacco advertising, promotion and sponsorship and assisting tobacco cessation measures. The supply reduction measures tackle illicit trade, sale to minors and support for alternative activities.[15,16]

### Mpower

This is a technical measures package to help countries implement and enforce tobacco control measures.[17] The six evidence-based components are as follows:

**M**onitor tobacco use and prevention policies—accurate measurement of the tobacco epidemic and wide dissemination of the information to bolster stakeholder support.[18]

**P**rotect people from tobacco smoke—smoke-free legislation and smoking bans to prevent harmful exposure to SHS.[19]

Offer help to quit tobacco use—providing health system support for programs aimed at tobacco cessation measures.[20]

Warn about the dangers of tobacco use—using various platforms to comprehensively increase awareness of the health risk posed by tobacco consumption.[21]

Enforce bans on advertising, promotion and sponsorship—guidelines to restrict direct and indirect advertising, promotion and sponsorship of tobacco products by the industry.[22]

Raise taxes on tobacco—providing disincentives by increasing the price of tobacco through higher taxes and raising government revenue.[23]

### Tobacco Taxation

A significant increase in the tax and price of tobacco products is the most cost-effective method to control the use of tobacco. This, in conjunction with public smoking prohibitions and advertising bans, ensures effectiveness of tobacco demand reduction measures. Evidence from all countries shows that higher prices deter initiation and encourage cessation. It also reduces the rates of relapse among those who have quit and reduces the consumption of current users.

A 10% price increase on a pack of cigarettes is expected to decrease demand of cigarettes by 4% in high-income countries and 5% in LMICs. Children, adolescents and adults in LMICs show a higher sensitivity to changes in price, allowing for focused interventions in these population groups.

The various types of taxes levied by the government can be an excise tax, value-added tax (VAT) or general sales tax or import duties. Of these, excise taxes uniquely apply to tobacco products and raise their price relative to that of other goods and services and hence are the most important. There are two types of excise taxes—specific, which is levied based on quantity (e.g. weight of tobacco), and ad valorem, which is levied based on value (e.g. percentage of retail price).[24]

### Smoke-Free Policies

Smoke-free policies are unique among the tobacco control policies, as they primarily affect nonsmokers and require widespread population-based support. There are two general types of smoke-free policies: those that are mandated by law and those that are voluntarily adopted.

California was the first state to ban smoking in workplaces, bars and restaurants in 1998.[25] The first country to introduce a comprehensive smoking ban was Ireland in 2004, which outlawed smoking in the workplace and pubs, bars and restaurants prior to the FCTC.[26]

Shortly after signing the treaty, New Zealand and Norway implemented similar policies. The first Latin American country to pass a nationwide smoke-free policy was Uruguay in 2006, and by 2011 seven others had followed, the latest being Argentina. Today, smoke-free policies are expanding and evolving from private indoor areas to include public outdoor areas like outdoor eating and drinking areas of bars and restaurants, parks, beaches, public transportation and prisons.[25] A review done by Frazer et al in 2010, updated in 2016, found consistent evidence of a positive impact of national smoke-free legislature on cardiovascular health outcomes and mortality associated with smoking-related diseases.[27]

### Plain Packaging

Plain packaging is different from other packaging and labeling measures, for example, large graphic health warnings. The WHO FCTC Articles 11 and 13 describe methods of implementation and a clear description of plain packaging, respectively. It is defined as "measures to restrict or prohibit the use of logos, colours, brand images or promotional information on packaging other than brand names and product names displayed in a standard colour and font style". It serves to reduce the attractiveness, eliminate advertisements and promotion through packaging and increase the visibility and effectiveness of health warnings.

In 2012, Australia was the first WHO member state to implement standardized packaging of tobacco products. Following this France, Hungary, New Zealand, Norway, the United Kingdom and Ireland also passed laws to implement this. Burkina Faso, Canada, Georgia, Romania, Slovenia, Thailand and Uruguay have passed enabling laws since then.[14]

### REFERENCES

1. World Health Organization. Factsheet—www.who.int/news-room/fact-sheets/detail/tobacco.

2. Global Burden of Disease 2017—https://vizhub.healthdata.org/gbd-compare/.

3. 10. Saleheen D, Zhao W, Rasheed A. Epidemiology and public health policy of tobacco use and cardiovascular disorders in low- and middle-income countries. Arterioscler Thromb Vasc Biol. 2014;34:1811–1819. https://doi.org/10.1161/ATVBAHA.114.303826.

4. World Health Organisation. Tobacco breaks hearts: Choose health, Not tobacco. 2018—https://apps.who.int/iris/bitstream/handle/10665/272675/WHO-NMH-PND-18.4-eng.pdf?ua=1.

5. Mathur MR, Prabhakaran D. Tobacco and CVD—A historical perspective. Global Heart. 2012;7(2):107–111.

6. National Cancer Institute and Centers for Disease Control and Prevention. Smokeless tobacco and public health: a global perspective. Bethesda, MD: U.S. Department of Health and Human Services, Centers for Disease Control and Prevention and National Instit.

7. Joseph P, Leong D, McKee M et al. Reducing the global burden of cardiovascular disease, Part 1: The epidemiology and risk factors. Circ Res. 2017;121(6):677–695. https://doi.org/10.1161/CIRCRESAHA.117.308903.

8. Rawal I, Salahuddin S, Roy A. Tobacco and cardiovascular disease. Ch—33;9–14 in Prabhakaran D, Anand S, Gaziano TA, et al., editors. Disease Control Priorities, Third Edition (Volume 5): Cardiovascular, Respiratory, and Related Disorders. Washington, DC: The International Bank for Reconstruction and Development/The World Bank; 2017 Nov 17.

9. Mathur MR, Singh N, Arora M. Tobacco use and cardiovascular diseases – Evidence, interventions and primary prevention. J Preventive Cardiol. 2011;1:66–72.

10. Matt GE, Quintana PJE, Destaillats H, Gundel LA, Sleiman M, Singer BC, et al. Thirdhand tobacco smoke: emerging evidence and arguments for a multidisciplinary research agenda. Environ Health Perspect. 2011;119:1218–1226. http://dx.doi.org/10.1289/ehp.1103.

11. Protano C, Vitali M. The new danger of thirdhand smoke: why passive smoking does not stop at secondhand smoke. Environ Health Perspect. 2011 Oct;119(10):A422. https://doi.org/10.1289/ehp.1103956.

12. MacDonald A, Middlekauff H.R. Electronic cigarettes and cardiovascular health: what do we know so far? Vascular Health Risk Manag. 2019;15:159–174.

13. World Health Organisation. Tobacco breaks hearts: Choose health, Not tobacco. 2018—https://apps.who.int/iris/bitstream/handle/10665/272675/WHO-NMH-PND-18.4-eng.pdf?ua=1.

14. World Health Organisation. Tobacco plain packaging products: global status update. 2018. https://apps.who.int/iris/bitstream/handle/10665/275277/WHO-NMH-PND-NAC-18.9-eng.pdf?ua=1.

15. World Health Organization. Framework convention on tobacco control: summary. June 2018. www.who.int/fctc/WHO_FCTC_summary.pdf?ua=1.

16. World Health Organization. Framework Convention on Tobacco Control—www.who.int/fctc/text_download/en/.

17. World Health Organization. MPOWER—www.who.int/cancer/prevention/tobacco_implementation/mpower/en/.

18. MPOWER: Monitor—www.who.int/tobacco/mpower/monitor/en/.

19. MPOWER: Protect—www.who.int/tobacco/mpower/protect/en/.

20. MPOWER: Offer—www.who.int/tobacco/mpower/offer/en/.

21. MPOWER: Warn—www.who.int/tobacco/mpower/warn/en/.

22. MPOWER: Enforce—www.who.int/tobacco/mpower/enforce/en/.

23. MPOWER: Raise taxes—www.who.int/tobacco/mpower/raise_taxes/en/.

24. World Health Organization. Tobacco Free Initiative | Taxation | www.who.int/tobacco/economics/taxation/en/.

25. Hyland A, Barnoya J, Corral J.E. Smoke-free air policies: past, present and future. BMJ Tob Control. 2012;21:154–161. doi:10.1136/tobaccocontrol-2011–050389.

26. Koh HK, Joossens LX, Connolly GN. Making smoking history worldwide. N Engl J Med. 2007;356:1496–1498. www.nejm.org/doi/pdf/10.1056/NEJMp068279?articleTools=true.

27. Frazer K, Callinan JE, McHugh J, et al. Legislative smoking bans for reducing harms from second hand smoke exposure, smoking prevalence and tobacco consumption. Cochrane Database of Systematic Reviews. 2016;2. Art. No.: CD005992. https://doi.org/10.

# 5.3 Diet

*Lindsay M. Jaacks, Arun K. Chopra, and Dorairaj Prabhakaran*

## CONTENTS

## INTRODUCTION

Few things in medicine, or even the media, evoke as much curiosity and debate as diet and its relationship to health. Diet is also one of the most important risk factors for cardiovascular disease (CVD). According to the Global Burden of Disease Study, in 2017, dietary risks accounted for 10.9 million deaths, with the leading dietary risk factor being high sodium intake, which alone accounted for an estimated 2.3 million deaths (1). Diets high in sugar-sweetened beverages show some of the most worrisome trends, with marked increases since 1990 (1). Yet some progress in improving the healthfulness of diets has been made over the past 20 years; in particular, there have been substantial reductions in the consumption of industrial trans fats (2).

Major public health-promoting foundations such as Resolve to Save Lives and Bloomberg Philanthropies have prioritized reducing sodium, trans fat, and sugar-sweetened beverage intake globally. The focus of this chapter is on public health approaches—primarily policies but also community-based interventions—to address these three dietary risk factors. Readers interested in the biological and epidemiological evidence linking other aspects of diet to CVD are referred to Chapter 48 ("Atherosclerotic Cardiovascular Disease") of *Present Knowledge in Nutrition* (3) and Chapter 33 ("Diet and Cardiovascular Disease") of *Tandon's Textbook of Cardiology* (4). These texts synthesize evidence on various aspects of diet, including the balance of macronutrients (carbo-hydrates, fats, and proteins) and the role of micronutrients in the development of CVD. In this chapter, we will discuss priority nutrients of concern for public health, and these are salt, trans and saturated fats, and sugar (Table 5.3.1).

## SODIUM

Sodium consumption over 2 grams per day (equivalent to 5 grams of salt) increases the risk of high blood pressure (e.g., hypertension). An estimated 1 in 10 deaths from CVD are attribut-able to high sodium intake (5). The consumption of salt is far too high in nearly all parts of the world—affecting low-, middle-, and high-income countries alike. The global mean intake of sodium was estimated to be 3.95 grams per day in 2010—close to 10 grams of salt (6). Out of 60 countries with data available in 2015, 27 (45%) reported mean population salt intake levels of 10 grams or more, more than double the World Health Organization (WHO) recommended daily salt intake limit of 5 grams (7). It is therefore not surprising that one of the targets set in the *Global Action Plan for the Prevention and Control of Noncommunicable Diseases 2013–2020* is a

## Table 5.3.1 Summary of Dietary Risks that Should Be Prioritized in Public Health Interventions Based on the Global Burden of Disease Study

| Dietary Risks | Minimum Risk Threshold | World Health Organization (WHO) Guidance |
| --- | --- | --- |
| Sodium | 24-h urinary sodium 1–5 g per day | SHAKE Technical Package for Salt Reduction (2016) |
| Trans fats | Consumption of trans fats 0–1% of total daily energy | REPLACE Trans Fat (2018) |
| Sugar-sweetened beverages | Consumption of sugar-sweetened beverages 0–5 g per day | Taxes on sugary drinks: Why do it? (2017) Guideline: Sugars intake for adults and Children (2015) |

DOI: 10.1201/b23266-8

30% relative reduction in mean population salt/sodium intake by 2025. As of 2015, 12 countries had reported reductions in population salt intake, 19 had reported reductions in salt content of foods, and 75 had a national salt reduction strategy (7). Finland, one of the first countries to implement a national salt reduction strategy (8), has achieved one of the greatest recorded reductions in mean population intake of salt: from 13 to 9.9 grams per day in men and from 10.5 to 6.8 grams per day in women between 1979 and 2007 (9, 10). Thus, there is some precedent for meeting this global target.

Sodium enters our diets mainly through two routes: (1) processed foods such as instant noodles and snack foods, which are increasingly available and affordable all over the world, and (2) discretionary salt added during cooking or at the table. What proportion of sodium enters the diet through these two routes differs between populations. Thus, priority strategies to reduce sodium also differ. If the primary route is through processed foods, industry reformulation should be prioritized. If the primary route is through discretionary salt added during cooking or at the table, education campaigns should be prioritized. In terms of what has been adopted in practice, consumer education is the most commonly used national salt reduction strategy, followed by food industry engagement to reformulate products and front-of-package labeling schemes (7). Other approaches could include legislation to establish a maximum sodium content of processed foods, sodium limits on publicly produced foods, sodium taxes (similar to sugar taxes), and warning labels for high-sodium foods.

In addition to Finland, one of the most widely cited success stories for population sodium reduction comes from the UK. Public Health England introduced voluntary salt targets for the food industry in 2006 (to be met by 2010), which were revised in 2009 and 2014. Between 2000–2001 and 2011, population salt intake declined by 15% and average adult systolic blood pressure declined by 3 mmHg and diastolic blood pressure declined by 1.5 mmHg (11, 12). However, mean population salt intake remains at 8.1 grams, which is above the UK target of 6 grams and the WHO target of 5 grams. Moreover, there was not a significant decline from 2008 to 2011 (12), suggesting that the reduction is waning over time and further action—such as legislative action rather than voluntary targets—is needed. Indeed, the latest evaluation of industry progress on meeting their voluntary pledges, conducted in 2017, suggests that just 52% of all salt targets were met by manufacturers and retailers (13).

In China, where most dietary sodium is from salt added during cooking rather than processed foods (14), population salt reduction efforts, implemented since at least 2007, have focused on education campaigns and the promotion of salt substitutes (15). For example, through the China Healthy Lifestyle for All campaign, salt control spoons were disseminated and are reportedly used by nearly 50% of those living in urban areas and nearly 30% of those living in rural areas (15, 16), and evidence suggests that use of the spoon is effective for reducing salt intake (17). However, while substantial reductions in mean population salt intake have been reported in China—29% reduction between 1991 and 2009 in one study (14) and 22% between 2000 and 2009–2011 in a second study (18)—mean levels still far surpass 5 grams per day. South Africa and Argentina also stand out as leaders in national salt reduction strategies, particularly in the shift from voluntary targets to legislative action (19).

Given current levels of sodium intake, nearly all would agree with the goal of a 30% reduction in population sodium intake, as well as the fact that people with hypertension and stroke—which is millions of people globally—should reduce sodium intake. However, what is not clear is whether people with low blood pressure, congestive heart failure, type 1 diabetes, and possibly other subpopulations should reduce sodium intake. Also unclear is whether an absolute goal of <2 grams per day should be recommended—some posit this is too low. This stems from the fact that observational studies—in particular, the Prospective Urban Rural Epidemiology (PURE) study, which is a cohort study of over 150,000 adults in 17 low-, middle-, and high-income countries, but also other cohorts (20)—have recently suggested a J-shaped curve between sodium intake and CVD with an increased risk when intake falls below 2.3–3 grams per day (21). However, not all studies have reported such a curve and instead find a linear association, even at levels of 1.5 grams per day (22, 23). A recent National Academies of Sciences, Engineering and Medicine report in the United States found no evidence of deficiency symptoms across nine sodium reduction trials, and thus established an adequate sodium intake level of 1.5 grams per day and confirmed a chronic disease risk reduction intake level of 2.3 grams per day (24). It is also worth noting that such low levels of sodium intake have not been achieved long-term in any free-living population. Moreover, evidence is starting to accumulate that it is in fact the sodium-to-potassium ratio that matters, rather than sodium alone (25). For now, the best approach may be to focus on reducing sodium intake to moderate levels (30% reduction of current levels) and promoting potassium-rich foods such as fruits, vegetables, and nuts.

## TRANS AND SATURATED FATS

Trans fat is naturally occurring in ruminant dairy and meat products (i.e., products from cows, goats, and sheep), but the majority of trans fat in global diets comes from industrially produced processed foods (e.g., bakery products and snacks) and fried foods produced using partially hydrogenated oils. Biscuits, for example, in some Middle East and Asian countries (e.g., Iran, Pakistan, and Lebanon) have up to 26.7 g trans fat per 100 g fat (2).

Trans fat intake that exceeds 1% of total energy intake is associated with a 21% increase in the risk of CVD and 28% increase in coronary heart disease mortality, accounting for more than 500,000 CVD deaths attributable annually to excess trans fat (26). This is especially concerning because replacing industrially produced trans fat with healthier fats is cheap and feasible without impacting the taste of food. Because of this, the number of success stories when it comes to eliminating industrially produced trans fat from the food supply is growing rapidly. The WHO REPLACE action program was launched in 2018 with a goal of achieving <1% of daily energy intake from industrially produced trans fat by 2023 and a complete ban on partially hydrogenated oils (27). In 2010, global mean trans fat intake was estimated to be 1.4% of daily energy intake, ranging from 0.2% in Barbados to 6.5% in Egypt (28).

As of the beginning of 2018, 28 countries had mandatory trans fat limits or bans already in place, and similar regulations came into place by the end of 2018 in six additional countries and were passed in a further 24 countries (29). The WHO predicts that these laws will help protect 3.2 billion individuals in 58 countries from excess trans fat by the end of 2021, with a majority of countries for which data are available already reporting trans fat intake <1% of daily caloric intake (29). A systematic review of 32 studies evaluating the impact of trans fat regulations found that bans were the most effective, economical, and equitable, resulting in trans fat being virtually eliminated, through voluntary industry reductions (20–38% reduction in trans fat intake) and labeling (30–74% reduction in trans fat intake) were also found to be effective (30). Following Denmark, which was the first country to ban trans fat in 2003, several countries, including the United States, Canada, Thailand, and South Korea, have followed suit. Prior to national implementation in the United States, an analysis that compared CVD events (hospitalizations for myocardial infarction or stroke) in counties of one state (New York) with trans fat restrictions versus those without such restrictions showed that three or more years after adopting the restrictions, the population experienced a 6.2% decrease in events relative to the population without the restrictions (31).

However, over 100 countries still need to take effective action, especially 11 of the 15 countries that account for two-thirds of the global mortality linked with trans fat consumption (18). In addition to trans fat limits or bans, other public health approaches to reducing trans fat intake include mandatory or voluntary trans fat labelling and reformulation; investing in adequate monitoring mechanisms and educating lay people regarding safer cooking practices such as avoiding reheated/reused oils; and a general reduction in the consumption of processed foods and fried foods. While there is some evidence that frying oil at high temperatures leads to modest increases in trans fat (approximately 3%) (32), this is relatively low compared to the amount of trans fat in partially hydrogenated oils (25–45% of the oil) (33).

Saturated fats continue to generate controversy. Most of the inconsistencies in the scientific literature can likely be attributed to substitutions. Cardiovascular benefits are observed when saturated fat is replaced with unsaturated fats, but not when it is replaced with refined carbohydrates and sugar (34). Thus, the 2017 Presidential Advisory from the American Heart Association (35) and the 2019 Consensus Report from the American Diabetes Association on nutrition therapy for adults with diabetes or prediabetes (36) both specifically recommend replacement of saturated fat with unsaturated fat, particularly polyunsaturated fat. Currently, the American Heart Association recommends restricting saturated fat to <6% of total energy intake, though it states, "The more important thing to remember is the overall dietary picture. Saturated fats are just one piece of the puzzle. In general, you can't go wrong eating more fruits, vegetables, whole grains and fewer calories" (37). In 2015, Canada's Heart & Stroke Foundation concluded that because the health effects of saturated fats could vary depending on the food source, it is best to recommend a healthy dietary pattern rather than a specific threshold or limit for saturated fat (38). They define a health dietary pattern as a diet that includes a variety of vegetables and fruits, whole grains, and proteins from various sources including beans, lentils, nuts, low-fat dairy or dairy alternatives (e.g., fortified soy milk), lean meats, poultry, and fish (38).

As mentioned earlier, experimental and cohort studies on substitution of nutrients conclude that isocalorically replacing saturated fat with polyunsaturated fat is beneficial, whereas replacing saturated fat with refined carbohydrates may in fact have deleterious effects (34). These sorts of observations are supported by experimental studies, which have demonstrated that there is a limited association between dietary saturated fat and plasma saturated fat, and in fact, increasing dietary carbohydrate appears to increase plasma palmitoleic acid (39)—a type of saturated fat associated with adverse cardiovascular outcomes. An analysis of the Nurses' Health Study and the Health Professionals Follow-Up Study found that isocaloric replacement of 5% of saturated fat with polyunsaturated fat, monounsaturated fat, or whole-grain carbohydrates was associated with a 25%, 15%, and 9% lower risk of coronary heart disease, respectively (40). Also of note is that the source of saturated fat seems to matter: saturated fat from dairy does not seem to have an adverse impact on CVD as opposed to saturated fat from meat, which does (41).

In terms of population-based strategies to reduce saturated fat, two widely cited studies are the Mauritius population-wide healthy lifestyle intervention program (42) and a Polish ecological study (43). In Mauritius, a pronounced decrease in blood cholesterol (5.5 mmol/l to 4.7 mmol/l from 1987 to 1992) was observed and was likely directly attributable to a change in the saturated fat content of a widely used cooking oil (from palm oil to soya oil) (42). In Poland, an ecological analysis that aimed to explain a sudden decrease in deaths from heart disease in the early 1990s found that the drop was largely explained by a shift from animal-based to plant-based dietary fat sources (animal-based foods are higher in saturated fat), as well as an increase in the supply of fresh fruit and vegetables (43).

There is strong evidence to support a predominantly plant-based diet, not only for the prevention of chronic diseases such as CVD but also to lower the environmental impact of diets (44). A recent analysis of the Nurses' Health Study and Health Professionals Follow-Up Study reported lower CVD and overall mortality on changing to a healthful plant-based diet in comparison to an unhealthy diet (whether plant- or meat-based) (45). This does not mean that animal foods need to be completely excluded from the diet. Omnivorous diets consisting primarily of plant-based foods but with some animal foods, particularly eggs, dairy, unprocessed poultry and meat, and fish, can also constitute a healthy diet.

As dietary cholesterol is generally not correlated with serum cholesterol (owing to regulation of biosynthesis and reabsorption) and has no definite correlation with CVD, many dietary guidelines, including, for example, the Dietary Guidelines for Americans (46), no longer specify a target for dietary cholesterol. An analysis of the PURE study including ~177,000 adults found no significant association between egg intake and lipoproteins or major CVD events (47). Even the American Heart Association now states, "Healthy individuals can include up to a whole egg or equivalent daily," and older individuals without dyslipidemia and vegetarians may include more eggs in their diets (48).

## SUGAR-SWEETENED BEVERAGES

Sugar-sweetened beverage taxes are recommended by international (e.g., WHO) and national institutes in order to meet recommendations for added sugar in the diet—less than 10% of total energy intake or about 12 teaspoons of sugar (49). It is estimated that a tax that increases prices by 20% will result in a reduction in consumption of about 20% (50). To date, the highest sugar-sweetened beverage taxes to be implemented have been in the Middle East: in 2017, the United Arab Emirates and Saudi Arabia introduced a 50% excise tax[1] on soft drinks and 100% excise tax on energy drinks, and similar taxes were also introduced in Qatar and Oman in 2019 (51). An additional 5% value-added tax (VAT) was introduced in Saudi Arabia on top of existing taxes in 2018 (51). Together, these taxes in Saudi Arabia resulted in a 41% reduction in sales of sugar-sweetened beverages in 2018 compared to pretax trends (2012–2106) (52). This is the largest observed reduction in sales of sugar-sweetened beverages to date, suggesting that higher taxes result in larger reductions. Other important policies aimed at tackling sugar include the Dietary Guidelines for Americans 2020–2025, which recommend avoiding all foods and beverages with added sugars in children under the age of 2 years (46). Given that taste preferences, including for sweet foods, develop at very young ages, this strategy will set kids up for healthier diets as they grow and develop.

Mexico stands out as an exemplar case study. In January 2014, Mexico began implementation of a 1 peso per liter (about 10% of 2013 prices) tax on nondairy beverages with added sugar. The Mexican Supreme Court decision in February 2015 concluded that the tax was constitutional and so it continues to be in place to this day. The impact of the tax on consumer purchases has been evaluated in several studies, finding reductions in purchases of taxed beverages ranging from 6% to 8% (53–55). A simulation study estimating the potential impact of Mexico's sugar-sweetened beverage tax on CVD events showed that a 10% reduction in sugar-sweetened beverage consumption with 39% calorie compensation would result in 20,400 fewer incident myocardial infarctions and strokes (56). A cost-effectiveness analysis of the tax suggests that the tax saved $3.98 per dollar spent on its implementation (57). Moreover, the tax raised over US$2.6 billion during the first two years of implementation (58).

Another modeling study in India found that a 20% sugar-sweetened beverage tax could reduce the prevalence of obesity by 3% and incidence of type 2 diabetes by 1.6% over a 10-year period (59). Since 2017, India has applied a 28% goods and services tax (a type of VAT) on all goods containing added sugar or other sweeteners, including sugar-sweetened beverages, with an additional 12% added to sugar-sweetened beverages, for a total of a 40% tax on sugar-sweetened beverages—the highest goods and services tax of any product in India (51). However, the impact of this tax on sales or consumption has not yet been evaluated.

## CONCLUDING RECOMMENDATIONS

Population-based approaches to improve the healthfulness of diets represent a critical aspect of CVD prevention. Polices and interventions should focus on overall dietary patterns and food-based approaches. The exceptions to this are trans fat, which should be eliminated, and sodium, which should be within the range of 3–5 g/day. Food-based recommendations that are shared across healthful dietary patterns include encouraging the consumption of whole grains, fruits, vegetables, nuts, legumes, and, for those who consume animal products, low-fat dairy products and fish. Governments have to step in to provide subsidies for growing healthy crops, adequate storage facilities and cool transport to avoid food waste; disseminate knowledge about healthy cooking practices; and monitor industry and smaller traders to check adherence to policies and regulations. As with many risky behaviors, education and awareness-raising interventions alone are insufficient to improve diets. Strong policies such as taxation and mandatary industry regulations have and will need to continue to play complementary roles.

## NOTE

1 A value-added tax (VAT) is a tax placed on a product whenever value is added across the supply chain, from production to point of sale. Thus, the cost of paying the tax ultimately falls on the consumer. This is in contrast to an excise tax, which is levied on a product at the point of manufacture.

## REFERENCES

1. Stanaway JD, Afshin A, Gakidou E, Lim SS, Abate D, Abate KH, et al. Global, regional, and national comparative risk assessment of 84 behavioural, environmental and occupational, and metabolic risks or clusters of risks for 195 countries and territories, 1990&#x2013;2017: a systematic analysis for the Global Burden of Disease Study 2017. Lancet. 2018;392(10159):1923–1994.
2. Wanders AJ, Zock PL, Brouwer IA. Trans fat intake and its dietary sources in general populations worldwide: a systematic review. Nutrients. 2017;9(8):840.
3. Erdman Jr JW, MacDonald IA, Zeisel SH. Present Knowledge in Nutrition, 10th edition. Ames, Iowa: John Wiley & Sons; 2012.
4. Jaacks LJ, Prabhakaran D. Chapter 33. Cardiovascular disease risk factors. diet and cardiovascular disease. In: Prabhakaran DK RK, Naik N, Kaul U, editors. Tandon's Textbook of Cardiology: Volume 2. 2. New Delhi: Wolters Kluwer Health (India); 2019. pp. 816–829.
5. Mozaffarian D, Fahimi S, Singh GM, Micha R, Khatibzadeh S, Engell RE, et al. Global sodium consumption and death from cardiovascular causes. N Engl J Med. 2014;371(7):624–634.
6. Powles J, Fahimi S, Micha R, Khatibzadeh S, Shi P, Ezzati M, et al. Global, regional and national sodium intakes in 1990 and 2010: a systematic analysis of 24 h urinary sodium excretion and dietary surveys worldwide. BMJ Open. 2013;3(12):e003733.
7. Trieu K, Neal B, Hawkes C, Dunford E, Campbell N, Rodriguez-Fernandez R, et al. Salt reduction initiatives around the world—a systematic review of progress towards the global target. PLoS One. 2015;10(7):e0130247.
8. European Commission. Collated information on salt reduction in the EU. Brussels: European Commission; 2008.

9. Laatikainen T, Pietinen P, Valsta L, Sundvall J, Reinivuo H, Tuomilehto J. Sodium in the finnish diet: 20-year trends in urinary sodium excretion among the adult population. Eur J Clin Nutr. 2006;60(8):965–970.

10. Pietinen P, Valsta LM, Hirvonen T, Sinkko H. Labelling the salt content in foods: a useful tool in reducing sodium intake in Finland. Public Health Nutr. 2008;11(4):335–340.

11. He FJ, Pombo-Rodrigues S, Macgregor GA. Salt reduction in England from 2003 to 2011: its relationship to blood pressure, stroke and ischaemic heart disease mortality. BMJ Open. 2014;4(4):e004549.

12. Sadler K, Nicholson S, Steer T, Gill V, Bates B, Tipping S, et al. National diet & nutrition survey: assessment of dietary sodium in adults (aged 19 to 64 years) in England, 2011. London: UK Department of Health; 2011.

13. Public Health England. Salt targets 2017: progress report. A report on the food industry's progress towards meeting the 2017 salt targets. London: Public Health England; 2018.

14. Du S, Batis C, Wang H, Zhang B, Zhang J, Popkin BM. Understanding the patterns and trends of sodium intake, potassium intake, and sodium to potassium ratio and their effect on hypertension in China. Am J Clin Nutr. 2014;99(2):334–343.

15. Shao S, Hua Y, Yang Y, Liu X, Fan J, Zhang A, et al. Salt reduction in China: a state-of-the-art review. Risk Manag Healthc Policy. 2017;10:17.

16. Xu JW, Yan LX, Zhang M, Chen X, Jiang Y, Wang L. Investigation on coverage of salt control spoon and oil control pot among Chinese resident households in 2010. Chinese J Health Educ. 2014;30(5):390–392.

17. Chen J, Tian Y, Liao Y, Yang S, Li Z, He C, et al. Salt-restriction-spoon improved the salt intake among residents in China. PLoS One. 2013;8(11):e78963.

18. Hipgrave DB, Chang S, Li X, Wu Y. Salt and sodium intake in China. JAMA. 2016;315(7):703–705.

19. Nghiem N, Blakely T, Cobiac LJ, Pearson AL, Wilson N. Health and economic impacts of eight different dietary salt reduction interventions. PLoS One. 2015;10(4):e0123915.

20. O'Donnell MJ, Yusuf S, Mente A, Gao P, Mann JF, Teo K, et al. Urinary sodium and potassium excretion and risk of cardiovascular events. JAMA. 2011;306(20):2229–2238.

21. O'Donnell M, Mente A, Rangarajan S, McQueen MJ, Wang X, Liu L, et al. Urinary sodium and potassium excretion, mortality, and cardiovascular events. N Engl J Med. 2014;371(7):612–623.

22. Cook NR, Appel LJ, Whelton PK. Lower levels of sodium intake and reduced cardiovascular risk. Circulation. 2014;129(9):981–989.

23. Cobb LK, Anderson CAM, Elliott P, Hu FB, Liu K, Neaton JD, et al. Methodological issues in cohort studies that relate sodium intake to cardiovascular disease outcomes. Circulation. 2014;129(10):1173–1186.

24. National Academies of Sciences, Engineering, and Medicine. Dietary Reference Intakes for Sodium and Potassium. Washington, DC: The National Academies Press; 2019. https://doi.org/10.17226/25353. Available from: https://nap.nationalacademies.org/catalog/25353/dietary-reference-intakes-for-sodium-and-potassium

25. Perez V, Chang ET. Sodium-to-potassium ratio and blood pressure, hypertension, and related factors. Adv Nutr. 2014;5(6):712–741.

26. Wang H, Naghavi M, Allen C, Barber RM, Bhutta ZA, Carter A, et al. Global, regional, and national life expectancy, all-cause mortality, and cause-specific mortality for 249 causes of death, 1980–2015: a systematic analysis for the Global Burden of Disease Study 2015. Lancet. 2016;388(10053):1459–1544.

27. World Health Organization. REPLACE Trans Fat: An Action Package to Eliminate Industrially-Produced Trans-Fatty Acids. Geneva: World Health Organization; 2018.

28. Micha R, Khatibzadeh S, Shi P, Fahimi S, Lim S, Andrews KG, et al. Global, regional, and national consumption levels of dietary fats and oils in 1990 and 2010: a systematic analysis including 266 country-specific nutrition surveys. BMJ. 2014;348:g2272.

29. World Health Organization. Countdown to 2023: WHO Report on Global Trans Fat Elimination 2020. Geneva: World Health Organization; 2020.

30. Downs SM, Bloem MZ, Zheng M, Catterall E, Thomas B, Veerman L, et al. The impact of policies to reduce trans fat consumption: a systematic review of the evidence. Current Developments in Nutrition. 2017;1(12).

31. Brandt EJ, Myerson R, Perraillon MC, Polonsky TS. Hospital admissions for myocardial infarction and stroke before and after the trans-fatty acid restrictions in New York. JAMA Cardiol. 2017;2(6):627–634.

32. Bhardwaj S, Passi SJ, Misra A, Pant KK, Anwar K, Pandey R, et al. Effect of heating/reheating of fats/oils, as used by Asian Indians, on trans fatty acid formation. Food Chem. 2016;212:663–670.

33. Tarrago-Trani MT, Phillips KM, Lemar LE, Holden JM. New and existing oils and fats used in products with reduced trans-fatty acid content. J Am Diet Assoc. 2006;106(6):867–880.

34. Hooper L, Martin N, Abdelhamid A, Davey Smith G. Reduction in saturated fat intake for cardiovascular disease. Cochrane Database Syst Rev. 2015;(6):CD011737.

35. Sacks FM, Lichtenstein AH, Wu JHY, Appel LJ, Creager MA, Kris-Etherton PM, et al. Dietary fats and cardiovascular disease: a presidential advisory from the American Heart Association. Circulation. 2017;136(3):e1–e23.

36. Evert AB, Dennison M, Gardner CD, Garvey WT, Lau KHK, MacLeod J, et al. Nutrition therapy for adults with diabetes or prediabetes: a consensus report. Diabetes Care. 2019;42(5):731–754.

37. American Heart Association. Saturated FAT: AHA Recommendation Dallas, Texas: American Heart Association; 2021. Available from: www.heart.org/en/healthy-living/healthy-eating/eat-smart/fats/saturated-fats.

38. Heart & Stroke Foundation. Position Statement on Saturated Fat, Heart Disease and Stroke. Ottawa, Canada: Heart & Stroke Foundation; 2015.

39. Volk BM, Kunces LJ, Freidenreich DJ, Kupchak BR, Saenz C, Artistizabal JC, et al. Effects of step-wise increases in dietary carbohydrate on circulating saturated fatty acids and palmitoleic acid in adults with metabolic syndrome. PLoS One. 2014;9(11):e113605.

40. Li Y, Hruby A, Bernstein AM, Ley SH, Wang DD, Chiuve SE, et al. Saturated fats compared with unsaturated fats and sources of carbohydrates in relation to risk of coronary heart disease: a prospective cohort study. J Am Coll Cardiol. 2015;66(14):1538–1548.

41. de Oliveira Otto MC, Mozaffarian D, Kromhout D, Bertoni AG, Sibley CT, Jacobs DR, Jr., et al. Dietary intake of saturated fat by food source and incident cardiovascular disease: the multi-ethnic study of atherosclerosis. Am J Clin Nutr. 2012;96(2):397–404.

42. Dowse GK, Gareeboo H, Alberti KGM, Zimmet P, Tuomilehto J, Purran A, et al. Changes in population cholesterol concentrations and other cardiovascular risk factor levels after five years of the non-communicable disease intervention programme in Mauritius. BMJ. 1995;311(7015):1255–1259.

43. Zatonski WA, McMichael AJ, Powles JW. Ecological study of reasons for sharp decline in mortality from ischaemic heart disease in Poland since 1991. BMJ. 1998;316(7137):1047.

44. Willett W, Rockstrom J, Loken B, Springmann M, Lang T, Vermeulen S, et al. food in the anthropocene: the EAT-Lancet Commission on healthy diets from sustainable food systems. Lancet. 2019;393(10170):447–492.

45. Shan Z, Li Y, Baden MY, Bhupathiraju SN, Wang DD, Sun Q, et al. Association between healthy eating patterns and risk of cardiovascular disease. JAMA Intern Med. 2020;180(8):1090–1100.

46. US Department of Agriculture. Dietary guidelines for Americans 2020–2025. Washington DC: US Department of Agriculture; 2020.

47. Dehghan M, Mente A, Rangarajan S, Mohan V, Lear S, Swaminathan S, et al. Association of egg intake with blood lipids, cardiovascular disease, and mortality in 177,000 people in 50 countries. Am J Clin Nutr. 2020;111(4):795–803.

48. Carson JAS, Lichtenstein AH, Anderson CAM, Appel LJ, Kris-Etherton PM, Meyer KA, et al. Dietary cholesterol and cardiovascular risk: a science advisory from the american heart association. Circulation. 2020;141(3):e39–e53.

49. World Health Organization. Sugars Intake for Adults and Children Guideline. Geneva: World Health Organization; 2015.

50. Powell LM, Chriqui JF, Khan T, Wada R, Chaloupka FJ. Assessing the potential effectiveness of food and beverage taxes and subsidies for improving public health: a systematic review of prices, demand and body weight outcomes. Obes Rev. 2013;14(2):110–128.

51. World Bank. Taxes on Sugar-Sweetened Beverages: International Evidence and Experiences Washington DC: World Bank; 2020.

52. Alsukait R, Wilde P, Bleich S, Singh G, Folta S. Evaluating Saudi Arabia's 50% carbonated drink excise tax: Changes in prices and volume sales. Econ Hum Biol. 2020;38:100868.

53. Colchero MA, Popkin BM, Rivera JA, Ng SW. Beverage purchases from stores in Mexico under the excise tax on sugar sweetened beverages: observational study. BMJ. 2016;352:h6704.

54. Colchero MA, Molina M, Guerrero-Lopez CM. After Mexico implemented a tax, purchases of sugar-sweetened beverages decreased and water increased: difference by place of residence, household composition, and income level. J Nutr. 2017;147(8):1552–1557.

55. Colchero MA, Rivera-Dommarco J, Popkin BM, Ng SW. In Mexico, evidence of sustained consumer response two years after implementing a sugar-sweetened beverage tax. Health Aff (Millwood). 2017;36(3):564–571.

56. Sánchez-Romero LM, Penko J, Coxson PG, Fernández A, Mason A, Moran AE, et al. Projected impact of Mexico's sugar-sweetened beverage tax policy on diabetes and cardiovascular disease: a modeling study. PLoS Med. 2016;13(11):e1002158.

57. Basto-Abreu A, Barrientos-Gutierrez T, Vidana-Perez D, Colchero MA, Hernandez FM, Hernandez-Avila M, et al. Cost-effectiveness of the sugar-sweetened beverage excise tax in Mexico. Health Aff (Millwood). 2019;38(11):1824–1831.

58. The Nutritional Health Alliance. Fact Sheet. Uncapping the Truth: The Mexican Sugar Sweetened Beverage Tax Works. Mexico: The Nutritional Health Alliance; 2016.

59. Basu S, Vellakkal S, Agrawal S, Stuckler D, Popkin B, Ebrahim S. Averting obesity and type 2 diabetes in India through sugar-sweetened beverage taxation: an economic-epidemiologic modeling study. PLoS Med. 2014;11(1):e1001582.

# 5.4 Physical Activity

*Shifalika Goenka, Prarthna Mukerjee, and Greg Heath*

## CONTENTS

## INTRODUCTION

Physical activity is considered a miracle drug, as it has wide-ranging benefits on cardiovascular diseases (CVDs) (1). The benefits are direct (effects on the heart) and indirect (positive effects on blood pressure, glucose, and lipids). The benefits of physical activity (PA) have been known for more than six decades after the seminal paper on the role of PA in lowering coronary heart disease (CHD) mortality by Jerry Morris (2). Despite widespread knowledge on the benefits of PA, its use by individuals is limited, and policymakers have not given enough attention to improving the PA of populations. This chapter will discuss the mechanisms by which PA is useful in preventing CVD, the current recommendations for individuals, and the policy landscape for enhancing PA.

### How Does Physical Activity Prevent Cardiovascular Disease?

PA lowers several cardiovascular risk factors in individuals. It is beneficial both in primary and secondary prevention of CVD. It acts through multiple mechanisms. PA reduces blood pressure and blood sugar and increases high-density lipoprotein cholesterol (HDL-C), thereby favorably altering the metabolic milieu (3, 4).

In terms of blood sugar regulation, PA intensifies insulin action, increases insulin sensitivity of the body and cells, and enhances glucose uptake of the muscles by almost fivefold. It does so both by insulin-dependent and insulin-independent mechanisms. All modes of exercise (aerobic, resistance) do this, and a combination has been shown to work even better (5).

Further, regular PA helps with weight loss and its maintenance. It decreases abdominal fat even in the absence of weight loss (4). In general, aerobic training has the potential to result in reductions of abdominal visceral fat by more than 30 cm² and 40 cm² (on computerized tomography [CT] scan) and also substantial reductions in ectopic fat (in the liver and heart) (6).

Several lines of investigation (cohort studies, primary and secondary prevention trials) demonstrate a dose-dependent relationship of PA with blood sugar, total cholesterol, hypertension, obesity, and waist circumference (4). Data from population-based cohort studies reveal that those participating in regular moderate PA (walking briskly for 2.5 hrs/wk) had a 30% lower risk of incident diabetes (7). Trials for the prevention of adult-onset diabetes mellitus have conclusively demonstrated that a structured PA intervention and dietary control that leads to a 5–10% loss of body weight can lower the incidence of diabetes by 58% at five years. This reduction in incidence was even better than that seen with metformin (8). Similarly, it is estimated that approximately 34% of the incident hypertension in populations can be prevented if adults moved to higher PA and fitness levels (9). PA has also been shown to impact lipoprotein lipids, especially with increases in blood levels of HDL-C, with modest lowering of serum triglycerides and low-density lipoprotein (LDL) cholesterol (10, 11). Table 5.4.1 summarizes the CVD benefits associated with PA.

DOI: 10.1201/b23266-9

**Table 5.4.1 Benefits and Adaptations Associated with Increased Levels of Physical Activity and the Prevention and Management of Cardiovascular Disease (12–14)**

| Predisposing Diseases/ Conditions | Potential Mechanisms |
|---|---|
| i. Hypertension | Prevents hypertension in normotensive adolescents and adults and decreases both systolic and diastolic blood pressure among adults with mild hypertension |
| ii. Type 2 diabetes | Increases insulin sensitivity and improves glucose tolerance through skeletal muscle adaptations |
| iii. Obesity | Prevents weight gain, maintains energy balance, and improves lean/fat body ratio |
| iv. Metabolic syndrome | Improves blood lipid profile with increased HDL blood cholesterol levels and lower LDL levels |
| v. Physical fitness levels | Increased cardiorespiratory fitness, muscle strength and endurance |
| vi. Vascular inflammation and atherosclerosis | Reduced blood concentrations of inflammatory biomarkers (e.g., C-reactive protein, lipoprotein-associated phospholipase A2, cytokines IL-1β, IL-6, and TNF-α) *TNF: Tumor necrosis factor; IL: Interleukin |
| **Physiologic benefits** | |
| i. Central and peripheral circulatory | Decreases resting heart rate, resting blood systolic pressure, myocardial oxygen demand, risk of myocardial ischemia, sympathetic tone, arterial stiffness |
| | Increases heart rate reserve, diastolic function, coronary circulation, myocardial perfusion, parasympathetic activity, endothelial function |
| ii. Skeletal muscle adaptations | Increased mitochondrial function (number and size); improved muscle fuel uptake (carbohydrates and free fatty acids); improved extraction of oxygen at the level of the muscle cell and production of energy (increased arterial/venous oxygen difference) |

HOW MUCH IS RECOMMENDED?

Daily regular PA has significant dose-dependent benefits for the prevention of CVD and its risk factors. Individuals who engaged in >150 minutes and >300 minutes of moderate-intensity leisure-time physical activity (LTPA) had 15% and 20% lower CHD, respectively, as compared to those who did less (15). Thus, the World Health Organization (WHO) guidelines 2020 on physical activity and sedentary behaviors recommend that adults (18–64 years) indulge in 150–300 minutes of moderate-intensity aerobic activity or 75–150 minutes of vigorous activity or a combination of both. Sitting needs to be decreased as much as possible. Further, adults should do muscle-strengthening exercises at least two or more days a week (12). Additional benefits accrue when moderate-intensity activity is more than 300 minutes per week or vigorous activity is more than 150 minutes per week. For older adults, the recommendations are the same as younger adults (150–300 minutes). In addition, at least three days a week, they should do various activities like balancing and strength training to enhance functional capacity to prevent falls.

It is important to note that the recommended amounts of PA are designed to be added to routine activities of daily living (e.g., casual walking or grocery shopping).

In terms of population-based approaches to promoting PA across the life course, the WHO "Global Action Plan for Physical Activity 2018–2030" (GAPPA) proposes four strategic ways to enhance the population PA levels. The four strategic methods are to create 1) active environments, 2) active societies, 3) active systems, and 4) active people (16). They stated their overall objective was "to ensure that all people have access to safe and enabling environments and to diverse opportunities to be physically active in their daily lives".

Creating active environments involves improving the environment for active transport, walking, and cycling, where people walk out of choice and not out of compulsion. Sidewalks need to be wide, with trees for shade to provide a pleasurable experience while walking. In the same vein, well-maintained, large public parks with safe and convenient access within a 0.5-km radius of every person will encourage people to be active across the life course. This is in line with the general GAPPA guiding principles of proportionate universality, equity, multisectoral action, human rights, and policy coherence across the sectors (16).

Individual countries like the United Kingdom address PA in their medical guidelines. The National Institute for Health and Care Excellence (NICE) recommends the promotion of PA through built or natural environments (17). Some of the key recommendations include the following. In the context of open spaces, they recommend that:

- open spaces and parks be within 0.5-km radius or walking distance
- open spaces and footpaths are maintained to a high standard
- there is shade and shelter for comfort
- seats with arms and backrests are sited at frequent intervals.

In the context of building construction, NICE suggests that building constructions should:

- ensure different parts of campus sites (worksites, hospitals, and universities) are linked by accessible walking and cycling routes
- improve the existing walking and cycling infrastructure by creating new through routes
- ensure staircases are wide, well designed and comfortable, lit and decorated, and given prominence.

There are other guidelines in the context of pedestrian crossings, curbs, pathways, schools, etc. They also emphasize seating be provided at regular intervals along pathways that are walking routes to encourage people to walk.

### Create Active Societies

Conduct national and local campaigns to raise awareness about the benefits of PA, motivating them along with site-specific actions and policies to make societies (people) active at worksites, schools, "walking only roads", etc. Community empowerment can increase PA. To cite an example, in Chennai, with a high burden of diabetes, some communities were imparted with education about the benefits of PA. They were motivated to clean up and renovate an existing park for walking and play. When evaluated a few years later, the PA had significantly gone up. At baseline, only 14.2% of the residents did some form of exercise more than three times a week, which subsequently increased to 58.7% [p < 0.001]. The number of subjects who walked more than three times a week increased from 13.8% at baseline to 52.1% during follow-up (18). A study of parks in Delhi showed that community action helped maintain the local parks and enhance their usage (19).

### Create Active Systems

Creating an active system needs strengthened policy frameworks, leadership, and governance systems at the national and sub-national levels to support the implementation of actions to increase PA in all sectors and reduce sedentary behaviors by multisectoral engagement, coordination, and policy coherence across sectors. Also necessary is a robust surveillance system on PA and a monitoring mechanism for the same. Adequate allocation of resources for research and evidence generation for PA and its promotion is needed to create active systems.

### Create Active People

This strategy aims to make PA socially desirable. This includes promoting programs of PA at various locations; tailoring programs for older adults, women, and children, and adopting whole-school approaches and whole-community approaches to develop and implement PA promotion strategies and programs.

### Public Transport

Users of public transport increase PA by more than 8–33 minutes/day. Public transport needs to be of adequate capacity and high quality, enticing people to use them out of choice. Transportation and travel policies should look at the seamless connection between different types of transport, for example, metro use in Delhi and then the ability to walk or cycle to destinations within a 2- to 3-km radius with ease and comfort (20). According to NICE, PA increases as the quality, capacity, and frequency of the public transport improves (17).

## CONCLUSIONS

Improvement of PA in populations through the multi-sectoral actions outlined will lower cardiovascular diseases in individuals and population. They also collaterally benefit several of the UN Sustainable Development Goals (SDGs). The PA interventions are aligned to several SDGs (4, 5, 10, 11, 13, 15, 16).

## REFERENCES

1. Pimlott N. The miracle drug. Can Fam Physician. 2010 May;56(5):407, 409.
2. Hallal PC, Bauman AE, Heath GW, Kohl HW, Lee I-M, Pratt M. Physical activity: more of the same is not enough. The Lancet. 2012 Jul;380(9838):190–191.
3. U.S. Department of Health and Human Services, National Institutes of Health, National Heart, Lung, and Blood Institute, National High Blood Pressure Education Program. The Seventh Report of the Joint National Committee on: Prevention, Detection, Evaluation, and Treatment of High Blood Pressure [Internet]. 2004. Available from: www.nhlbi.nih.gov/files/docs/guidelines/jnc7full.pdf
4. NG B, Prud'homme D. Adult obesity clinical practice guidelines: physical activity in obesity management. 2020. Available from: https://obesitycanada.ca/wp-content/uploads/2021/05/9-Physical-Activity-v3-with-links.pdf
5. Colberg SR, Sigal RJ, Yardley JE, Riddell MC, Dunstan DW, Dempsey PC, et al. Physical activity/exercise and diabetes: a position statement of the American Diabetes Association. Dia Care. 2016 Nov;39(11):2065–2079.
6. Ismail I, Keating SE, Baker MK, Johnson NA. A systematic review and meta-analysis of the effect of aerobic vs. resistance exercise training on visceral fat: Exercise for visceral fat. Obesity Reviews. 2012 Jan;13(1):68–91.
7. Jeon CY, Lokken RP, Hu FB, van Dam RM. Physical activity of moderate intensity and risk of type 2 diabetes: a systematic review. Diabetes Care. 2007 Mar 1;30(3):744–752.
8. Knowler WC, Barrett-Connor E, Fowler SE, Hamman RF, Lachin JM, Walker EA, et al. Reduction in the incidence of type 2 diabetes with lifestyle intervention or metformin. N Engl J Med. 2002 Feb 7;346(6):393–403.
9. Carnethon MR, Evans NS, Church TS, Lewis CE, Schreiner PJ, Jacobs DR, et al. Joint associations of physical activity and aerobic fitness on the development of incident hypertension: coronary artery risk development in young adults. Hypertension. 2010 Jul;56(1):49–55.
10. Clarke J, Janssen I. Sporadic and Bouted Physical Activity and the Metabolic Syndrome in Adults. Medicine & Science in Sports & Exercise. 2014 Jan;46(1):76–83.
11. Di Blasio A, Bucci I, Ripari P, Giuliani C, Izzicupo P, Di Donato F, et al. Lifestyle and high density lipoprotein cholesterol in postmenopause. Climacteric. 2014 Feb;17(1):37–47.
12. Organisation mondiale de la santé. WHO guidelines on physical activity and sedentary behaviour. S.l.: s.n.; 2020.
13. Powell KE, King AC, Buchner DM, Campbell WW, DiPietro L, Erickson KI, et al. The scientific foundation for the physical activity guidelines for Americans, 2nd edition. J Phys Act Health. 2018 Dec 17;1–11.
14. Alves AJ, Viana JL, Cavalcante SL, Oliveira NL, Duarte JA, Mota J, et al. Physical activity in primary and secondary prevention of cardiovascular disease: Overview updated. WJC. 2016;8(10):575.
15. Sattelmair J, Pertman J, Ding EL, Kohl HW, Haskell W, Lee I-M. Dose response between physical activity and risk of coronary heart disease: a meta-analysis. Circulation. 2011 Aug 16;124(7):789–795.
16. Organisation mondiale de la santé, editor. Global action plan on physical activity 2018–2030: more active people for a healthier world. Geneva: World health organization; 2018.
17. National Institutes of Health and Care Excellence. NICE guideline [NG90] Physical activity and the environment [Internet]. 2018. Available from: www.nice.org.uk/guidance/ng90/chapter/Recommendations#public-open-spaces
18. Mohan V, Shanthirani CS, Deepa M, Datta M, Williams OD, Deepa R. Community empowerment—a successful model for prevention of non-communicable diseases in India—the Chennai Urban Population Study (CUPS-17). J Assoc Physicians India. 2006 Nov;54:858–862.
19. Unpublished data. A situational analysis of park in Delhi, WHO SEARO.
20. Devarajan R, Prabhakaran D, Goenka S. Built environment for physical activity—An urban barometer, surveillance, and monitoring. Obesity Reviews [Internet]. 2020 Jan [cited 2021 Aug 19];21(1). Available from: https://onlinelibrary.wiley.com/doi/10.1111/obr.12938

# 5.5 Cardiovascular Disease, Overweight, and Obesity

## *Shared Strategies for Prevention and Management*

*Johanna Ralston, Piyu Sharma, and Panniyammakal Jeemon*

## CONTENTS

## INTRODUCTION

Obesity may be defined as a chronic relapsing disease—as well as a risk factor for other noncommunicable diseases—which affects an increasing number of people globally (1). There has been a marked increase in the prevalence of overweight and obesity in the last four decades. Obesity ranged from around 3% in men and over 6% in women in 1975 to 11% of men and 15% of women in 2016 and overweight from 20% in men and under 23% in women in 1975 to 39% in both men and women in 2016 (2).

Obesity has become one of the main drivers of cardiovascular disease (CVD) (3) and in some respects has displaced tobacco as the main risk factor that triggers a host of cardiovascular (CV)-related issues. The management of CVD will often require addressing the weight of a patient, and while some measures have been successful in preventing or managing obesity, the relative absence of a consistent comprehensive approach (4) is one of the reasons that obesity rates are still rising. The following infographics show current numbers of people across four categories of overweight and obesity (Figure 5.5.1) and the association between ischemic heart disease (IHD) and high body mass index (BMI) (Table 5.5.1).

Trends are even more concerning among children and adolescents; a study analyzing worldwide trends in BMI from 1975 to 2016 concluded that although rising BMI trends for children and adolescents have plateaued in many high-income countries (HICs), they have accelerated in parts of Asia.

The problem is only growing more serious with many low- and middle-income countries (LMICs), where the incidence is growing most rapidly, while the number of people living with obesity has become more equally distributed across LMICs and HICs, as noted in the following chart (Figure 5.5.2) among men and women above age 20.

The estimated cost burden of high BMI to health services globally is around US$990 billion per year, which is 13% of total healthcare expenditure. Obesity also incurs indirect costs such as reduced quality of life, productivity, and life years lost. Both direct and indirect costs together decrease the well-being and the economic output of a country (5).

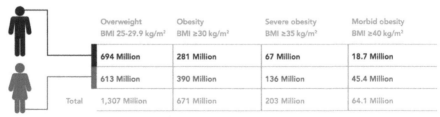

| | Overweight BMI 25-29.9 kg/m² | Obesity BMI ≥30 kg/m² | Severe obesity BMI ≥35 kg/m² | Morbid obesity BMI ≥40 kg/m² |
|---|---|---|---|---|
| | 694 Million | 281 Million | 67 Million | 18.7 Million |
| | 613 Million | 390 Million | 136 Million | 45.4 Million |
| Total | 1,307 Million | 671 Million | 203 Million | 64.1 Million |

Source: NCD Risc Collaboration, 2017²

**Figure 5.5.1** Estimated number of adults over 20 years old living with obesity globally, 2016.

*Source*: NCD Risk Factor Collaboration (2017) and World Obesity Federation (2020).

DOI: 10.1201/b23266-10

## Table 5.5.1 Estimated Number of Ischemic Heart Disease Cases Attributable to High BMI

|  | Men | Women | Total |
|---|---|---|---|
| *Global* | *3.5 m* | *8.2 m* | *11.7 m* |
| African Region | 0.2 m | 0.3 m | 0.5 m |
| Region of the Americas | 0.4 m | 1.1 m | 1.5 m |
| Southeast Asian Region | 0.2 m | 0.5 m | 0.7 m |
| European Region | 1.1 m | 2.6 m | 3.6 m |
| Eastern Mediterranean Region | 0.8 m | 1.6 m | 2.4 m |
| Western Pacific Region | 0.9 m | 2.1 m | 3.0 m |

World Obesity Federation. *2020 Atlas. Obesity: Missing the 2025 Targets* (2nd edition). London: WOF 2020.

|  |  | Men |  | Women |
|---|---|---|---|---|
| 1 | United States of America | 42.9 m | United States of America | 46.8 m |
| 2 | China | 33.2 m | China | 36.2 m |
| 3 | Brazil | 13.4 m | India | 21.3 m |
| 4 | India | 12.3 m | Brazil | 19.6 m |
| 5 | Russian Federation | 9.7 m | Russian Federation | 17.6 m |
| 6 | Mexico | 9. 4m | Mexico | 14.0 m |
| 7 | Germany | 8.2 m | Egypt | 11.6 m |
| 8 | United Kingdom | 6.9 m | Turkey | 11.1 m |
| 9 | Turkey | 6.5 m | Iran | 9.1 m |
| 10 | Egypt | 6.3 m | Indonesia | 7.8 m |
| 11 | Iran | 5.6 m | United Kingdom | 7.7 m |
| 12 | France | 5.3 m | South Africa | 7.4 m |
| 13 | Italy | 5.0 m | Germany | 7.3 m |
| 14 | Spain | 4.6 m | Pakistan | 6.3 m |
| 15 | Canada | 4.3 m | Nigeria | 5.8 m |
| 16 | Saudi Arabia | 4.2 m | France | 5.6 m |
| 17 | Indonesia | 4.2 m | Italy | 5.3 m |
| 18 | Argentina | 3.9 m | Ukraine | 5.3 m |
| 19 | Ukraine | 3.7 m | Algeria | 4.7 m |
| 20 | Poland | 3.6 m | Colombia | 4.7 m |

**Figure 5.5.2**   Countries with the largest number of adults over 20 years old living with obesity, 2016.

*Source:* NCD Risk Factor Collaboration (2017) and World Obesity Federation (2020).

OBESITY BACKGROUND

While there has always been some level of overweight or excess adiposity, the most striking feature of obesity is the rapid increase that began in the 1970s and 1980s (6). A constellation of factors led to this, including in the United States and Europe the changes in agricultural subsidies which catalyzed dramatic changes in the production and availability of low-cost and energy-dense (though often nutrient-poor) food, increases in portion sizes, and concurrent saturation of the food system with cheap sweetening agents such as high fructose corn syrup.

There are multiple upstream and downstream determinants of obesity which form a complex causal pathway of interaction. Upstream determinants are those factors which are not in the control of the individual but have a significant impact on the more direct determinants of the health of an individual. The increased supply of cheap, palatable, energy-dense foods and more persuasive and pervasive food marketing are dominant drivers of the obesity epidemic. The obesogenic drivers within the food and physical activity environments, taxation regimes, regulation of the marketplace, and social and economic policies set the conditions under which businesses and individuals operate and have distal effects on obesity. The distal effects might convert to higher obesity prevalence through psychosocial and behavioral effects. At one end of the spectrum rates of childhood obesity have increased tenfold over the past four decades, while at the other, efforts to address obesity among adults have met with some success, but with an intractable challenge at the higher BMI rates, which continue to rise, and in weight regain, which continues to be the norm rather than the exception.

The migration of cheaper food products occurred over a longer timeframe to LMICs, facilitated by trade agreements between and among high-, middle-, and low-income countries. Such transformations have been linked to dramatic changes in the availability of what are now called ultra-processed foods, reduced diversification of crops driven by subsidies, and a push for cheaper food, which helped address hunger but distorted the kinds of diets people ate. Other factors influencing the increase in overweight and obesity worldwide include a shift from active to sedentary transport and work; air quality and urbanization that have inhibited physical activity and also accelerated CVD and chronic pulmonary disease; and a host of genetic, biological, and social factors that continue to be discovered.

The INTERHEART study, a global case-control study conducted in 52 countries, identified waist-to-hip ratio as one of the nine risk factors attributable to myocardial infarction (MI). They found that waist-to-hip-ratio shows a graded and significant association with MI worldwide as compared to BMI, the more conventional measure (7). The INTERSTROKE study, a study assessing risk factors for ischemic and intracerebral hemorrhagic stroke in 22 countries globally, identified waist-to-hip ratio as one of the ten risk factors attributable to 90% of the risk of stroke (8). This points to the need to improve how overweight and obesity are measured and the impact that changes in measurement are likely to have on reinforcing the association between adiposity and CVD. Of particular concern is the recognition that alongside the dramatic increase in CVD prevalence and mortality in LMICs, the increase in rates of obesity is highest in LMICs, where the systems and skills required to address them are particularly poorly equipped to do so.

Moreover, the rise in overweight and obesity is occurring alongside undernutrition, and the double burden of malnutrition (DBM) is seen in the same communities, families, and even individuals, given that stunting associated with undernutrition predisposes the individual to having obesity. Further, a mother's weight before, during, and after pregnancy has an impact on the weight of the child, making the fact that close to one-sixth of all women of reproductive age (18–49) are living with obesity even more concerning, especially given that most women of reproductive age live in LMICs.

## CHILDHOOD OBESITY

At the heart of the obesity challenge, and one of the drivers of ever-earlier manifestations of CVD and drivers, including diabetes, is the emergence of childhood obesity across the globe. As of 2016, it was estimated that 42 million children under the age of five had overweight or obesity (Table 5.5.2),

**Table 5.5.2 Percentage and Numbers of Children Ages 5–19 Years Living with Obesity: Regional and Global Estimates for 2010 and 2016 and Predicted 2025**

| WHO Regions | 2010 | 2016 | 2025 | Estimated Numbers in 2025 |
|---|---|---|---|---|
| *Global* | *4.9%* | *6.8%* | *10.5%* | *205.5 m\** |
| African Region | 1.8% | 2.8% | 5.2% | 23.5 m |
| Region of the Americas | 12.5% | 14.4% | 18.1% | 42.0 m |
| Southeast Asian Region | 6.2% | 8.2% | 12.0% | 26.4 m |
| European Region | 6.9% | 8.6% | 11.2% | 18.4 m |
| Eastern Mediterranean Region | 1.7% | 3.0% | 6.3% | 32.0 m |
| Western Pacific Region | 5.6% | 9.6% | 16.9% | 61.8 m |

\*Includes 1.3 m outside WHO regions (primarily Taiwan, Hong Kong, and North Korea).

*Source:* NCD Risk Factor Collaboration (2017) and World Obesity Federation (2020).

and the World Health Organization (WHO) reports that 75% lived in Asia and Africa (9). The likelihood of children with obesity becoming adults with obesity is high, and the impact of having obesity as a child extends to inequities in educational attainment and long-term quality of life.

In 2014, the WHO director general established the Ending Childhood Obesity Commission to mobilize expertise and support for addressing childhood obesity. The commission convened experts from low-, middle- and high-income countries to address the challenge and propose an integrated series of solutions. This integrated approach, which had previously been identified as central to addressing obesity by expert groups, including the Foresight report in 2007, was in some respects modeled after tobacco control in tackling a health issue across multiple domains. The recommendations of the commission (10) were sixfold:

- Promote intake of healthy foods—Improve intake of healthy foods while at the same time reducing access to and marketing of unhealthy foods and beverages.

- Promote physical activity—This includes publicly supported programs to increase physical activity and decrease sedentary behaviors.

- Preconception and pregnancy care—Prevent noncommunicable diseases (NCDs) through integrated preconception, prenatal, and antenatal care.

- Early childhood diet and physical activity—Support healthy diets and physical activity in early childhood, starting with breastfeeding and encouraging access to physical activity.

- Health, nutrition, and physical activity for school-age children—Utilize education channels to promote and integrate nutrition and physical activity among school-age children.

- Weight management—Provide family-based, multicomponent, lifestyle weight management services for children and young people who are obese.

The commission's recommendations were adopted in 2017 and implemented with varying degrees of success. Fiscal policies such as a tax on sugary drinks and consumer initiatives, including adoption of front-of-pack labeling, originally started in Chile, and as of 2020 the models underway in over 30 countries have, in general, seen successful implementation, while consistent integration of school-based policies have been fragmented and DBM approaches are also mixed. Overcoming barriers to successfully addressing childhood obesity includes greater adoption of a life-course approach, improved stakeholder alignment, and improved narrative of obesity as a disease and a driver of other disease (11).

## MANAGEMENT AND RESEARCH

Individual-level and large-scale environment-level changes are required in conjunction to tackle the burden of overweight and obesity. Community engagement and supportive environments are often needed to aid people in making healthier food choices and engaging in regular physical activity. Issues surrounding availability, accessibility, and affordability of both food choice and physical activity need to be addressed for sustained change of lifestyle measures at the population level. Regulation of the food industry and policy measures like taxation of sugar-sweetened beverages and calorie-dense foods are some effective strategies to tackle obesity at the population level.

The WHO Global Strategy on Diet adopted by the World Health Assembly (WHA) in 2004 outlined the actions needed to support healthy diets and regular physical activity by governments. It called for stakeholder engagement at the global, national, and local level. Most important, it has served as a foundation for specific strategies on sugar, salt, trans fats, and other factors which contribute to CVD and obesity.

Lifestyle interventions, pharmacotherapy, and bariatric surgery are individual-level options for management of obesity with a reasonable body of evidence. Regular recording of food intake, physical activity, and weight via a personal diary or an mHealth application and goal settings can help in self-monitoring moderate levels of weight loss. The key components of dietary advice are healthy food choices and portion control. For individuals with severe metabolic disorders, exercise regimens can be tailored to the cardiorespiratory health of the individuals.

Pharmacotherapy may be used as an adjunct in individuals with BMI >30kg/m$^2$ or in individuals with BMI 27–29 kg/m$^2$ and an existing comorbid condition. Centrally acting noradrenergic agents can be used for short-term management. A few drugs may be used long-term (lorcaserin, orlistat), but their long-term efficacy and effect on CV health are yet to be determined (12).

Bariatric surgery is indicated for individuals with BMI ≥40 kg/m² or presence of a comorbid condition like hypertension, type 2 diabetes, or nonalcoholic fatty liver or heart disorders in conjunction with BMI >35 kg/m². The procedures show larger weight reduction as compared to the measures outlined earlier but carry a higher cost and require surgical revisions during follow-up. Of note, the COVID-19 pandemic reinforced that individuals with severe obesity are more likely to experience complications of COVID-19 and are more likely to die from the disease, reinforcing that while obesity is a driver of CVD, the underlying poor health of populations with high rates of obesity and CVD also places them at risk for morbidity and mortality associated with communicable diseases for reasons that are still emerging.

Several gaps exist in our understanding of the obesity epidemic despite the growing body of research evidence. Prior to successfully tackling this 'wicked problem' (13), we need to evolve our understanding of obesity from a complicated system to a complex adaptive system (CAS) with feedback, interactions, and compensatory behavior, and with it our approach to the problem. As public health professionals, it is vital to be open to uncertainty and unpredictability in our interventions and aim to find sustainable approaches. The difference between a complicated and complex system is an important one. A complicated system has many parts which interact in a linear predictable fashion, whereas a complex system has multiple unintended consequences and contains feedback loops (14) and displays emergent properties—'it is more than the sum of its parts.'

Nationally representative surveys may help identify secular trends prevalent in different countries. They can also be used to gain a better understanding of the impact and effectiveness of national and state-level policy interventions for obesity prevention and control. There is strong evidence to suggest a significant reduction in the risk of diabetes and CVDs by weight loss in overweight and obese individuals. But further research is needed to demonstrate risk reduction in CV events and mortality by weight loss in these individuals. Cluster randomized trials can be conducted to better understand the impact of behavior change strategies in individuals with overweight and obesity at the population level. Pre-/post-evaluations with data collected at several time points and quasi-experimental designs such as interrupted time series analysis can help attain a clear understanding of the impact of health policies.

## CONCLUSION

While the association between CVD and obesity has been well documented and is tied in large part to wider trends in how people eat, move, and live, the pandemic of 2020 has drawn urgent attention to the dual challenges of CVD and obesity across the globe and especially in LMICs (15). Thus, a whole-of-society approach is needed to effectively prevent and manage both childhood and adult obesity, particularly in the many middle-income countries where rates are rising most rapidly. Of promise are comprehensive approaches for CVD, including the WHO technical package HEARTS (Healthy lifestyle counselling, Evidence-based treatment, Access to medicines, Team-based care, and Systems for monitoring) and the World Obesity Federation's ROOTS (Recognize obesity as both disease and risk factor, Obesity monitoring, Obesity through the life course, Treat obesity, and Systems-based approaches). Obesity and CVD both require stepping beyond single-silo approaches, and there is significant potential for alignment across the respective strategies.

## REFERENCES

1. Bray GA, Kim KK, Wilding JPH; World Obesity Federation. Obesity: a chronic relapsing progressive disease process. A position statement of the world obesity federation. Obes Rev. 2017 Jul;18(7):715–723. https://doi.org/10.1111/obr.12551. Epub 2017 May 10. PMID: 28489290.
2. NCD Risk Factor Collaboration (NCD-RisC). Trends in adult body-mass index in 200 countries from 1975 to 2014: a pooled analysis of 1698 population-based measurement studies with 19·2 million participants. Lancet. 2016 Apr 2;387(10026):1377–1396. https://doi.org/10.1016/S0140–6736(16)30054-X. Erratum in: Lancet. 2016 May 14;387(10032):1998. PMID: 27115820.
3. Powell-Wiley TM, Poirier P, Burke LE, Després JP, Gordon-Larsen P, Lavie CJ, Lear SA, Ndumele CE, Neeland IJ, Sanders P, St-Onge MP; American Heart Association council on lifestyle and cardiometabolic health; council on cardiovascular and stroke nursing; council on clinical cardiology; council on epidemiology and prevention; and stroke council. obesity and cardiovascular disease: a scientific statement from the American Heart Association. Circulation. 2021 May 25;143(21):e984–e1010.

3. Hubert HB, Feinleib M, McNamara PM, Castelli WP; Obesity as an independent risk factor for cardiovascular disease: a 26-year follow-up of participants in the Framingham heart study. Circulation. 1983;67:968–977. https://doi.org/10.1161/01.CIR.67.5.968. [PubMed]

4. Foresight. Tackling obesities: future choices—project report. The Stationery Office, London. 2007. www.foresight.gov.uk/Obesity/obesity_final/Index.html

5. Roth G, Johnson C; Global, regional, and national burden of cardiovascular diseases for 10 causes, 1990 to 2015. J Am College Cardiology. 2017 July: 1–25.

6. Rodgers A, Woodward A, Swinburn B, Dietz W; Prevalence trends tell us what did not precipitate the US obesity epidemic. Lancet. 2018;3(4):E162–E16.

7. Yusuf S, Hawken S, Ôunpuu S, et al; On behalf of the interheart study investigators. Obesity and the risk of myocardial infarction in 27 000 participants from 52 countries: a case-control study. Lancet. 2005;366:1640–1649. https://doi.org/10.1016/S0140-6736(05)67663-5

8. O'Donnell MJ, Xavier D, Liu L, et al; On behalf of the interstroke investigators. Risk factors for ischaemic and intracerebral haemorrhagic stroke in 22 countries (the INTERSTROKE study): a case-control study. The Lancet. 2010;376(9735):112–123. https://doi.org/10.1016/S0140-6736(10)60834-3

9. Dinsa GD, Goryakin Y, Fumagalli E, Suhrcke M; Obesity and socioeconomic status in developing countries: a systematic review. Obes. Rev. 2012;13:1067–1079. https://doi.org/10.1111/j.1467-789X.2012.01017.x. [PMC free article] [PubMed] [CrossRef] Google Scholar.

10. World Health Organization: Report of the Commission on Ending Childhood Obesity. 2015. https://apps.who.int/iris/bitstream/handle/10665/204176/9789241510066_eng.pdf (accessed 21/09/2021)

11. Ralston J, Brinsden H, Buse K, Candeias V, Caterson I, Hassell T, Kumanyika S, Nece P, Nishtar S, Patton I, Proietto J, Salas XR, Reddy S, Ryan D, Sharma AM, Swinburn B, Wilding J, Woodward E; Time for a new obesity narrative. Lancet. 2018 Oct 20;392(10156):1384–1386. https://doi.org/10.1016/S0140-6736(18)32537-6. Epub 2018 Oct 10. PMID: 30316458.

12. Jeemon P, Sivasubramonian S; Obesity and cardiovascular disease. Cardiovascular disease risk factors. Textbook of Cardiology. In Prabhakaran D, Kumar RK, Naik N (Eds.). Tandon's text book of cardiology. Wolters Kluwer India Pvt Ltd. 2019

13. Rutter H; The single most important intervention to tackle obesity. Int J Public Health. 2012;57:657–658.

14. Swinburn BA, Kraak VI, Allender S, et al; The global syndemic of obesity, undernutrition, and climate change: *The Lancet* Commission report. Lancet 2019;393:791–846.

15. Lobstein T; COVID-19 and obesity: the 2021 Atlas. World obesity federation. www.worldobesityday.org/assets/downloads/COVID-19-and-Obesity-The-2021-Atlas.pdf (accessed 10.04.2021)

# 5.6 Alcohol

*Monika Arora, Neha Jain, and Sven Andreasson*

## CONTENTS

## INTRODUCTION

Alcohol has become an inseparable part of many individuals' social lives. Attractive marketing tactics by the manufacturers (1) and inadequate or lack of stringent control policies (2, 3) have contributed towards increased uptake and easy availability of alcohol. Moreover, conflicting reports and evidence about the degree of benefits or negative health impacts of consuming alcohol have hindered public health professionals' efforts to delineate the harms of excessive alcohol use.

In this chapter, we outline the current levels of alcohol consumption worldwide and describe known deleterious effects on health and ongoing programmatic efforts to reduce alcohol consumption.

## GLOBAL BURDEN OF ALCOHOL CONSUMPTION

In 2016, a high prevalence of alcohol consumption was reported from high socio-demographic index (SDI) countries, where the prevalence was 72% in females and 83% in males. In comparison, 8.9% of females and 20% of males were alcohol consumers in low- and middle-income countries (LMICs) (4). Furthermore, the population average of standard drinks consumed daily was also higher for high SDI countries than for LMICs.

Alcohol affects human physiology either through years of consumption, acute intoxication, or dependence (4). It has been linked with approximately 230 International Classification of Diseases, 10th edition (ICD-10) three-digit disease categories, including 40 diseases that would not prevail without alcohol (5). Alcohol has been ascribed as a crucial factor in deaths due to infectious diseases, intentional and unintentional injuries, digestive diseases, and several noncommunicable diseases (NCDs) (3). In 2016, it was the seventh leading risk factor for both death and disability-adjusted life years (DALYs). According to the Global Burden of Disease (GBD) study, there has been a constant rise in the number of deaths attributed to alcohol use over the last two decades. According to a World Health Organization (WHO) report, the total number of deaths increased (in absolute numbers) by more than 5% between 2010 and 2016 (3). In 2017, nearly 2.8 million deaths were attributed to alcohol or related factors, accounting for 5% of all deaths globally. Also, more than 107 million DALYs were caused by alcohol in the same year (6).

Furthermore, alcohol was also responsible for 7.2% of all premature mortality in 2016, with 13.5% of all deaths among those aged 20-39. Gender is also a determinant of alcohol-attributed diseases, death, and DALYs, wherein all three are usually higher for men than for women. This excess adverse outcome is partly due to the higher consumption of alcohol by men than by women and because men more frequently engage in other risky lifestyle choices such as tobacco consumption (7) and unhealthy diet (8). Leading causes for alcohol-attributable deaths among men are unintentional injuries and digestive and infectious diseases. In women, the leading causes of alcohol-attributable deaths are cardiovascular diseases (CVDs), followed by digestive diseases and unintentional injuries.

Socioeconomic status (SES) is a significant determinant of alcohol-related burden, wherein it unequivocally impacts people belonging to lower SES more (3). This can be attributed to multiple factors such as access to quality health care (9) and clustering of other risk factors (10). Furthermore, compared by income groups, a higher overall burden of death was observed in LMICs compared to high-income countries. When the burden of alcohol-attributed death was classified according to the underlying cause, deaths due to alcohol-attributed infectious diseases were

DOI: 10.1201/b23266-11

more common in LMICs and deaths due to alcohol- attributed cancer were more common in high- and middle-income countries (11).

In addition to health impacts, alcohol is known to have a severe economic burden. In a middle-income country such as India, it was estimated that direct and indirect costs from alcohol-related conditions would equate to USD 1.87 trillion between the years 2011 and 2050 (12), amounting to approximately 1.45% of the gross domestic product (GDP) per year of the Indian economy. This societal burden of alcohol includes the health system's cost, out-of-pocket expenditure, and productivity losses.

## PREGNANCY AND ALCOHOL CONSUMPTION

Fetal alcohol syndrome (FAS) is a combination of abnormalities (physical, behavioral, and learning) that occur in babies of mothers who drank alcohol during their pregnancy (13). The global prevalence of alcohol use during pregnancy is estimated to be 9.8%, and the prevalence of FAS in the general population is estimated to be 14.6 per 10,000 people. Besides, 1 in every 67 women who consumed alcohol during pregnancy would deliver a child with FAS. This translates to about 119,000 children born every year with FAS (14).

## SECONDHAND EFFECT OF ALCOHOL

While sufficient data are available on the direct burden of alcohol on the health, social, and economic aspects of the population and individuals, little focus is accorded to the harms of alcohol on the nondrinking people who may be affected in myriad ways. Road traffic injuries due to car accidents and drunk driving, sexual assault, domestic violence, negative impact on children, and lost productivity are some of the secondhand impacts of consuming alcohol. Also, the economic burden of secondhand effects is more extensive as compared to the burden on the consumer (15). According to the GBD, close to 9% of all road traffic injuries can be attributed to alcohol. In numbers, the highest prevalence of such deaths occurs in middle-income countries, with nearly 40,000 deaths in 2017 (6).

## ALCOHOL AND YOUTH

The ramifications of alcohol consumption are well-evidenced in adolescents and young adults. The brain of an individual develops until the age of 25 years (16). Alcohol use during this period negatively affects the brain (17). Studies also suggest that heavy drinking during adolescence and young adulthood is associated with lower neurocognitive functioning during the young adult years and particularly with impairment of attention and visio-spatial skills (17).

## ALCOHOL AND CARDIOVASCULAR DISEASES

The WHO lists four main behavioral risk factors that put an individual at an increased risk from CVDs and other NCDs, which include alcohol (18). In its Global Action Plan for prevention and control of NCDs, the WHO called for a 10% relative reduction in the harmful use of alcohol between 2013 and 2020 (19).

People with moderate consumption, with no binge episodes, appear to have a lower risk of ischemic heart disease (IHD). The protective effect of moderate alcohol consumption on IHD has been challenged, as the evidence is based entirely on nonrandomized studies (20). The debate over the role of low to moderate alcohol use and risk of myocardial infarction arises from inconsistent results from several studies. Most studies that demonstrate CVD protection by alcohol come from high-income countries (HICs), particularly the white population. These studies have shown that those who consume low to moderate levels of alcohol have lower rates of heart attacks as compared to those who abstain or drink high amounts of alcohol (J-curve). In specific populations like the South Asians, such a protection has not been demonstrated (21, 22). The reasons for this include difference in ethnicities, binge drinking, and drinking before meals as a cultural norm in HICs, higher smoking prevalence among those who consume alcohol, and differences in alcohol dehydrogenase type. Furthermore, India is an LMIC, and alcohol intake is much higher in low SES areas, which has long been recognized as a risk factor for CVD. While drinking patterns vary in different cultures, low SES in a country such as India is generally associated with more harmful patterns of drinking, e.g. binge drinking, which is recognized as a risk factor for CVD (23).

In summary the widely held J-shaped effect of alcohol consumption on health has not been entirely disproved, but what is clear is that there is heterogeneity in its effects because of several reasons, including ethnic variations and variations in alcohol consumption patterns. Perhaps the moderate consumption of alcohol is not protective as widely believed, but also that there is no evidence of severe harm specifically in terms of coronary heart disease.

## HARMS VS. BENEFITS

Given that the evidence for a protective effect, based on observational studies, is weak, contrary to popular opinion, alcohol appears to be not good for the heart. No randomized controlled trials (RCTs) of alcohol consumption have been conducted so far. This is a major limitation, as observational studies cannot prove causation. The main reasons for this are problems with confounding and misclassification.

Confounding is a serious problem in observational studies in this field (24). In addition to the distribution of traditional cardiac risk factors, low-dose alcohol consumption in western countries appears to be a marker of general well-being (25, 26). Studies on heart disease or mortality in non-western cultures, on the other hand, find no reduced risk from low-dose consumption (22, 27, 28). In fact, in a study done on Indian men, it was found that alcohol users were 1.4 times more likely to have coronary heart disease as compared to lifetime abstainers (22). This suggests that alcohol consumption, and especially moderate consumption, is related to sociocultural factors and might be a sign of adjustment to prevailing norms, rather than the cause of reduced risk.

A frequent problem is misclassification, which often causes moderate drinkers to appear healthy in comparison with abstainers. The best-known example of this is referred to as the "sick quitter effect" whereby former drinkers are mixed in with lifetime abstainers. Because people who give up alcohol have significantly worse health profiles, this procedure contaminates the abstainer reference group and makes the moderate drinkers "look good" by comparison. When lifetime intake of alcohol among current abstainers or near abstainers is calculated, no benefit on mortality is found among moderate drinkers compared with abstainers (29).

In the absence of clinical RCTs, genetic (Mendelian) randomization studies are perhaps the strongest available study design to assess the effects of alcohol consumption, particularly for chronic disease-related outcomes. In these studies (30), individuals with a genetic predisposition to consume less alcohol have lower, not higher, mortality rates from coronary heart disease. This effect is seen in all drinking categories, including those with low and moderate consumption. In summary: research in the latest decade has led to major reversals in the perception of alcohol in relation to health in general and CVD in particular. These developments have prompted health authorities in a number of countries, e.g. the Netherlands (31), England (32), and Australia (33), to lower their guidelines for low-risk drinking.

## CLINICAL PRACTICES

Given what we now know, what advice is appropriate for clinicians or public health professionals to advise patients or the public? Classification of alcohol drinkers on the basis of their consumption habit is given in Table 5.6.1. Here are four categories of alcohol consumption:

- **Abstainers**: should be commended and not advised to start drinking.

- **Moderate drinkers**: patients describing low-risk consumption and are not pregnant or suffering from disorders where alcohol is contraindicated (such as several of the cardiovascular disorders): while not protective, alcohol in moderate amounts poses little harm. By "moderate" is meant a maximum of ten standard drinks per week and a maximum of four standard drinks on a single occasion. A standard drink contains 12 grams of ethanol and is found in a 30-40 mL per serving of spirits or 120 mL per serving of table wine.

- **Heavy drinkers**: advise to reduce to a maximum of ten drinks/week, with an offer of support if this is difficult.

- **Binge drinkers**: advise to plan drinking to a maximum of four standard drinks on any occasion and to consume these slowly; no more than one drink per hour.

## Table 5.6.1 Classification of Alcohol Drinkers (34)

| Abstainers | Fewer than 12 Drinks in a Lifetime |
|---|---|
| Moderate drinkers | **For women**: More than 3 drinks but no more than 7 drinks per week*<br>**For men**: More than 3 drinks but no more than 14 drinks per week* |
| Heavy drinkers | **For women**: More than 7 drinks per week*<br>**For men**: More than 14 drinks per week* |
| Binge drinkers | **For women**: Having 4 or more drinks in a two-hour period in the past 30 days<br>**For men**: Having 5 or more drinks in a two-hour period in the past 30 days |

* On average over the past one year.

## NEED FOR ACTION: FRAMEWORK CONVENTION FOR ALCOHOL CONTROL

The harms of alcohol are well documented, with recent evidence stating that no alcohol level is indeed safe for consumption. In 2010, the World Health Assembly adopted the global strategy to control the NCDs, which included reducing the harmful use of alcohol (19). However, recent reports suggest that very few countries are implementing comprehensive strategic measures to do the same. Notably, few countries are implementing effective regulation of alcohol marketing (2). Policy measures such as increase in the legal age to drink alcohol lead to less drinking in adolescence and development of more moderate drinking patterns and less frequent harmful drinking patterns as adults (35, 36). Studies have found that policy measures that target the general population rather than the underage population, alcohol consumption rather than impaired driving, and raising prices have a stronger association with a reduction in binge drinking (37). However, research on the effectiveness of alcohol policy measures are more commonly conducted in HICs, and there is a need to understand the context of LMICs on the success of different policy measures. From the evidence that exists, limiting the physical availability of alcohol, raising prices, and banning advertisements had a positive impact on alcohol control (38). Hence, stringent, comprehensive, and uniform policies are required to effectively control the negative impacts of alcohol use. Now is the time to call for a Framework Convention for Alcohol Control (FCAC) to counter supportive alcohol environments and promote comprehensive health-promoting policies to promote cardiovascular health (39). To achieve this, stricter regulation of the alcohol industry is necessary.

## REFERENCES

1. Smith LA, Foxcroft DR. The effect of alcohol advertising, marketing and portrayal on drinking behaviour in young people: Systematic review of prospective cohort studies. BMC Public Health. 2009 Feb 6;9(1):1–11.
2. World Health Organization. Non-communicable diseases: progress monitor 2020. World Health. Geneva; 2020.
3. World Health Organisation. Global Status Report on Alcohol and Health. 2018.
4. Griswold MG, Fullman N, Hawley C, Arian N, Zimsen SRM, Tymeson HD, et al. Alcohol use and burden for 195 countries and territories, 1990–2016: A systematic analysis for the Global Burden of Disease Study 2016. Lancet. 2018;392(10152):1015–1035.
5. Rehm, Ph.D. J, Borges G, Gmel G, Graham K, Grant B, Parry C, et al. The comparative risk assessment for alcohol as part of the Global Burden of Disease 2010 Study: What changed from the last study? Int J Alcohol Drug Res. 2013 May 1;2(1).
6. Institute for Health Metrics and Evaluation. Global health data. GBD Results Tool | GHDx [Internet]. Available from: http://ghdx.healthdata.org/gbd-results-tool
7. Gubner NR, Delucchi KL, Ramo DE. Associations between binge drinking frequency and tobacco use among young adults. Addict Behav. 2016 Sep 1;60:191–196.
8. Fawehinmi TO, Ilomäki J, Voutilainen S, Kauhanen J. Alcohol consumption and dietary patterns: The FinDrink study. PLoS One. 2012 Jun 12;7(6).
9. Adler NE, Newman K. Socioeconomic disparities in health: pathways and policies. Health Aff. 2002;21(2):60–76.
10. Bellis MA, Hughes K, Nicholls J, Sheron N, Gilmore I, Jones L. The alcohol harm paradox: Using a national survey to explore how alcohol may disproportionately impact health in deprived individuals. BMC Public Health. 2016 Feb 18;16(1).
11. Hammer JH, Parent MC, Spiker DA, World Health Organization. Global status report on alcohol and health 2018 [Internet]. Vol. 65, Global status report on alcohol. 2018. pp. 74–85. Available from: http://www.who.int/substance_abuse/publications/global_alcohol_report/msbgsruprofiles.pdf%0Ahttp://www.ncbi.nlm.nih.gov/pubmed/29355346
12. Jyani G, Prinja S, Ambekar A, Bahuguna P, Kumar R. Health impact and economic burden of alcohol consumption in India. Int J Drug Policy [Internet]. 2019 Jul 1 [cited 2020 Mar 20];69:34–42. Available from: http://www.ncbi.nlm.nih.gov/pubmed/31055044
13. Riley EP, Mattson SN, Thomas JD. Fetal alcohol syndrome. In: Encyclopedia of Neuroscience. Elsevier Ltd; 2009. pp. 213–220.
14. Popova S, Lange S, Probst C, Gmel G, Rehm J. Estimation of national, regional, and global prevalence of alcohol use during pregnancy and fetal alcohol syndrome: a systematic review and meta-analysis. Lancet Glob Heal. 2017 Mar 1;5(3):e290–e299.

15. Andréasson S, Chikritzhs T, Dangardt F, Holder H, Naimi T, Stockwell and T. Alcohol and society: second hand effects of alcohol consumption [Internet]. 2015. Available from: http://iogt.org/wp-content/uploads/2015/03/Alcohol_and_society2015_en.pdf#page=6

16. Arain M, Haque M, Johal L, Mathur P, Nel W, Rais A, et al. Maturation of the adolescent brain. Neuropsychiatr Dis Treat [Internet]. 2013 [cited 2020 Mar 19]; Available from: http://dx.doi.org/10.2147/NDT.S39776

17. Squeglia LM, Jacobus J, Tapert SF. The effect of alcohol use on human adolescent brain structures and systems. In: Handbook of Clinical Neurology. Elsevier B.V.; 2014. pp. 501–510.

18. WHO. Global action plan for the prevention and control of noncommunicable diseases 2013-2020. World Heal Organ [Internet]. 2013;102. Available from: http://apps.who.int/iris/bitstream/10665/94384/1/9789241506236_eng.pdf

19. World Health Organisation. Global Action Plan for Prevention and Control of Non Communicable Diseases 2013-2020 [Internet]. 2013 [cited 2020 Feb 25]. Available from: www.who.int

20. Stockwell T, Zhao J, Panwar S, Roemer A, Naimi T, Chikritzhs T. Do "moderate" drinkers have reduced mortality risk? A systematic review and meta-analysis of alcohol consumption and all-cause mortality. Stud. Alcohol Drugs. 2016;77.

21. Leong DP, Smyth A, Teo KK, McKee M, Rangarajan S, Pais P, et al. Patterns of alcohol consumption and myocardial infarction risk: observations from 52 countries in the INTERHEART case-control study. Circulation [Internet]. 2014 Jul 29 [cited 2021 Feb 26];130(5):390–398. Available from: https://pubmed.ncbi.nlm.nih.gov/24928682/

22. Roy A, Prabhakaran D, Jeemon P, Thankappan KR, Mohan V, Ramakrishnan L, et al. Impact of alcohol on coronary heart disease in Indian men. Atherosclerosis [Internet]. 2010 Jun [cited 2020 Mar 19];210(2):531–535. Available from: http://www.ncbi.nlm.nih.gov/pubmed/20226461

23. Degerud E, Ariansen I, Ystrom E, Graff-Iversen S, Høiseth G, Mørland J, et al. Life course socioeconomic position, alcohol drinking patterns in midlife, and cardiovascular mortality: Analysis of Norwegian population-based health surveys. Rehm J, editor. PLOS Med [Internet]. 2018 Jan 2 [cited 2020 Mar 19];15(1):e1002476. Available from: https://dx.plos.org/10.1371/journal.pmed.1002476

24. Stockwell T, Greer A, Fillmore K, Chikritzhs T, Zeisser C. How good is the science? BMJ (Online). Br Med J Pub Group. 2012;344:30.

25. Naimi TS, Brown DW, Brewer RD, Giles WH, Mensah G, Serdula MK, et al. Cardiovascular risk factors and confounders among nondrinking and moderate-drinking U.S. adults. Am J Prev Med [Internet]. 2005 May [cited 2020 Mar 19];28(4):369–373. Available from: http://www.ncbi.nlm.nih.gov/pubmed/15831343

26. Hansel B, Thomas F, Pannier B, Bean K, Kontush A, Chapman MJ, et al. Relationship between alcohol intake, health and social status and cardiovascular risk factors in the urban Paris-Ile-De-France Cohort: Is the cardioprotective action of alcohol a myth. Eur J Clin Nutr [Internet]. 2010 Jun [cited 2020 Mar 19];64(6):561–568. Available from: http://www.ncbi.nlm.nih.gov/pubmed/20485310

27. Zhou X, Li C, Xu W, Hong X, Chen J. Relation of alcohol consumption to angiographically proved coronary artery disease in Chinese men. Am J Cardiol. 2010 Oct 15;106(8):1101–1103.

28. Schooling CM, Wenjie S, Ho SY, Chan WM, Tham MK, Ho KS, et al. Moderate alcohol use and mortality from ischaemic heart disease: A prospective study in older Chinese people. PLoS One [Internet]. 2008 Jun 4 [cited 2020 Mar 19];3(6):e2370. Available from: http://www.ncbi.nlm.nih.gov/pubmed/18523644

29. Ortolá R, García-Esquinas E, López-García E, León-Muñoz LM, Banegas JR, Rodríguez-Artalejo F. Alcohol consumption and all-cause mortality in older adults in Spain: an analysis accounting for the main methodological issues. Addiction [Internet]. 2019 Jan 1 [cited 2020 Mar 19];114(1):59–68. Available from: http://www.ncbi.nlm.nih.gov/pubmed/30063272

30. Holmes M V., Dale CE, Zuccolo L, Silverwood RJ, Guo Y, Ye Z, et al. Association between alcohol and cardiovascular disease: mendelian randomisation analysis based on individual participant data. BMJ. 2014 Jul 10;349.

31. Kromhout D, Spaaij CJK, De Goede J, Weggemans RM, Brug J, Geleijnse JM, et al. The 2015 Dutch food-based dietary guidelines. Eur J Clin Nutr. Nature Publishing Group. 2016;70:869–878.

32. Department of Health. UK chief medical officers' alcohol guidelines review. 2016. Available from: https://assets.publishing.service.gov.uk/government/uploads/system/uploads/attachment_data/file/545739/GDG_report-Jan2016.pdf

33. Australian Government, National Health and Medical Research Council. Australian guidelines to reduce health risks from drinking alcohol. 2019. Available from: https://www.nhmrc.gov.au/health-advice/alcohol

34. National Center for Health Statistics, Centers for Disease Control and Prevention (CDC). Adult alcohol use – glossary [Internet]. [cited 2021 Feb 26]. Available from: https://www.cdc.gov/nchs/nhis/alcohol/alcohol_glossary.htm

35. O'Malley PM, Wagenaar AC. Effects of minimum drinking age laws on alcohol use, related behaviors and traffic crash involvement among American youth: 1976-1987. J Stud Alcohol. 1991;52(5):478–491.

36. Toumbourou JW, Kypri K, Jones SC, Hickie IB. Should the legal age for buying alcohol be raised to 21 years? Med J Aust. 2014 Jun 2;200(10):568–570.

37. Xuan Z, Blanchette J, Nelson TF, Heeren T, Oussayef N. The alcohol policy environment and policy subgroups as predictors of binge drinking measures among US adults. Am J Public Health [Internet]. 2015 Apr 1 [cited 2021 Feb 26];105(4):816–822. Available from: https://pubmed.ncbi.nlm.nih.gov/25122017/

38. Cook WK, Bond J, Greenfield TK. Are alcohol policies associated with alcohol consumption in low- and middle-income countries? Addiction [Internet]. 2014 [cited 2021 Feb 26];109(7):1081–1090. Available from: /pmc/articles/PMC4107632/

39. Casswell S, Thamarangsi T. Reducing harm from alcohol: call to action. Vol. 373, The Lancet. Elsevier; 2009. pp. 2247–2257.

# 5.7 Hypertension

*Arun Pulikkottil Jose and Neil R. Poulter*

## CONTENTS

## BACKGROUND

### Reason for Concern

Raised blood pressure (BP) is the leading risk factor for morbidity and mortality worldwide.[1] According to the Global Burden of Disease Study, in 2017, raised systolic BP was responsible for 10.4 million (9.39–11.5) deaths and 218 million (198–237) disability adjusted life years (DALYs) across the globe.[1] A disease that largely affected high-income countries (HICs) in the past has now been shown to affect low-income and middle-income countries (LMICs) disproportionately.[2] A pooled analysis of trends in BP from 1975 to 2015 in 200 countries revealed that the highest levels of BP shifted from HICs to LMICs over the last four decades.[3] The absolute number of hypertensive individuals worldwide increased from 594 million in 1975 to 1.13 billion in 2015, a large proportion of which was contributed by LMICs.[3] A meta-analysis of population-based studies in 45 LMICs showed that one in three adults suffered from hypertension.[4] While most HICs have been experiencing a relative decline in the prevalence of hypertension, LMICs have witnessed an upward trend.[2,3] It is estimated that over three-quarters of the world's hypertensive population will be living in LMICs by 2025.[5]

### Estimates May Be Deceiving

The actual burden of hypertension may be a lot larger than what is estimated. Hypertension is often described as a "silent killer", and rightly so. Individuals often present to the healthcare system only after the onset of overt complications and irreversible target organ damage. Hypertension follows the epidemiological "iceberg phenomenon of disease" principle, according to which a majority of hypertensive individuals remain undetected by the health system. This is further complicated by the fact that those who are aware remain inadequately treated with poor BP control. The hypertension care cascade has been classically described to follow the "rule of halves". According to this principle, it is assumed that half of all hypertensives are aware of their disease status, half of those aware are on treatment and only half of those treated are being adequately treated or have their BP under control. A recent analysis of 1.1 million adults from 44 LMICs revealed that there are considerable losses to care at each level of the hypertension care cascade.[6] Among those with hypertension, only 39.2% (38.2–40.3) were aware, 29.9% (28.6–31.3) received treatment, and a mere 10.3% (9.6–11.0) achieved BP control.[6] Screening status was also abysmal, with almost a third of hypertensive individuals never having a BP ever recorded.[6] Studies have shown that wide disparities exist between HICs and LMICs not only in prevalence and absolute numbers but also in awareness, treatment, and control levels.[2] A systematic analysis of population-based studies from 90 countries showed that HICs had double the proportions of awareness and treatment and four times the proportion of BP control as compared with LMICs.[2] While HICs showed improvement at all levels of the care cascade between 2000 and 2010, LMICs showed a smaller percentage increase in awareness and treatment levels and a decrease in control levels.[2]

DOI: 10.1201/b23266-12

A Preventable Cause of Death

Hypertension is a preventable disease with numerous well-known risk factors and few emerging potential risk factors. These are usually classified as either being modifiable or non-modifiable. Non-modifiable risk factors include increasing age, ethnicity, family history, gender, and genetic predisposition, while modifiable risk factors include unhealthy diet, physical inactivity, obesity, excessive visceral fat, alcohol abuse, and psychological stress, among others.[7] Lifestyle modifications have been undervalued and poorly advocated despite there being strong evidence for their role in reducing BP (Table 5.7.1).[8] There is mounting evidence to suggest that novel risk factors such as noise pollution, certain persistent organic pollutants, and short- and long-term exposure to air pollution are associated with hypertension.[9–11] Prevalence of hypertension in LMICs is further augmented by conditioning upstream factors such as globalization, increasing urbanization, rural-to-urban migration, population aging, and economic and nutritional transitions.[7] Apart from its direct association with BP, sociodemographic factors have also been seen to be associated with poor performance in the hypertension cascade in LMICs.[6] A country's performance in the care cascade was found to be positively related to gross domestic product (GDP) per capita, with poorest performance being in the sub-Saharan region.[6] Many countries performed poorly relative to their predicted performance based on GDP per capita, indicating potential for improvement in healthcare.[6] Weak health infrastructure, poor access, high illiteracy rates, poverty, high costs of drugs, bad dietary habits, and skewed national health priorities have been found to contribute to the poor performance in LMICs.[7]

Public Health Approaches to Prevention and Management of Hypertension

It is useful to view and analyze the current healthcare system and the various interventions for hypertension according to the levels described in the Innovative Care for Chronic Conditions Framework (ICCCF) set out by the World Health Organization (WHO).[13] The three strata described are the micro-, meso-, and macro-levels.[12] The micro-level comprises strategies targeting patient behavior and interaction between the patient and the health system, the meso-level deals with interventions related to healthcare organization and community-based activities, and the macro-level pertains to health policy.[12] Table 5.7.2 lists the various public health interventions for controlling hypertension. A clear distinction between these levels is not always possible, and considerable interaction exists among them. Prevention and control strategies for hypertension usually comprise one or more interventions implemented through a targeted or population-based approach in a complementary and mutually reinforcing manner.[13]

*Micro-Level Interventions*

Interventions at this level include those that target patients, families, and their interactions with the health system. Interactions at the micro-level are often ignored while instituting interventions.[12] Hypertension, like other chronic illnesses, mandates behavioral modifications for which

## Table 5.7.1 **Lifestyle Modifications to Prevent and Manage Hypertension**

| Intervention | Recommendation | Expected Systolic BP Reduction (range) |
|---|---|---|
| **Weight reduction** | Maintain ideal BMI (20–25kg/m²). | 5–20 mmHg per 10 kg weight loss |
| **Dietary Approaches to Stop Hypertension (DASH) eating plan** | Eat a diet rich in fruit, vegetables, and low-fat dairy products. Eat less saturated and total fat. | 8–14 mmHg |
| **Dietary sodium restriction** | Reduce dietary sodium intake to <100 mmol/day <2.4 g sodium or <6 g salt (sodium chloride). | 2–8mmHg |
| **Physical activity** | Regular aerobic physical activity, e.g. brisk walking for at least 30 min most days. | 4–9 mmHg |
| **Alcohol moderation** | Men ≤21 units per week. Women ≤14 units per week. | 2–4 mmHg |

*Source:* The Seventh Report of the Joint National Committee on Prevention, Detection, Evaluation, and Treatment of High Blood Pressure[11]

## Table 5.7.2 Public Health Strategies to Control Hypertension

| WHO ICCCF Strata | Interventions |
| --- | --- |
| Micro-level | Interventions that target patients, families, and their interactions with the health system |
| Meso-level | • Team-based care and task redistribution<br>• Health coaching and self-management<br>• Physician training<br>• Information systems and health technology<br>• Screening<br>• Pharmacotherapy and related issues<br>• Community engagement and participation |
| Macro-level | Health policy interventions that target health system changes, dietary interventions, and tobacco legislations |

the patient, as well as their families, need to be committed and motivated throughout their life. Effective and quality interactions between the patient and the health system are necessary to ensure adherence to lifestyle advice, treatment regimens, and follow-up schedules.[13] While designing any initiative for hypertension control, it is important to ensure that the health team has the time and necessary skills for effective communication, health education, and behavioral interventions. Creating an environment in which patients feel free to discuss concerns and where the health team has the time and resources to support and encourage efforts made by patients is critical for effective BP control.[13] It is important for the patient to develop lifelong quality relationships with the health team and feel involved in their own treatment decisions.[12] A randomized controlled trial conducted in Iran found a significant improvement in medication adherence, self-efficacy, and importantly, hypertension outcomes (SBP CI: $-1.02$, $-0.31$; P: 0.00) and DBP (CI: $-1.32$, $-0.49$: P: 0.00) among patients treated by physicians that underwent communication training.[13] Shared decision making, wherein patients play an active role in clinical decision making along with the physician, has also been shown to improve medication adherence and hypertension control and augments the need to focus on micro-level interactions.[14,15]

### *Meso-Level Interventions*

i.  **Team-based care and task redistribution:** Health systems in most LMICs are overburdened, lacking the manpower and infrastructure to handle the large number of hypertensive individuals.[16] Team-based care and task redistribution are some of the strategies used to improve health system efficiency. Team-based care focuses on patient-centered care by a health team consisting of the patient, physician, and other health professionals such as nurses, community health workers, dieticians, pharmacists, and physician assistants, with specific roles defined for every member.[17] Task redistribution is the sharing or shifting of certain tasks conventionally handled by the physician to non-physician health workers.[17] Apart from reducing costs, these strategies helps free up time for the physician to manage complex patient care problems and allows other health staff to spend adequate time in risk communication, imparting lifestyle advice and ensuring continuity of care between different levels of the health system.[14,18] A systematic review and meta-analysis of 100 clinical trials found team-based care to be the most effective intervention for reducing BP.[19] Team-based care with medication titration by a non-physician healthcare worker had the greatest reduction in systolic BP [$-7.1$ mmHg (95% CI: $-8.9$, $-5.2$; p<0.001)] or physician [$-6.2$ mmHg (95% CI: $-8.1$, $-4.2$; p<0.001)] as compared to health coaching, home BP monitoring, provider training, audit and feedback, and electronic decision support systems.[19] Allaying previous concerns regarding its effectiveness in LMICs, a recent systematic review and meta-analysis of 63 studies done in various LMICs (including 32 randomized controlled trials) concluded that task sharing was an effective option for BP control, showing an effective reduction in BP (average mean difference in systolic BP of $-4.85$ mm Hg [$-6.12$ to $-3.57$; $I^2$ =76%]) across various task-sharing models involving different groups of healthcare workers.[20]

ii. **Health coaching and self-management:** Health coaching is described as a focused process of educating and motivating patients to improve lifestyle modification and adherence to medication.[21] Empowering patients with knowledge required to monitor and manage BP can help motivate them to internalize lifestyle modification advice, improve medication adherence, and access the health system when necessary. A meta-analysis found significant reductions of systolic BP through health coaching (−3.9 mmHg [−5.4, −2.3]) and home BP monitoring (−2.7 mmHg [−3.6, −1.7]).[19] Trial evidence from the UK has shown self-monitoring coupled with self-titration using an individualized titrating algorithm to result in better BP reductions as compared to usual care patients at high risk for cardiovascular disease (CVD) (difference of 9.2 mmHg [5.7, 12.7] systolic and 3.4 mmHg [1.8, 5.0] diastolic BP between intervention and control groups).[22] However, this may need further validation in diverse and larger samples of individuals before consideration as a public health intervention in LMICs.

Nevertheless, the practice of self-management of hypertension through education and self-monitoring of BP at home is an important part of hypertension control and should be recommended as an important adjunct to routine office care.[14,23] It could result in fewer visits and decreased health expenditure, while allowing health resources to be focused on patients who need urgent attention, thereby playing an important role in LMICs where access to healthcare is poor.

iii. **Physician training:** Primary care physicians are often the first point of contact for hypertension patients. They are involved in health education, detection, initiation of therapy, and ensuring BP control. However, formal medical education is designed and structured around acute care, with poor focus on chronic condition management that requires specialized knowledge and emphasis on preventive aspects.[13] Moreover, physicians rarely receive structured continuing medical education or retraining in basic skills after completion of their professional training.[24] Physician therapeutic inertia due—at least in part—to inadequate knowledge in hypertension management contributes to poor BP control and suboptimal treatment outcomes.[15] Data from the U.S. National Ambulatory Medical Care Survey showed that physicians failed to initiate treatment in over 80% of the cases that required it.[25,26] This is further complicated by frequent updates and ambiguous treatment guidelines that differ in diagnostic criteria, BP targets, and pharmacotherapy options.[26] Structured physician training to fill gaps in knowledge and to regularly update them on new evidence can play an important role in BP control, especially in LMICs.[27,28] A cluster randomized trial in Germany found that patients of physicians who received structured training, feedback on target-level attainment, and reminders for treatment intensification achieved better and earlier BP control as compared to patients of physicians in the control group that received no intervention.[27] Physician inertia was also significantly lesser among trained physicians.[27]

iv. **Information systems and health technology:** Rapidly advancing information systems and technology have led to the evolution of several of its applications to improve hypertension care. One of the earliest uses of telemedicine was telemonitoring of home BP, in which home BP readings are directly transmitted to the health professional.[15] This has been shown to improve quality of life, produce significant reductions in BP, and have a high degree of acceptance.[29] A meta-analysis of randomized controlled trials found that home BP telemonitoring improved office systolic BP by 4.71 mmHg [(6.18, 3.24); P < 0.001] and diastolic BP by 2.45 mmHg [(3.33, 1.57); P < 0.001] as compared to usual care.[30] Another early application was the use of telephonic interventions to deliver lifestyle advice and titrate medication, thereby reducing costs and saving physician time.[15] Today, plenty of mobile applications have become available to help improve adherence and deliver health education, most of which have been found effective in improving BP control.[15,31,32]

Apart from patient-centered applications, health technology has been used to promote evidence-based clinical practice among physicians and help in task redistribution through clinical decision support systems. Nurse care coordinators, trained in the use of these systems, have been shown to be able to successfully screen, assess risk, and improve BP control even in low-resource settings, making it an effective option to be considered in LMICs that have a scarcity of physicians.[32] A trial of a mobile phone–based electronic clinical decision support system at a community health center in India using a mixed service delivery model (involving a care coordinator and physician) resulted in reductions of −14.6 mmHg (95% CI: −15.3, −13.8) systolic and −7.6 mmHg (CI: −8.0, −7.2) diastolic BP at 18 months of follow-up.[32]

With improvement in internet connectivity, widespread use of smartphones, advancements in technology, and improved technology literacy among the general public, telemedicine is another intervention that could play an important role in improving BP control in LMICs where access to healthcare is a significant problem.[18,33,34]

v. **Screening:** Increasing screening activities is an important public health measure to improve hypertension control. Screening not only plays an important role in improving detection rates and initiating treatment early but also serves as an opportunity to raise awareness regarding hypertension among patients. Screening strategies for hypertension include mass, targeted, or opportunistic approaches. Although some LMICs, such as India, have embarked on the resource-intensive universal screening strategy,[35] under low-resource settings that prevail in most LMICs, targeted and opportunistic screening could prove a more reasonable option. Opportunistic screening is recommended as a cost-effective intervention, especially in regions where access to healthcare is poor and every interaction with the health system is an opportunity to raise awareness and screen and treat hypertension.[36] The volunteer-driver BP screening campaign of the International Society of Hypertension called the "May Measurement Month" (Box 5.7.1) is an interesting example of opportunistic screening.[37]

vi. **Pharmacotherapy and related issues:** A recent meta-analysis by the Blood Pressure Lowering Trialist Collaboration that included 348,854 participants from 48 trials revealed that over an average four years of follow-up, there was a 10% reduction in relative risk of major cardiovascular events with each 5 mmHg reduction in systolic BP.[38] The risks for stroke, ischemic heart disease, heart failure, and death from CVD were reduced by 13%, 7%, 14%, and 5%, respectively.[38] Despite there being strong evidence for the benefits of pharmacotherapy and the availability of effective medications, less than 50% of adults with hypertension receive BP-lowering medication, while those that are prescribed medication often have poor adherence.[6] Little or no attention is given to the recommended ideal characteristics (Table 5.7.3) for drug therapy in hypertension.[39]

---

**BOX 5.7.1 MAY MEASUREMENT MONTH: AN EXAMPLE OF A COST-EFFECTIVE OPPORTUNISTIC BP SCREENING CAMPAIGN**

A remarkable volunteer-driven BP screening campaign of the International Society of Hypertension called the "May Measurement Month" has successfully screened over 4.2 million individuals globally in three years and has detected approximately 900,000 individuals with untreated or inadequately treated hypertension and is a strong testimony to the importance of opportunistic screening in controlling hypertension.[37] Since its inception in 2017, the campaign has screened individuals from over 90 countries across the globe. The 2019 campaign alone measured BP of approximately half a million people who had never measured BP before.[37] Over half a million individuals were found to be hypertensive, and one-third of a million participants were found to have either untreated or inadequately treated hypertension.[37] For countries where systematic screening is difficult, volunteer-driven opportunistic screening initiatives such as the May Measurement Month offer an inexpensive method to raise awareness and detect hypertension in LMICs. Findings from such campaigns can also inform macro-level interventions and formulation of appropriate health system–level policies.

---

## Table 5.7.3 Ideal Characteristics of Drug Treatment

1. Treatment should be evidence-based in relation to morbidity/mortality prevention.
2. Use a once-day regimen, which provides 24h blood pressure control.
3. Treatment should be affordable and/or cost-effective relative to other agents.
4. Treatments should be well-tolerated.
5. Evidence of benefits of use of medication in populations to which it is to be applied.

*Source:* 2020 International Society of Hypertension global hypertension practice guidelines[39]

Most patients require drugs from more than one class of antihypertensive agents to lower BP.[40] This is reflected in recent guideline recommendations to initiate therapy with two drugs for most patients (United States (US), European Society for Hypertension (ESH), and International Society for Hypertension (ISH)). Therapy-related factors contributing to non-adherence include its long-term nature, need for multiple pills, multiple daily doses, and need for frequent adjustment of dosing.[41] The fear of up-titrating dosages or adding a new class of drug in uncontrolled hypertension is also cited as a reason for physician inertia.[42] Single-pill combinations containing low-dose multiple BP-lowering drugs can counter some of these issues and improve BP control and treatment adherence. Results from the TRIUMPH study showed that a larger proportion of hypertensive patients achieved target BP with fixed low-dose triple combination pills as compared with usual care.[43] The cardiovascular polypill, which includes statins and aspirin in addition to antihypertensives, has the additional potential benefit of reducing overall cardiovascular risk.[44,45] Evidence from the PolyIran study shows that the cardiovascular polypill was effective in preventing major cardiovascular events and improving adherence without an increase in side effects.[46] In LMICs where adherence to medication and access to healthcare is poor, single-pill combination strategies are available and affordable and may be an effective solution.

Ethnic differences can even influence the effectiveness and final choice of anti-hypertensive agents.[47] A systematic review of current hypertension treatment guidelines found that only one LMIC had its own country-specific hypertension guideline, while all others used HIC guidelines adopted without checking whether they would be implementable in local settings.[48] No guidelines met the criteria of validity, reliability, clinical applicability, clinical flexibility, or socioeconomic and ethical-legal contextualization to justify their use in LMICs.[49] This is an important issue that needs to be addressed while formulating context-specific strategies for hypertension control. A noteworthy effort in this direction is the latest ISH guidelines that provide a practical format contextualized to resource settings and made easy to use by clinicians as well as nurses and community health workers.[38]

**vii. Community engagement and participation:** Hypertension care needs to be modeled around the needs of the community, and it is important to engage stakeholders from the community during design and implementation. Empowering the community and ensuring their participation while planning hypertension care models through community engagement can help make interventions socially, culturally, and economically appropriate and have the potential to improve its access and acceptability.[18] This is particularly important while designing health education and behavioral interventions for lifestyle modification, which have better chances of success if tailored to local cultural and social settings. In addition, using community resources for delivery of interventions such as awareness and screening activities can encourage community involvement and alleviate some of the burden on the health system. While clinical success has not been documented yet, participatory community outreach projects in South Africa and the United States have shown varying degrees of success in improving health behaviors and development of culturally appropriate health education material.[49,50]

## Macro-Level Interventions

Policy interventions usually target multiple levels of the ICCCF framework and have a direct or indirect impact on patients, their families, the community, and the way the health system is organized. It could range from policies to strengthen health systems through improving availability of resources, including trained manpower, consistent financing, intersectoral coordination, and infrastructure changes, to those that target population-level changes such as taxes and regulations to reduce sodium or alcohol consumption. Policy-level interventions in hypertension have traditionally targeted health system–level changes that include task redistribution, team-based care, telemedicine, and screening strategies described earlier, as well as population-level dietary interventions.

Dietary interventions in hypertension have primarily focused on strategies to reduce the consumption of sodium. Most national and international scientific bodies advocate a population-level reduction in salt intake to prevent and control hypertension.[51] The WHO identifies reduction in salt intake as one of the most cost-effective interventions to improve population health outcomes and estimates that approximately 2.5 million deaths could be averted by following the recommendation of limiting individual-level daily intake to <5 grams and a 30% reduction in global salt intake by 2025.[52] The WHO SHAKE technical package assists its member states in development, implementation, and monitoring of population salt reduction strategies.[53] As of 2015, over 75 countries have implemented national salt reduction initiatives such as food product reformulation, pricing interventions, food procurement policies, restricted marketing, on-package nutrition information, and information campaigns.[54,55] Many of these initiatives have been successful in effectively reducing population-level salt intake without any adverse events.[55] Insufficient potassium intake and altered sodium-to-potassium ratio have also been found to be strongly associated with BP.[52,56] A recent study conducted in Peru on replacement of regular salt with potassium-enriched substitutes has shown to reduce BP (–1.29 mmHg [–2.17, –0.41] systolic; –0.76 mmHg [–1.39, –0.13] diastolic BP) and hypertension incidence (reduced risk of 51% [29%, 66%]), supporting salt substitution as a possible population-level strategy.[57] Other dietary interventions to lower the incidence of hypertension include policies to reduce consumption and advertisement of unhealthy foods rich in trans fats and sugars and increase the availability and affordability of healthy food such as fruits and vegetables.[58]

### Conclusion and Way Forward

Public health approaches employed in hypertension have conventionally focused on improving awareness, treatment, and BP control through health promotion strategies, dietary interventions, health system reforms, and innovations in hypertension management. These strategies have been found to be most effective when delivered in a multilevel integrated and complementary manner.[15,20] Despite there being multiple interventions to choose from, development and success of population-level interventions for BP control in LMICs have remained a challenge. Population-level interventions for non-communicable diseases have traditionally faced stiff competition from those for the control of infectious diseases, which have and still remain the focus in many LMICs. However, with the relative increase in the importance of the former, BP control interventions should form a vital and integral component of a country's health plan.

One important reason for this could be the dependence on evidence generated elsewhere to guide hypertension care practices and policy in LMICs. Differences in socioeconomic conditions, health policies, availability of drugs, and local lifestyle are often ignored while designing interventions for hypertension. There is an urgent need for collaboration between professional organizations, involvement of relevant stakeholders, consideration of country-specific socioeconomic settings, and performing high-quality LMIC-specific studies.[48] It is also important for countries to share implementation experiences in order to understand the effectiveness of existing interventions. A systematic review comparing effectiveness of hypertension control interventions found sparse information available from LMICs.[19]

It is vital to address gaps in epidemiological data regarding awareness, treatment, and control levels, as well as the incidence of complications due to hypertension. Economic analyses to evaluate losses due to hypertension and its complications could be a helpful tool in garnering political support to promote research, prompt health systems change, and ensure continued financing for population-level interventions. A possible solution could be the maintenance of hypertension registries that could help generate evidence and guide health policy in the long run. Countries also have to address effects of upstream factors such as urbanization, globalization, and climate change and institute efforts to keep them under check.

To conclude, there is no universally applicable plan to control hypertension. Every country needs to devise coordinated, collaborative, and context-specific efforts that address multiple levels of the healthcare system in order to effectively reduce the burden caused by hypertension and its complications. The disparate burden and increasing trends of hypertension in LMICs warrant urgent public health responses.

### REFERENCES

1. Stanaway JD, Afshin A, Gakidou E, et al. Global, regional, and national comparative risk assessment of 84 behavioural, environmental and occupational, and metabolic risks or clusters of risks for 195 countries and territories, 1990–2017: A systematic analysis for the Global Burden of Disease Study 2017. *Lancet.* 2018;392(10159):1923–1994. doi:10.1016/S0140-6736(18)32225-6
2. Mills KT, Bundy JD, Kelly TN, et al. Global disparities of hypertension prevalence and control. *Circulation.* 2016;134(6):441–450. doi:10.1161/CIRCULATIONAHA.115.018912
3. Zhou B, Bentham J, Di Cesare M, et al. Worldwide trends in blood pressure from 1975 to 2015: a pooled analysis of 1479 population-based measurement studies with 19·1 million participants. *Lancet.* 2017;389(10064):37–55. doi:10.1016/S0140-6736(16)31919-5

4. Sarki AM, Nduka CU, Stranges S, Kandala NB, Uthman OA. Prevalence of hypertension in low- and middle-income countries: A systematic review and meta-analysis. *Med (United States)*. 2015;94(50). doi:10.1097/MD.0000000000001959

5. Kearney PM, Whelton M, Reynolds K, Muntner P, Whelton PK, He J. Global burden of hypertension: analysis of worldwide data. *Lancet*. 2005;365(9455):217–223. doi:10.1016/s0140-6736(05)17741-1

6. Geldsetzer P, Manne-Goehler J, Marcus ME, et al. The state of hypertension care in 44 low-income and middle-income countries: a cross-sectional study of nationally representative individual-level data from 1·1 million adults. *Lancet*. 2019;394(10199):652–662. doi:10.1016/S0140-6736(19)30955-9

7. Ibrahim MM, Damasceno A. Hypertension in developing countries. *Lancet*. 2012;380(9841):611–619. doi:10.1016/S0140-6736(12)60861-7

8. Program NHBPE. *The seventh report of the joint national committee on prevention, detection, evaluation, and treatment of high blood pressure*. National Heart, Lung, and Blood Institute (US); 2004. www.ncbi.nlm.nih.gov/pubmed/20821851. Accessed November 2, 2020.

9. Münzel T, Sørensen M. Noise pollution and arterial hypertension. *Eur Cardiol Rev*. 2017;12(1):26–29. doi:10.15420/ecr.2016:31:2

10. Park SH, Lim J eun, Park H, Jee SH. Body burden of persistent organic pollutants on hypertension: a meta-analysis. *Environ Sci Pollut Res*. 2016;23(14):14284–14293. doi:10.1007/s11356-016-6568-6

11. Giorgini P, Di Giosia P, Grassi D, Rubenfire M, D. Brook R, Ferri C. Air pollution exposure and blood pressure: An updated review of the literature. *Curr Pharm Des*. 2015;22(1):28–51. doi:10.2174/1381612822666151109111712

12. World Health Organization. *Innovative care for chronic conditions: Building blocks for action: Global report*. 2002. www.who.int/chp/knowledge/publications/icccglobalreport.pdf. Accessed April 21, 2020.

13. Carey RM, Muntner P, Bosworth HB, Whelton PK. Prevention and control of hypertension: JACC health promotion series. *J Am Coll Cardiol*. 2018;72(11):1278–1293. doi:10.1016/j.jacc.2018.07.008

14. Schoenthaler A, Chaplin WF, Allegrante JP, et al. Provider communication effects medication adherence in hypertensive African Americans. *Patient Educ Couns*. 2009;75(2):185–191. doi:10.1016/j.pec.2008.09.018

15. The World Health Report 2006: Working Together for Health—World Health Organization—Google Books. https://books.google.co.in/books?hl=en&lr=&id=taYsDwAAQBAJ&oi=fnd&pg=PR13&ots=9eo92rCdy-&sig=LAXSrRDRfpfJvDT_o9c8u_tqgaE&redir_esc=y#v=onepage&q&f=false. Accessed May 5, 2020.

16. Whelton PK, Carey RM, Aronow WS, et al. 2017 ACC/AHA/AAPA/ABC/ACPM/AGS/APhA/ASH/ASPC/NMA/PCNA guideline for the prevention, detection, evaluation, and management of high blood pressure in adults: A report of the american college of cardiology/American heart association task force on clinical practice guidelines. *J Am Coll Cardiol*. 2018;71(19):e127–e248. doi:10.1016/j.jacc.2017.11.006

17. Vedanthan R, Bernabe-Ortiz A, Herasme OI, et al. Innovative approaches to hypertension control in low- and middle-income countries. *Cardiol Clin*. 2017;35(1):99–115. doi:10.1016/j.ccl.2016.08.010

18. Mills KT, Obst KM, Shen W, et al. Comparative effectiveness of implementation strategies for blood pressure control in hypertensive patients: A systematic review and meta-analysis. *Ann Intern Med*. 2018;168(2):110–120. doi:10.7326/M17-1805

19. Anand TN, Joseph LM, Geetha A V., Prabhakaran D, Jeemon P. Task sharing with non-physician health-care workers for management of blood pressure in low-income and middle-income countries: a systematic review and meta-analysis. *Lancet Glob Heal*. 2019;7(6):e761–e771. doi:10.1016/S2214-109X(19)30077-4

20. Wolever RQ, Simmons LA, Sforzo GA, et al. A systematic review of the literature on health and wellness coaching: defining a key behavioral intervention in healthcare. *Glob Adv Heal Med*. 2013;2(4):38–57. doi:10.7453/gahmj.2013.042

21. McManus RJ, Mant J, Haque MS, et al. Effect of self-monitoring and medication self-titration on systolic blood pressure in hypertensive patients at high risk of cardiovascular

disease: The TASMIN-SR randomized clinical trial. *JAMA—J Am Med Assoc.* 2014;312(8): 799–808. doi:10.1001/jama.2014.10057

22. Reboussin DM, Allen NB, Griswold ME, et al. Systematic Review for the 2017 ACC/AHA/ AAPA/ABC/ACPM/AGS/APhA/ASH/ASPC/NMA/PCNA guideline for the prevention, detection, evaluation, and management of high blood pressure in adults: A report of the American college of cardiology/american heart association task force on clinical practice guidelines. *J Am Coll Cardiol.* 2018;71(19):2176–2198. doi:10.1016/j.jacc.2017.11.004

23. Medical Association A. *Blood pressure measurement training research report | AMA.* 2019.

24. Krousel-Wood M, Joyce C, Holt E, et al. Predictors of decline in medication adherence: Results from the cohort study of medication adherence among older adults. *Hypertension.* 2011;58(5):804–810. doi:10.1161/HYPERTENSIONAHA.111.176859

25. Rehan HS, Grover A, Hungin APS. Ambiguities in the guidelines for the management of arterial hypertension: Indian perspective with a call for global harmonization. *Curr Hypertens Rep.* 2017;19(2). doi:10.1007/s11906-017-0715-4

26. Lüders S, Schrader J, Schmieder RE, Smolka W, Wegscheider K, Bestehorn K. Improvement of hypertension management by structured physician education and feedback system: Cluster randomized trial. *Eur J Prev Cardiol.* 2010;17(3):271–279. doi:10.1097/ HJR.0b013e328330be62

27. Sharma A, Jose AP, Pandey N, et al. A collaborative model for capacity building of primary care physicians in the management of hypertension in India. *J Hum Hypertens.* 2019;33(8):562–565. doi:10.1038/s41371-019-0213-z

28. Omboni S, Ferrari R. The role of telemedicine in hypertension management: Focus on blood pressure telemonitoring. *Curr Hypertens Rep.* 2015;17(4):1–13. doi:10.1007/s11906-015-0535-3

29. Omboni S, Gazzola T, Carabelli G, Parati G. Clinical usefulness and cost effectiveness of home blood pressure telemonitoring: Meta-analysis of randomized controlled studies. *J Hypertens.* 2013;31(3):455–468. doi:10.1097/HJH.0b013e32835ca8dd

30. Nobian A, Retno W, Bambang Budi S. Mobile phone-based intervention in hypertension management. *Int J Hypertens.* 2019;2019. doi:10.1155/2019/9021017

31. Ajay VS, Jindal D, Roy A, et al. Development of a smartphone-enabled hypertension and diabetes mellitus management package to facilitate evidence-based care delivery in primary healthcare facilities in India: The mpower heart project. *J Am Heart Assoc.* 2016;5(12). doi:10.1161/JAHA.116.004343

32. Piette JD, Datwani H, Gaudioso S, et al. Hypertension management using mobile technology and home blood pressure monitoring: Results of a randomized trial in two low/middle-income countries. *Telemed e-Health.* 2012;18(8):613–620. doi:10.1089/tmj.2011.0271

33. Beratarrechea A, Lee AG, Willner JM, Jahangir E, Ciapponi A, Rubinstein A. The impact of mobile health interventions on chronic disease outcomes in developing countries: A systematic review. *Telemed e-Health.* 2014;20(1):75–82. doi:10.1089/tmj.2012.0328

34. Jose AP, Prabhakaran D. World hypertension day: Contemporary issues faced in India. *Indian J Med Res.* 2019;149(5):567–570. doi:10.4103/ijmr.IJMR_549_19

35. Bovet P, Chiolero A, Paccaud F, Banatvala N. Screening for cardiovascular disease risk and subsequent management in low and middle income countries: Challenges and opportunities. *Public Health Rev.* 2015;36(1). doi:10.1186/s40985-015-0013-0

36. Beaney T, Schutte AE, Stergiou GS, et al. May measurement month 2019: The global blood pressure screening campaign of the international society of hypertension. *Hypertension.* 2020;76(2):333–341. doi:10.1161/HYPERTENSIONAHA.120.14874

37. Blood pressure-lowering is even more beneficial than previously thought. www.escardio.org/The-ESC/Press-Office/Press-releases/Blood-pressure-lowering-is-even-more-beneficial-than-previously-thought. Accessed October 27, 2020.

38. Unger T, Borghi C, Charchar F, et al. 2020 International Society of Hypertension global hypertension practice guidelines. *J Hypertens.* 2020;38(6):982–1004. doi:10.1097/ HJH.0000000000002453

39. Cushman WC, Ford CE, Einhorn PT, et al. Blood pressure control by drug group in the antihypertensive and lipid-lowering treatment to prevent heart attack trial (ALLHAT). *J Clin Hypertens.* 2008;10(10):751–760. doi:10.1111/j.1751-7176.2008.00015.x

40. Burnier M, Egan BM. Adherence in hypertension: A review of prevalence, risk factors, impact, and management. *Circ Res*. 2019;124(7):1124–1140. doi:10.1161/CIRCRESAHA.118.313220

41. Faria C, Wenzel M, Lee KW, Coderre K, Nichols J, Belletti DA. A narrative review of clinical inertia: focus on hypertension. *J Am Soc Hypertens*. 2009;3(4):267–276. doi:10.1016/j.jash.2009.03.001

42. Webster R, Salam A, De Silva HA, et al. Fixed low-dose triple combination antihypertensive medication vs usual care for blood pressure control in patients with mild to moderate hypertension in Sri Lanka a randomized clinical trial. *JAMA—J Am Med Assoc*. 2018;320(6):566–579. doi:10.1001/jama.2018.10359

43. Lafeber M, Spiering W, Visseren FLJ, Grobbee DE. Multifactorial prevention of cardiovascular disease in patients with hypertension: the cardiovascular polypill. *Curr Hypertens Rep*. 2016;18(5):1–7. doi:10.1007/s11906-016-0648-3

44. Cimmaruta D, Lombardi N, Borghi C, Rosano G, Rossi F, Mugelli A. Polypill, hypertension and medication adherence: The solution strategy? *Int J Cardiol*. 2018;252:181–186. doi:10.1016/j.ijcard.2017.11.075

45. Roshandel G, Khoshnia M, Poustchi H, et al. Effectiveness of polypill for primary and secondary prevention of cardiovascular diseases (PolyIran): a pragmatic, cluster-randomised trial. *Lancet*. 2019;394(10199):672–683. doi:10.1016/s0140-6736(19)31791-x

46. Ojji DB, Mayosi B, Francis V, et al. Comparison of Dual Therapies for Lowering Blood Pressure in Black Africans. *N Engl J Med*. 2019;380(25):2429–2439. doi:10.1056/NEJMoa1901113

47. Owolabi M, Olowoyo P, Miranda JJ, et al. Gaps in hypertension guidelines in low- and middle-income versus high-income countries: A systematic review. *Hypertension*. 2016;68(6):1328–1337. doi:10.1161/HYPERTENSIONAHA.116.08290

48. Bradley HA, Puoane T. Prevention of hypertension and diabetes in an urban setting in South Africa: Participatory action research with community health workers. *Ethn Dis Winter*. 2007;17(1):49–54.

49. Balcazar HG, Byrd TL, Ortiz M, Tondapu SR, Chavez M. A randomized community intervention to improve hypertension control among mexican americans: using the promotoras de salud community outreach model. *J Health Care Poor Underserved*. 2009;20(4):1079–1094. doi:10.1353/hpu.0.0209

50. Jose AP, Prabhakaran D. Salt reduction at a population level: To do or not to do? *Natl Med J India*. 2016;29(5):253–256.

51. World Health Organization. Salt reduction. www.who.int/news-room/fact-sheets/detail/salt-reduction. Published April 29, 2020. Accessed May 9, 2020.

52. World Health Organization. *The SHAKE technical package for salt reduction*. 2016.

53. Trieu K, Neal B, Hawkes C, et al. Salt reduction initiatives around the world—A systematic review of progress towards the global target. DeAngelis MM, ed. *PLoS One*. 2015;10(7):e0130247. doi:10.1371/journal.pone.0130247

54. McLaren L, Sumar N, Barberio AM, et al. Population-level interventions in government jurisdictions for dietary sodium reduction. *Cochrane Database Syst Rev*. 2016;(9). doi:10.1002/14651858.CD010166.pub2

55. Perez V, Chang ET. Sodium-to-potassium ratio and blood pressure, hypertension, and related factors. *Adv Nutr*. 2014;5(6):712–741. doi:10.3945/an.114.006783

56. Bernabe-Ortiz A, Sal y Rosas VG, Ponce-Lucero V, et al. Effect of salt substitution on community-wide blood pressure and hypertension incidence. *Nat Med*. 2020;26(3):374–378. doi:10.1038/s41591-020-0754-2

57. Jose AP, Shridhar K, Prabhakaran D. Diet, nutrition and cardiovascular disease: The role of social determinants. *Proc Indian Natl Sci Acad*. 2018;84(4):945–953. doi:10.16943/ptinsa/2018/49451

# 5.8 Diabetes

*Dorothy Lall, Ram Jagannathan, and K.M. Venkat Narayan*

## CONTENTS

## INTRODUCTION

The cataclysmic increase in type 2 diabetes mellitus (T2DM) is a significant healthcare burden globally (1). According to the recent global update by the International Diabetes Federation (IDF), 463 million (9.3%) adults aged 20–79 years were living with diabetes in 2019, with a projected rise to 578 million (10.2%) by the year 2030 (2). T2DM is diagnosed based on plasma glucose criteria, either fasting plasma glucose or a 2-h plasma glucose value during a 75-g oral glucose tolerance test (OGTT). The development of T2DM is preceded by an intermediate stage of prediabetes characterized by an impaired glucose tolerance (IGT) or impaired fasting glucose (IFG) in which blood glucose is elevated but is below the threshold for diabetes (3). Both diabetes and prediabetes are important, well-established risk factors for cardiovascular disease (CVD) (4). The previous history of gestational diabetes is also associated with an increased risk of both diabetes and CVD (5).

This chapter discusses public health approaches to prevent and control T2DM as a critical component of CVD prevention and control. We begin by identifying from the literature the current understanding of the risk factors of diabetes, its pathophysiology, and contextual factors driving the epidemic. We then identify evidence-based public health approaches, with relevant examples, for the control of this epidemic.

## CURRENT UNDERSTANDING OF RISK FACTORS FOR T2DM

A plethora of risk factors is associated with an increase in the probability of developing diabetes. They are broadly classified as non-modifiable, those that cannot change, and modifiable, those that can be changed.

DOI: 10.1201/b23266-13

## Non-Modifiable Risk Factors

Prominent among the non-modifiable risk factors are age, positive family history of diabetes, ethnicity, a history of gestational diabetes, and polycystic ovarian syndrome. T2DM is known to aggregate in families (6). The lifetime risk at 80 years of age for T2DM is estimated to be 38% if one parent has T2DM (7) and 60% by the age of 60 years if both parents are affected (8). Family studies, including those involving monozygotic or dizygotic twins, indicate that the heritability of T2DM exceeds 50% (9, 10). Ethnicity is also a major contributory factor in the development of diabetes. Though all ethnic groups are at risk of T2DM, certain non-white groups, such as Indo-Asians, Native Americans, and African Americans, appear to have a particularly strong predisposition (11, 12).

## Role of Genes and the Environment

Genome-wide association studies (GWAS) have implicated around 250 genomic regions associated with the development of T2DM (13). However, there is no clear evidence of causal associations; instead, multiple causations and a complex interplay between genes and the environment seem to be the underlying mechanism of phenotypic expression (14). This concept is broadly referred to as a "gene × environment interaction," in which the "gene" is usually one or more DNA variants, and the "environment" refers to risk factors (15).

## Modifiable Risk Factors

Modifiable risk factors include overweight and obesity, low birth weight, in utero undernutrition, physical inactivity and sedentary behavior, dietary habits, smoking, increased psychological stress, and sleep irregularities.

## Overweight and Obesity

Overweight and obesity, defined by an excess body mass index (BMI), is the single most important independent risk factor for diabetes (risk ratio [RR] 7.19, 95% confidence interval [CI]: 5.74, 9.0 for obesity and 2.9, 95% CI: 2.42, 3.72 for overweight) (16). Obesity (BMI >30) results in insulin resistance as well as β-cell dysfunction. Low-grade inflammation, a persistent state of glucolipotoxicity in obesity, results in oxidative stress and the progressive destruction of β-cells (17). However, obesity, as defined by BMI, has poor sensitivity, especially among Asian Indians. Corroborative evidence from epidemiological studies showed that visceral adiposity or abdominal fat, more than just raised BMI, is strongly associated with T2DM in South Asians (18). Increasing evidence points to the role of ectopic hepatic fat and low muscle mass as independent risk factors for diabetes (19). However, among Asian and African ethnicities, diabetes commonly occurs among those with normal weight or even underweight (20, 21). Apart from the differences in fat distribution, a predominance of inadequate insulin secretion among Asians may be responsible for this association (20, 22).

## Low Birth Weight and in Utero Undernutrition

Pooled estimates of 132,180 individuals found low birth weight associated with an increased risk of T2DM (odds ratio [OR] 1.32 [95% CI: 1.06, 1.64]) (23). However, the mechanisms for this are not completely clear. Barker et al. postulate that diabetes in adult life is a long-term consequence of in utero undernutrition (24), while others suggest that rapid weight gain in small babies (defined as metabolic stunting) results in diabetogenic disturbances throughout life, predisposing individuals to the development of diabetes (25). The association is also attributed to the "thrifty phenotype" in which low birth weight due to poor intrauterine growth followed by rapid childhood weight gain due to nutritional transition and physical inactivity promotes the development of obesity and associated metabolic complications (26).

## Physical Inactivity and Sedentary Behavior

There is a strong association between physical inactivity and diabetes that may, in part, be mediated by overweight and obesity. According to a meta-analysis, an increase in physical activity lowered the risk of developing T2DM by 35% compared to a sedentary lifestyle (27). Sedentary behavior (e.g., television time), independent of physical activity, is also associated with a higher risk of diabetes (28).

## Unhealthy Diets

Many studies have evaluated associations between food groups and single foods, micro- and macro-nutrients, alcohol and beverages, diet quality, and the incidence of diabetes. Several reviews find strong support for the benefit of whole grain products and total fiber intake on the incidence of T2DM (29). The adverse association of white rice, processed meat products, and sugar-sweetened beverages with the incidence of T2DM have also been reported (30, 31).

### Smoking

A meta-analysis of 84 studies showed a relative risk of 1.37 (95% CI: 1.33–1.42) for T2DM among smokers compared to those who had never smoked (32). Smoking is known to cause endovascular damage, endothelial dysfunction, and inflammation, all of which contribute to poor insulin sensitivity and β-cell dysfunction.

### Sleep and Stress

Sleep is known to regulate a plethora of metabolic functions of the body. While the exact mechanisms remain unclear, the association of less sleep and poor sleep quality with T2DM is well established (33). Studies suggest that obesity is, in this association's pathway, mediated by an imbalance in hormones such as leptin and ghrelin (34).

## CURRENT UNDERSTANDING OF THE PATHOPHYSIOLOGY IN THE DEVELOPMENT OF TYPE 2 DIABETES

Hyperglycemia that characterizes diabetes occurs due to defects in insulin secretion, insulin action, or both (3). The normoglycemic state is regulated by a feedback loop between insulin-sensitive tissues and insulin release from β-cells (35). Insulin resistance, associated with adiposity and the progressive destruction of β-cell function, results in impaired feedback loops causing persistent hyperglycemia. Progressive deterioration of β-cell function accounts for the evolving nature of the disease from prediabetes to diabetes. Advancing age contributes to diminishing β-cell function as the body is unable to replace these cells. Mechanisms currently known to cause β-cell dysfunction include glucotoxicity, lipotoxicity, hepatic and pancreatic steatosis, oxidative stress, inflammatory stress, and amyloid deposition (17). Studies in Pima Indians indicate that in susceptible individuals, insulin resistance is the predominant mechanism for the development of diabetes, usually present before the β-cell function declines (36). Whereas in Asian Indians, evidence suggests that early poor insulin secretion, more than insulin resistance, may be the primary driving factor (37, 38).

## CONTEXTUAL FACTORS FOR DIABETES

The presence or absence of the previously mentioned risk factors is set in the social and economic context of where people live and work. These context-specific circumstances are shaped by the distribution of money, power, lifestyle, healthcare facilities, and resources at local, national, and global levels. Data from the United States, for example, indicate that the incidence of diabetes varies seven-fold across counties and is associated with county-level income, poverty, unemployment, healthcare access, food, and exercise availability (39). The social determinants of health go beyond the individual to account for the influence of local environments, public policies, and industry on health. Globalization, vested commercial interests, and unplanned urbanization are believed to have fueled the epidemics of diabetes, obesity, and CVDs (40).

### Globalization and Commercial Determinants

Globalization has been described as the process of increasing economic, political, and social interdependence and global integration as capital traded goods, persons, ideas, and values diffuse across boundaries (41). The impact of globalization on the growth of diabetes, obesity, and other non-communicable diseases (NCDs) is mediated through countries' economic growth and their influence on household incomes and prices of goods. More direct effects of globalization are the changes in local diets towards processed, packaged foods, shifts in transportation, and the production and marketing of tobacco and alcohol (42). Commercial determinants of health have been defined as "strategies and approaches used by the private sector to promote products and choices that are detrimental to health" (43). There is a growing awareness that large multinationals influence the consumption landscape through aggressive marketing strategies, lobbying, and extensive supply chains. Through the manufacture, sale, and promotion of tobacco, alcohol, and ultra-processed food and drink, transnational corporations are major drivers of NCDs (44).

## Unplanned Urbanization and Socioeconomic Conditions

The movement of people to urban centers is a global phenomenon. However, the pace of urbanization, often unplanned, especially in low- and middle-income countries (LMICs), is unprecedented over the past few decades. Unplanned urbanization and the change in lifestyles have adverse effects on health (45) and are associated with diabetes and other NCDs (46, 47). Poverty, poor housing, and low education are associated with a two-fold higher risk of diabetes, especially in high-income countries (48, 49). In LMICs, however, the distribution of diabetes is more ubiquitous across the socioeconomic spectrum, possibly indicating an ongoing transition (50).

## PUBLIC HEALTH APPROACHES TO PREVENTION AND CONTROL OF DIABETES

Diabetes is clearly a complex problem with multiple factors at various levels (e.g., individual, family, society, environment) that need to be addressed to effectively control this epidemic (Figure 5.8.1). The public health approach to the control of diabetes needs nothing less than a "whole of society" engagement, including civil society, patients, family, schools, governments, media, and industry (51). Further, multisectoral action will be required across health, education, agriculture, transport, communication, urban planning, recreation, law and order, environment, labor, employment, industry, and trade sectors. Adopting health in all policies (HiA) will enable governments to address the determinants of diabetes comprehensively. The framework of social determinants of health developed by Dahlgren and Margaret Whitehead (52) is relevant to understand the various levels of influences and consider the multiple levels at which prevention and control of diabetes need to be enacted (Figure 5.8.1).

## INDIVIDUAL-LEVEL TARGETED APPROACH

### Early Identification: Screening

As a public health approach, screening has been adopted by many countries, as it enables early detection and prompt initiation of prevention or treatment. In the absence of screening for diabetes, it is estimated that about 50% of T2DM and over 90% of prediabetes remain undetected (2). However, mass screening through testing is expensive, and the yield of persons who access care even after detection is usually poor (53). Instead, a strategy of two-stage screening, first identifying those at high risk and then testing blood glucose levels, yields better results (54). The most cost-effective strategy for early detection remains opportunistic screening that is done when a person presents to a health facility independent of the primary complaint (55).

### Prevention and Care for Diabetes at the Primary Level

Studies have shown that low-cost prevention can be effectively delivered to those at high risk of diabetes with substantial benefit (56). Primary care facilities, closest to people's homes, are best

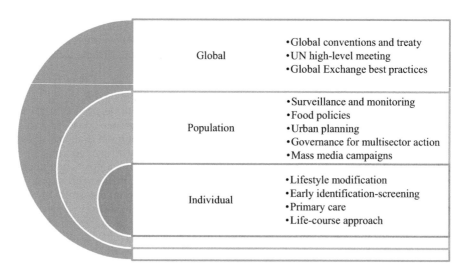

**Figure 5.8.1** Public health approaches to the prevention and control of diabetes.

suited for the care of persons with diabetes, as this facilitates continuity of care (57). There are challenges in caring for persons with diabetes, especially as most healthcare delivery systems are traditionally geared towards acute diseases (58, 59). Primary care needs redesigning to respond to the needs of persons with chronic diseases, such as continuity of care, both relational and informational; coordination between levels of care; and a much greater focus on empowering families to self-manage the condition (60). Models of chronic care such as the Wagner et al. model (61) may be useful for redesigning with adaptations relevant to the LMIC context (62). The chronic care model by Wagner et al. identifies six essential elements that encourage high-quality chronic disease care: the community, the health system, self-management support, delivery system design, decision support, and clinical information systems. Continuous quality improvement with attention to local context will be required, and evidence suggests that it results in improving CVD risk among people with diabetes (63, 64).

### Life-Course Approach

The life-course approach recognizes opportunities to prevent and control diseases at key stages of life, from preconception through pregnancy, infancy, childhood, and adolescence, through to adulthood (65). Mitigating poor nutrition influences during the preconception and antenatal periods requires education, awareness, and access to good nutrition. Encouraging exclusive breastfeeding has a protective effect and lowers the risk of developing diabetes in adult life (66). Measures to ensure physical activity and healthy diets in childhood, both at home and in school, are important preventive measures (67).

### Support for Lifestyle Modification

Systematic reviews and meta-analysis of lifestyle interventions on body weight and glycemic levels are effective and cost-effective (68, 69). Interventions included in these reviews are typically based on a targeted approach for those with IGT or at high risk and include strategies to motivate the adoption of healthy lifestyles (70). There is evidence from LMICs to support lifestyle modification interventions, although from fewer studies (56, 71). For example, Brazil offers physical activity classes in community settings, at no cost to participants, in 4000 Brazilian municipalities in more than 80% of cities in the country. This is integrated with primary care and is organized at the healthcare facilities (72). Technology-based innovations such as text messaging and mobile-based apps to deliver lifestyle modification messages are promising and may have the potential to motivate persons to adopt health-promoting lifestyles (73, 74).

## POPULATION-LEVEL: MULTISECTORAL ACTION

### Surveillance and Monitoring

Surveillance of disease is an important public health measure that involves the collection of information regarding the burden of disease and its risk factors and quality of care and costs among those with the disease. Analysis of this information is crucial to guide and inform timely action. For example, in the United States, the division of Diabetes Translation of the Centers for Disease Control and Prevention (CDC) supports the national and state surveillance system using several different data sources (75). These data have highlighted the burden of diabetes, its trends, and also initiatives to document and improve the quality of care for people with diabetes (76). The World Health Organization (WHO) STEPS surveillance and the global monitoring framework provide guidance for establishing robust information systems necessary for timely action (77).

### Urban Planning and Built Environment

Cities are at the forefront of the diabetes epidemic, and therefore, attention to the design of cities is required to facilitate healthy lifestyles, especially physical activity. Planned walking spaces, cycling tracks, and the availability of adequate public transport are some measures cities can take to tackle this epidemic (78). Many countries have taken this agenda of creating livable cities that promote physical activity seriously through the formation of the network for healthy cities (79). Copenhagen is an example where the bicycle account, a status report on public mobility on bicycles, is routinely consulted for policy decisions. Barcelona provides a good example of reclamation of spaces for public use by reducing urban traffic by 21% and freeing up close to 60% of road areas for reuse as "citizen spaces" such as cycle paths, widened pavements, and small public spaces for various activities (80). The Ciclovia and Cicloruta programs in Bogota, Colombia, are two well-known initiatives that have successfully promoted physical activity in complex urban settings (81). The streets in the city are temporarily closed to motorized vehicles to encourage walking and other recreational activities. The city also has an extensive bicycle path network, the largest in Latin America, connecting public transport to many destinations in the city (82).

### Mass Media Campaigns and Community-Based Initiatives

Targeting large sections of society with well-designed, focused messages in short or sustained campaigns over periods of time has been variably effective (83). The appeal of this public health approach lies in the fact that a large number of people can be reached at a relatively low cost. In particular, Latin America has had several successful mass media campaigns, such as the Agita São Paulo program and the Muévete Bogotá to encourage physical activity (84, 85). However, providing information through mass media alone may be inadequate if not accompanied by an enabling environment to promote the desired behavior change. For example, healthy diets have to be inexpensive for people to choose them over unhealthy diets.

### Food Policies

Persuading individuals to favor healthy dietary choices is complex and challenging since economic and sociocultural environments influence dietary habits in addition to individual likes and dislikes. Policies that influence food choices are crucial to achieving population-level success. Specific approaches such as sustained, focused media and education campaigns; mandatory nutrition labeling on packaged foods; subsidies for healthy foods, fruits, and vegetables; taxation for less healthy food/sweetened beverages; and policies that favor eco-friendly public transportation are effective (74).

### Governance to Enable Multisectoral Action

The determinants of diabetes can be effectively addressed only through multisectoral action involving sectors other than health (86). Governance structures to enable these multisectoral actions are required. Iran provides an example in the setting up of a National Non-Communicable Diseases Committee (INCDC) through multisectoral mechanisms and partnerships of all sectors in the Ministry of Health and other related sector ministries, organizations, non-governmental organizations (NGOs), and communities. In Brazil, ministries of sports and education collaborate to encourage increased physical activity in schools and have made shifts in the types of food purchased for the school food program (87).

## GLOBAL POLICY LEVEL

Global policies such as the WHO Framework Convention on Tobacco Control (WHO FCTC) are one way to ensure countries' sustained commitment to the fight against diabetes. High-level UN General Assembly meetings are another way to garner global attention and commitment to a global health issue. The UN General Assembly has held three high-level meetings on the NCD problem to review the global and national progress achieved in putting measures in place to prevent NCDs. It is challenging to sustain countries' commitment to NCDs compared to communicable diseases, especially since the threats are not obvious and immediate (88).

Even though progress is slow, the use of frameworks and scorecards for monitoring has the potential to support countries (89). Global exchange of best practices such as the best buys suggested by the WHO has also been effective in engaging countries (90).

## CONCLUSION

Diabetes is an important risk factor for CVD that has globally escalated in the last few decades to attain epidemic proportions. Diabetes is a complex problem caused by multiple factors and requires a public health approach that is multipronged in its levels of influence. Individual, population, and global policies all have critical roles to play in the control of the twin epidemics of T2DM and CVD.

# REFERENCES

1. World Health Organization. Classification of diabetes mellitus [Internet]. Licence: CC BY-NC-SA 3.0 IGO. Geneva; 2019. Available from: https://linkinghub.elsevier.com/retrieve/pii/S0140673677927350

2. International Diabetes Federation. IDF Diabetes Atlas [Internet]. 9th ed. International Diabetes Federation. Brussels, Belgium; 2019. Available from: https://diabetesatlas.org/upload/resources/material/20200106_152211_IDFATLAS9e-final-web.pdf

3. American Diabetes Association. Classification and diagnosis of diabetes: Standards of medical care in diabetes—2019. Diabetes Care [Internet]. 2019 Jan 17;42(Supplement 1):S13–28. Available from: http://care.diabetesjournals.org/lookup/doi/10.2337/dc19-S002

4. Huang Y, Cai X, Mai W, Li M, Hu Y. Association between prediabetes and risk of cardiovascular disease and all cause mortality: Systematic review and meta-analysis. BMJ. 2016;355.

5. Kramer CK, Campbell S, Retnakaran R. Gestational diabetes and the risk of cardiovascular disease in women: A systematic review and meta-analysis. Diabetologia [Internet]. 2019 Jun 7;62(6):905–914. Available from: http://link.springer.com/10.1007/s00125-019-4840-2

6. Rotter JI, Rimoin DL. The genetics of the glucose intolerance disorders. Am J Med [Internet]. 1981 Jan 1 [cited 2020 May 1];70(1):116–126. Available from: https://linkinghub.elsevier.com/retrieve/pii/0002934381904186

7. Zimmet P, Magliano D, Matsuzawa Y, Alberti G, Shaw J. The metabolic syndrome: A global public health problem and a new definition. J Atherosclerosis Thrombosis. 2005;12:295–300.

8. Raji A, Seely EW, Arky RA, Simonson DC. Body fat distribution and insulin resistance in healthy Asian Indians and Caucasians. J Clin Endocrinol Metab. 2001;86(11):5366–5371.

9. Medici F, Hawa M, Ianari A, Pyke DA, Leslie RDG. Concordance rate for type II diabetes mellitus in monozygotic twins: Actuarial analysis. Diabetologia. 1999;42(2):146–150.

10. Poulsen P, Ohm Kyvik K, Vaag A, Beck-Nielsen H. Heritability of type II (non-insulin-dependent) diabetes mellitus and abnormal glucose tolerance—A population-based twin study. Diabetologia. 1999;42(2):139–145.

11. Wilson SE, Rosella LC, Lipscombe LL, Manuel DG. The effectiveness and efficiency of diabetes screening in Ontario, Canada: a population-based cohort study. BMC Public Health [Internet]. 2010;10(1):506. Available from: www.biomedcentral.com/1471-2458/10/506

12. Rosella LC, Mustard CA, Stukel TA, Corey P, Hux J, Roos L, et al. The role of ethnicity in predicting diabetes risk at the population level. Ethn Heal. 2012 Aug 1;17(4):419–437.

13. Langenberg C, Lotta LA. Genomic insights into the causes of type 2 diabetes. Vol. 391, The Lancet. Lancet Publishing Group; 2018. p. 2463–2474.

14. Gujral UP, Narayan KMV, Pradeepa RG, Deepa M, Ali MK, Anjana RM, et al. Comparing type 2 diabetes, prediabetes, and their associated risk factors in Asian Indians in India and in the U.S.: The CARRS and MASALA studies. Diabetes Care. 2015 Jul 1;38(7):1312–1318.

15. Franks PW, Pearson E, Florez JC. Gene-environment and gene-treatment interactions in type 2 diabetes: Progress, pitfalls, and prospects. Vol. 36, Diabetes Care. American Diabetes Association; 2013. pp. 1413–1421.

16. Abdullah A, Peeters A, de Courten M, Stoelwinder J. The magnitude of association between overweight and obesity and the risk of diabetes: A meta-analysis of prospective cohort studies. Diabetes Res Clin Pract. 2010 Sep 1;89(3):309–319.

17. Cerf ME. Beta cell dysfunction and insulin resistance. Front Endocrinol (Lausanne). 2013;4(MAR):1–12.

18. Björntorp P. Metabolic implications of body fat distribution. Diabetes Care. 1991;14(12):1132–1143.

19. Cunningham SA, Kramer MR, Narayan KMV. Incidence of childhood obesity in the United States. N Engl J Med [Internet]. 2014 Jan 30 [cited 2020 Jun 11];370(5):403–411. Available from: www.nejm.org/doi/10.1056/NEJMoa1309753

20. Gujral UP, Weber MB, Staimez LR, Narayan KMV. Diabetes among non-overweight individuals: an emerging public health challenge [Internet]. Vol. 18, Current Diabetes Reports. Current Medicine Group LLC 1; 2018 [cited 2020 Mar 17]. p. 60. Available from: www.ncbi.nlm.nih.gov/pubmed/29974263

21. Yoon KH, Lee JH, Kim JW, Cho JH, Choi YH, Ko SH, et al. Epidemic obesity and type 2 diabetes in Asia. Lancet. 2006;368(9548):1681–1688.

22. Narayan KMV, Kanaya AM. Why are South Asians prone to type 2 diabetes? A hypothesis based on underexplored pathways. Vol. 63, Diabetologia. Springer; 2020. pp. 1103–1109.

23. Harder T, Rodekamp E, Schellong K, Dudenhausen JW, Plagemann A. Birth weight and subsequent risk of type 2 diabetes: A meta-analysis. Am J Epidemiol [Internet]. 2007 Apr 15 [cited 2020 May 2];165(8):849–857. Available from: www.ncbi.nlm.nih.gov/pubmed/17215379

24. Barker DJP, Hales CN, Fall CHD, Osmond C, Phipps K, Clark PMS. Type 2 (non-insulin-dependent) diabetes mellitus, hypertension and hyperlipidaemia (syndrome X): relation to reduced fetal growth. Diabetologia. 1993 Jan;36(1):62–67.

25. Stettler N, Stallings VA, Troxel AB, Zhao J, Schinnar R, Nelson SE, et al. Weight gain in the first week of life and overweight in adulthood: A cohort study of European American subjects fed infant formula. Circulation [Internet]. 2005 Apr 19 [cited 2020 Mar 22];111(15):1897–1903. Available from: www.ncbi.nlm.nih.gov/pubmed/15837942

26. Prentice AM. The emerging epidemic of obesity in developing countries. Int J Epidemiol. 2006;35(1):93–99.

27. Aune D, Norat T, Leitzmann M, Tonstad S, Vatten LJ. Physical activity and the risk of type 2 diabetes: A systematic review and dose-response meta-analysis. Eur J Epidemiol. 2015 Jul 1;30(7):529–542.

28. Wilmot EG, Edwardson CL, Achana FA, Davies MJ, Gorely T, Gray LJ, et al. Sedentary time in adults and the association with diabetes, cardiovascular disease and death: Systematic review and meta-analysis. Diabetologia [Internet]. 2012 Nov [cited 2020 Mar 22];55(11):2895–2905. Available from: www.ncbi.nlm.nih.gov/pubmed/22890825

29. Mozaffarian D. Dietary and Policy Prioritites for CVD, diabetes and obesity—A comprehensive RV. Circulation. 2017;133(2):187–225.

30. Bhavadharini B, Mohan V, Dehghan M, Rangarajan S, Swaminathan S, Rosengren A, et al. White rice intake and incident diabetes: A study of 132,373 participants in 21 countries. Diabetes Care. 2020;43(11):2643–2650.

31. Neuenschwander M, Ballon A, Weber KS, Norat T, Aune D, Schwingshackl L, et al. Role of diet in type 2 diabetes incidence: Umbrella review of meta-analyses of prospective observational studies. BMJ. 2019;366.

32. Pan A, Wang Y, Talaei M, Hu FB, Wu T. Relation of active, passive, and quitting smoking with incident type 2 diabetes: A systematic review and meta-analysis. Lancet Diabetes Endocrinol. 2015;3(12):958–967.

33. Grandner MA, Seixas A, Shetty S, Shenoy S. Sleep duration and diabetes risk: Population trends and potential mechanisms. Vol. 16, Current Diabetes Reports. Current Medicine Group LLC 1; 2016. p. 106.

34. Taheri S, Lin L, Austin D, Young T, Mignot E. Short sleep duration is associated with reduced leptin, elevated ghrelin, and increased body mass index. PLoS Med. 2004;1(3):210–217.

35. Stumvoll M, Goldstein BJ, van Haeften TW. Type 2 diabetes: principles of pathogenesis and therapy. Lancet [Internet]. 2005 Apr;365(9467):1333–1346. Available from: https://linkinghub.elsevier.com/retrieve/pii/S014067360561032X

36. Weyer C, Bogardus C, Mott DM, Pratley RE. The natural history of insulin secretory dysfunction and insulin resistance in the pathogenesis of type 2 diabetes mellitus. J Clin Invest. 1999;104(6):787–794.

37. Staimez LR, Weber MB, Ranjani H, Ali MK, Echouffo-Tcheugui JB, Phillips LS, et al. Evidence of reduced β-cell function in Asian Indians with mild dysglycemia. Diabetes Care [Internet]. 2013 Sep [cited 2020 Mar 17];36(9):2772–2778. Available from: www.ncbi.nlm.nih.gov/pubmed/23596180

38. Staimez LR, Deepa M, Ali MK, Mohan V, Hanson RL, Narayan KMV. Tale of two Indians: Heterogeneity in type 2 diabetes pathophysiology. Diabetes Metab Res Rev [Internet]. 2019 Nov 1 [cited 2020 Mar 17];35(8):e3192. Available from: www.ncbi.nlm.nih.gov/pubmed/31145829

39. Cunningham SA, Patel SA, Beckles GL, Geiss LS, Mehta N, Xie H, et al. County-level contextual factors associated with diabetes incidence in the United States. Ann Epidemiol [Internet]. 2018 Jan 1 [cited 2020 Jun 22];28(1):20–25.e2. Available from: https://pubmed.ncbi.nlm.nih.gov/29233722/

40. Gassasse Z, Smith D, Finer S, Gallo V. Association between urbanisation and type 2 diabetes: An ecological study. BMJ Glob Heal. 2017;2(4):1–8.

41. Yach D, Bettcher D. The globalization of public health, I: Threats and opportunities. Am J Public Health. 1998;88(5):735–738.

42. Beaglehole R, Yach D. Globalisation and the prevention and control of non-communicable disease: The neglected chronic diseases of adults. Lancet. 2003;362(9387):903–908.

43. Kickbusch I, Allen L, Franz C. The commercial determinants of health. Lancet Glob Heal [Internet]. 2016;4(12):e895–e896. http://dx.doi.org/10.1016/S2214-109X(16)30217-0

44. Moodie R, Stuckler D, Monteiro C, Sheron N, Neal B, Thamarangsi T, et al. Profits and pandemics: Prevention of harmful effects of tobacco, alcohol, and ultra-processed food and drink industries. Lancet [Internet]. 2013;381(9867):670–679. http://dx.doi.org/10.1016/S0140-6736(12)62089-3

45. Vlahov D, Freudenberg N, Proietti F, Ompad D, Quinn A, Nandi V, et al. Urban as a determinant of health. J Urban Heal. 2007;84(SUPPL. 1):16–26.

46. Cheema A, Adeloye D, Sidhu S, Sridhar D, Chan KY. Urbanization and prevalence of type 2 diabetes in Southern Asia: A systematic analysis. J Glob Health. 2014;4(1).

47. Ebrahim S, Kinra S, Bowen L, Andersen E, Ben-Shlomo Y, Lyngdoh T, et al. The effect of rural-to-urban migration on obesity and diabetes in india: A cross-sectional study. PLoS Med. 2010;7(4).

48. Krishnan S, Cozier YC, Rosenberg L, Palmer JR. Socioeconomic status and incidence of type 2 diabetes: Results from the black women's health study. Am J Epidemiol. 2010;171(5):564–570.

49. Everson SA, Maty SC, Lynch JW, Kaplan GA. Epidemiologic evidence for the relation between socioeconomic status and depression, obesity, and diabetes. J Psychosomat Res. Elsevier Inc.; 2002. pp. 891–895.

50. Patel SA, Cunningham SA, Tandon N, Narayan KMV. Chronic diseases in India-ubiquitous across the socioeconomic spectrum. JAMA Netw Open. 2019;2(4):e190404.

51. UN General Assembly. Political declaration of the high-level meeting of the general assembly on the prevention and control of non-communicable diseases. A/RES/66/2. Vol. 49777; 2012. https://doi.org/10.1007/BF03038934

52. Dahlgren G, Whitehead M. European strategies for tackling social inequities in health: Levelling up Part 2 [Internet]. 2007 [cited 2020 Jan 23]. Available from: www.euro.who.int

53. Ali MK, Siegel KR, Chandrasekar E, Tandon N, Montoya PA, Mbanya J-C, et al. Diabetes: An update on the pandemic and potential solutions. In Prabhakaran D, Anand S, Gaziano TA, et al., editors. Cardiovascular, Respiratory, and Related Disorders. 3rd edition. Washington (DC): The International Bank for Reconstruction and Development/The World Bank; 2017 Nov 17. Chapter 12. Available from: https://www.ncbi.nlm.nih.gov/books/NBK525150/ doi:10.1596/978-1-4648-0518-9_ch12.

54. Johnson EL, Feldman H, Butts A, Billy CDR, Dugan J, Leal S, et al. Standards of medical care in diabetes—2019 abridged for primary care providers. Clin Diabetes. 2019 Jan 1;37(1):11–34.

55. Kahn R, Alperin P, Eddy D, Borch-Johnsen K, Buse J, Feigelman J, et al. Age at initiation and frequency of screening to detect type 2 diabetes: a cost-effectiveness analysis. Lancet [Internet]. 2010 Apr 17 [cited 2021 Jan 7];375(9723):1365–1374. Available from: www.thelancet.com/article/S0140673609621620/fulltext

56. Weber MB, Ranjani H, Staimez LR, Anjana RM, Ali MK, Narayan KMV, et al. The Stepwise approach to diabetes prevention: results from the D-CLIP randomized controlled trial. Diabetes Care [Internet]. 2016 Oct [cited 2020 Jan 23];39(10):1760–1767. Available from: http://care.diabetesjournals.org/lookup/suppl/doi:10.2337/dc16-1241/-/DC1

57. World Health Organization. World health report 2008 "primary health care: Now more than ever." Geneva; 2008.

58. Lall D, Engel N, Devadasan N, Horstman K, Criel B. Challenges in primary care for diabetes and hypertension: an observational study of the Kolar district in rural India. BMC Health Serv Res [Internet]. 2019 Dec 18;19(1):44. Available from: https://bmchealthservres.biomedcentral.com/articles/10.1186/s12913-019-3876-9

59. Mohan V, Venkataraman K, Kannan A. Challenges in diabetes management with particular reference to India. Int J Diabetes Dev Ctries [Internet]. 2009;29(3):103. Available from: www.ijddc.com/text.asp?2009/29/3/103/54286

60. European Observatory on Health Systems and Policies Series. Caring for people with chronic conditions: A health system perspective [Internet]. Nolte EE, McKee M, editors.

England: Mc Graw Hill; 2008. Available from: www.euro.who.int/__data/assets/pdf_file/0006/96468/E91878.pdf

61. Wagner EH, Austin BT, Von KM. Organizing care for patients with chronic illness. MilbankQ1996. 1996;74(4):511.

62. Lall D, Engel N, Devadasan N, Horstman K, Criel B. Models of care for chronic conditions in low/middle-income countries: a 'best fit' framework synthesis. BMJ Glob Heal. 2018;3:1–12. https://doi.org/10.1136/bmjgh-2018-001077

63. Shah MK, Kondal D, Patel SA, Singh K, Devarajan R, Shivashankar R, et al. Effect of a multicomponent intervention on achievement and improvements in quality-of-care indices among people with Type 2 diabetes in South Asia: the CARRS trial. Diabet Med. 2020 Nov;37(11):1825–1831. doi: 10.1111/dme.14124. Epub 2019 Sep 28. PMID: 31479537; PMCID: PMC7051882.

64. Ali MK, Singh K, Kondal D, Devarajan R, Patel SA, Shivashankar R, et al. Effectiveness of a multicomponent quality improvement strategy to improve achievement of diabetes care goals. Ann Intern Med [Internet]. 2016 Sep 20 [cited 2020 Jun 22];165(6):399. Available from: http://annals.org/article.aspx?doi=10.7326/M15-2807

65. Ben-Shlomo Y, Kuh D. A life course approach to chronic disease epidemiology: conceptual models, empirical challenges and interdisciplinary perspectives. Int J Epidemiol. 2002;31.

66. Health Organization Regional Office for Europe W. Good maternal nutrition the best start in life [Internet]. 2016 [cited 2020 Jan 23]. Available from: www.euro.who.int/pubrequest

67. Mikkelsen B, Williams J, Rakovac I, Wickramasinghe K, Hennis A, Shin HR, et al. Life course approach to prevention and control of non-communicable diseases. BMJ. 2019 Jan 28;364.

68. Ivette Galaviz K, Beth Weber M, Straus A, Sonya Haw J, Venkat Narayan K, Kumail Ali M. Global diabetes prevention interventions: A systematic review and network meta-analysis of the real-world impact on incidence, weight, and glucose. Diabetes Care [Internet]. 2018 [cited 2020 Jan 23];41. Available from: http://care.diabetesjournals.org/lookup/suppl/

69. Alouki K, Delisle H, Bermúdez-Tamayo C, Johri M. Lifestyle interventions to prevent type 2 diabetes: A systematic review of economic evaluation studies. J Diabetes Res, 2016;2016:2159890. https://doi.org/10.1155/2016/2159890

70. The Diabetes Prevention Program (DPP) Research Group. Lifestyle balance. Diabetes Care. 2002;25(12):2165–2171.

71. Shirinzadeh M, Afshin-Pour B, Angeles R, Gaber J, Agarwal G. The effect of community-based programs on diabetes prevention in low- and middle-income countries: A systematic review and meta-analysis. Vol. 15, Globalization and Health. BioMed Central Ltd.; 2019.

72. Carvalho Malta D, Barbosa da Silva J. Policies to promote physical activity in Brazil. Lancet [Internet]. 2012 [cited 2020 Jan 23];380:195–196. Available from: http://portal.saude.gov.br/portal/saude/

73. Prabhakaran D, Ajay VS, Tandon N. Strategic opportunities for leveraging low-cost, high-impact technological innovations to promote cardiovascular health in India. Ethn Dis [Internet]. 2019 Feb 21 [cited 2020 Jan 23];29(Suppl 1):145–152. Available from: http://mdiabetes.nhp.

74. Afshin A, Babalola D, Mclean M, Yu Z, Ma W, Chen CY, et al. Information technology and lifestyle: A Systematic evaluation of internet and mobile interventions for improving diet, physical activity, obesity, tobacco, and alcohol use. J Am Heart Assoc. 2016 Sep 1;5(9).

75. Desai J, Geiss L, Mukhtar Q, Harwell T, Benjamin S, Bell R, et al. Public health surveillance of diabetes in the United States. J Public Health Manag Pract [Internet]. 2003 Nov [cited 2020 Mar 23];Suppl:S44–51. Available from: www.ncbi.nlm.nih.gov/pubmed/14677330

76. Saaddine JB, Engelgau MM, Beckles GL, Gregg EW, Thompson TJ, Narayan KMV. A diabetes report card for the United States: Quality of care in the 1990s. Ann Intern Med [Internet]. 2002 Apr 16 [cited 2020 Jun 22];136(8):565. Available from: http://annals.org/article.aspx?doi=10.7326/0003-4819-136-8-200204160-00005

77. NCDs. Monitoring and surveillance of non-communicable diseases [Internet]. [cited 2020 Mar 23]. Available from: www.who.int/ncds/surveillance/en/

78. Pasala SK, Rao AA, Sridhar GR. Built environment and diabetes. Int J Diabetes Dev Ctries. 2010;30(2):63–68.

79. WHO European Healthy Cities Network. EuroHealthNet [Internet]. [cited 2020 Mar 23]. Available from: https://eurohealthnet.eu/media/events/who-european-healthy-cities-network

80. World Health Organization. Regional Office for Europe. Towards more physical activity in cities: transforming public spaces to promote physical activity – a key contributor to achieving the Sustainable Development Goals in Europe. World Health Organization. Regional Office for Europe; 2018. Available from: https://apps.who.int/iris/handle/10665/345147.

81. Torres A, Sarmiento OL, Stauber C, Zarama R. The Ciclovia and Cicloruta programs: promising interventions to promote physical activity and social capital in Bogotá, Colombia. Am J Public Health [Internet]. 2013 Feb 9 [cited 2020 Jun 23];103(2):e23–e30. Available from: www.ncbi.nlm.nih.gov/pubmed/23237179

82. Parra D, Gomez L, Pratt M, Sarmiento OL, Mosquera J, Triche E. Policy and built environment changes in Bogotá and their Importance in health promotion. Indoor Built Environ [Internet]. 2007 Aug 27 [cited 2020 Jun 24];16(4):344–348. Available from: http://journals.sagepub.com/doi/10.1177/1420326X07080462

83. Wakefield MA, Loken B, Hornik RC. Use of mass media campaigns to change health behaviour. Lancet. 2010;376(9748):1261–1271.

84. Matsudo V, Matsudo S, Andrade D, Araujo T, Andrade E, de Oliveira LC, et al. Promotion of physical activity in a developing country: The Agita São Paulo experience. Public Health Nutr [Internet]. 2002 Feb [cited 2020 Jun 24];5(1a):253–261. Available from: https://pubmed.ncbi.nlm.nih.gov/12027292/

85. Gámez R, Parra D, Pratt M, Schmid TL. Muévete Bogotá: promoting physical activity with a network of partner companies. Promot Educ [Internet]. 2006 Jun 25 [cited 2020 Jun 23];13(2):138–143. Available from: http://journals.sagepub.com/doi/10.1177/10253823060130020109

86. Siegel K, Narayan KMV, Kinra S. Finding a policy solution to India's diabetes epidemic. Health Affairs. 2008;27:1077–1090.

87. Coitinho D, Monteiro CA, Popkin BM. What Brazil is doing to promote healthy diets and active lifestyles. Public Health Nutr. 2002 Feb;5(1a):263–267.

88. Bergman M, Jagannathan R, Narayan KMV. Nexus of COVID-19 and diabetes pandemics: Global public health lessons. Diabetes Res Clin Pract [Internet]. 2020 Jun;164(January):108215. Available from: https://linkinghub.elsevier.com/retrieve/pii/S0168822720304654

89. Allen LN, Nicholson BD, Yeung BYT, Goiana-da-Silva F, Mahecha Matsudo S, Rodrigues Matsudo V, et al. Implementation of non-communicable disease policies: A geopolitical analysis of 151 countries. Lancet Glob Heal. 2020;14(4):265–272.

90. Narayan KMV, Echouffo-Tcheugui JB, Mohan V, Ali MK. Global prevention and control of type 2 diabetes will require paradigm shifts in policies within and among countries. Health Aff. 2012;31(1):84–92.

# 5.9 Lipids

*Samuel S. Gidding and Arun K. Chopra*

CONTENTS

## INTRODUCTION

Dyslipidemia—either isolated high low-density lipoprotein cholesterol (LDL-c)—or metabolic dyslipidemia—high triglycerides (TG)/low high-density lipoprotein-cholesterol (HDL-c) phenotype associated with obesity, metabolic syndrome, and diabetes—has long been associated with premature atherosclerotic heart disease (ASCVD). Though clinical management of dyslipidemia primarily concerns LDL-c reduction, from the public health standpoint, it is useful to think of these two phenotypes separately, as their etiologies, both from a genetic and environmental perspective, are distinct, as is the focus of dietary treatment. Lowering saturated fats is the target for isolated LDL-c; excess caloric intake, particularly dietary sugar, is the target for metabolic dyslipidemia.

Elevated LDL-c is considered causal for ASCVD (1). Evidence for this comes from a wide range of studies, including basic science models of atherosclerosis development, observational epidemiologic studies relating elevated cholesterol early in life with future ASCVD, mendelian randomization studies showing the association of lifelong elevation of LDL-c with ASCVD events, and LDL-c reduction clinical trials showing reduction of ASCVD events linearly associated with achieved LDL-c reduction. Familial hypercholesterolemia (FH), an autosomal dominant genetic condition, provides a natural model for the impact of isolated and lifelong elevation of LDL-c on ASCVD events. For metabolic dyslipidemia, the elevated TG/HDL-c ratio is associated with a discordant increase in the number of LDL particles compared to the calculated LDL-c value, reflected in a higher apolipoprotein B level than would be expected for the calculated LDL-c, increasing the risk for ASCVD (2).

Evidence-based guidelines for lipid treatment have been published and are based on strong clinical trial evidence, conducted in primary and secondary prevention settings, for those above 50 years of age (3, 4). Treatment recommendations for younger individuals are based on natural history and epidemiologic data, basic science, and mendelian randomization studies of genetic variants associated with dyslipidemia.

It is useful to think about lipid values in four groups: optimal (no intervention needed), borderline (lifestyle intervention), elevated (likely requires pharmacologic intervention), and severe (requires intervention early in life, likely a genetic cause). A categorization of lipid values is presented in Table 5.9.1, including values for non-HDL-c and apolipoprotein B, which may also be helpful in risk stratification.

This chapter will review early (prevention of risk factor development), primary, and secondary prevention strategies for the management of dyslipidemia from both public health and clinical perspectives. Distinct approaches to high LDL-c and metabolic dyslipidemia will be discussed, along with clinical management and treatment goals, as they support the public health approach. Lifestyle management will be presented in relation to earlier prevention; however, lifestyle

DOI: 10.1201/b23266-14

## Table 5.9.1 Dyslipidemia Classification (lipid and protein values in mg/dL)

| Lipid | Optimal | Borderline | Elevated | Severe/Genetic Etiology |
|---|---|---|---|---|
| LDL-c | <100 | 100–129 | 130–189 | 190 |
| Non HDL-c | <130 | 130–159 | 160–219 | 220 |
| TG | <100 | 100–299 | 300–999 | 1000 |

Abbreviations

ApoB: apolipoprotein B

LDL-c: low density lipoprotein cholesterol

Non HDL-c: non-high density lipoprotein cholesterol

TG: triglycerides

## Table 5.9.2 Dyslipidemia Management Strategies

| | Elevated LDL-c | Metabolic Dyslipidemia |
|---|---|---|
| Early Prevention | Reduce dietary saturated fat, either primarily or with substitution of polyunsaturated fats<br>Eliminate trans fats<br>Increase dietary fiber | Appropriate caloric intake to maintain a normal body mass index<br>Reduce added sugars and complex carbohydrates<br>Participate in moderate physical activity to improve fitness |
| Primary prevention | Statin treatment to reduce LDL-c to <100 mg/dL (adults) or <130 mg/dL (children)<br>Add further medications if needed | Statin treatment to reduce LDL-c to <100 mg/dL (adults) or <130 mg/dL (children)<br>Add further medications if needed<br>Consider pharmacologic fish oil preparations (4 g/day) for TGs 500–1000 mg/dL<br>Consider routine estimation of Apo B in lipid profile |
| Secondary prevention | Reduce LDL-c to <70 mg/dL (or to <55 mg/dL in high-risk situations) | Reduce LDL-c to <70 mg/dL (or to <55 mg/dL in high-risk situations) |

Abbreviations

LDL-c: low density lipoprotein cholesterol

TG: triglycerides

management remains part of primary and secondary prevention efforts. An overview of prevention strategies is presented in Table 5.9.2.

## ISOLATED HIGH LDL-C

High LDL-c is caused by genetic predisposition and diet (1). The most common genetic cause is polygenic inheritance, an unfavorable combination of the many common genes associated with small increments in LDL-c elevation. Examples include variants related to cholesterol absorption, apolipoprotein E, and proprotein convertase subtilisin/kexin type 9 (PCSK9). High saturated fat and trans fat intake, in the absence of low carbohydrate intake, causes elevated LDL-c by decreasing hepatic LDL-c receptor production. Less LDL is scavenged from the circulation, and there is a subsequent increase in plasma LDL-c. The general population increase with aging is unexplained; in women, menopause is associated with a jump in LDL-c.

LDL-c increases with age; in women, menopause is a key transition point; however, a less common but important genetic cause of premature ASCVD is FH, an autosomal dominant condition with a frequency of about 1:200–300 in the general population (5). FH genetic variants cause extreme, lifelong elevation of LDL-c by adversely impacting LDL receptor function. FH may be diagnosed by genetic testing or the presence of severely elevated LDL-c (≥190 mg/dL), a positive family history of premature ASCVD or severe cholesterol elevation, and, occasionally, the presence of xanthoma or corneal arcus. FH is underdiagnosed worldwide; <10% of patients have been identified, with a particularly large gap in low- and middle-income countries. Cascade screening of first-degree relatives of genetically confirmed cases and population-based cholesterol screening in youth are strategies to improve FH diagnosis rates.

## Early Prevention

Diet remains the most important public health strategy to prevent the development of high LDL-c in the general population (6, 7). Dietary intervention is based on population-based observations that directly relate ASCVD rates to dietary habits of a given population, particularly saturated fat, trans fat, and cholesterol intake. Population-based alterations in dietary composition for these components are strongly associated with changes in ASCVD rates. Epidemiologic dietary data are supported by intervention trials in humans showing a change in LDL-c with a reduction in saturated fat, cholesterol, or trans fat content and animal studies showing changes in measurable atherosclerosis related to changes in diet, though robust clinical trial data demonstrating lower mortality with reductions in saturated fats and cholesterol are lacking. The sole reduction of saturated fat has been mired by controversy, particularly in the recent past. Saturated fat replacement with polyunsaturated fat appears most beneficial. Dietary cholesterol plays a lesser role in determining serum cholesterol than saturated and trans fats.

Several dietary patterns worldwide have been associated with lower ASCVD event rates, including the Mediterranean diet and Oriental diets typical in China and Japan in the twentieth century prior to the influx of Western dietary influences (6, 7). Unifying features of these diets include the use of fish and lean poultry as sources of animal protein; high intake of legumes, fruits, and vegetables; and use of poly-unsaturated fats as sources of added dietary fat, as opposed to the use of saturated fat or trans fats. Public health strategies raising awareness about the harmful effects of dietary saturated fat, elimination of trans fats in the food supply, and education of the use of saturated vegetable fats (coconut and palm oil) in the food supply have contributed to reductions in both total cholesterol and ASCVD in many countries.

## Primary Prevention

Statin medications have revolutionized primary prevention of ASCVD and are the first-choice medications for those with elevated LDL-c (3, 4). Initiation of high-intensity statins is recommended for LDL-c $\geq$190 mg/dL, the level associated with FH, beginning at 8–10 years of age. In adults, initiation of statins at LDL-c 130–190 mg/dL is based on age and risk stratification algorithms published in evidence-based guidelines, with older patients and those with higher risk recommended for treatments at lower LDL-c levels. Region-, country-, and race-specific risk scores would be desirable and should be a public health priority, as ASCVD rates vary by country, as does associated risk factor prevalence. In meta-analyses of primary prevention trials, the greatest therapeutic benefit is achieved by those who are younger and have the highest baseline LDL-c.

Most statins are available as generic medications, with rosuvastatin, pitavastatin, and atorvastatin having the highest potency and simvastatin, fluvastatin, pravastatin, and lovastatin having lower potency. Statins are generally safe but are associated with rhabdomyolysis (rare), a slightly increased risk of developing diabetes (in those at risk for diabetes), and muscle pain and cramping. In those who are statin intolerant or who do not achieve LDL-c goals, ezetimibe is the second-choice medication. PCSK9 inhibitors are potent reducers of LDL-c but are expensive and not available universally; thus far, they have not been evaluated in primary prevention in conditions other than FH.

## Secondary Prevention

The highest risk group for ASCVD are those with prevalent ASCVD, as event rates are substantially higher than in those who have not yet experienced ASCVD (3, 4). Clinical trial evidence suggests that the lower achieved LDL-c, the better. Thus, LDL-c targets are lower for this group, 70 mg/dL generally and 55 mg/dL for those with familial hypercholesterolemia, and the treatment options remain high-dose statins and ezetimibe. Another drug that has recently been approved is bempedoic acid, which may be used in addition to maximally tolerated doses of statins and/or ezetimibe, in case these targets aren't achieved, especially as a cheaper option than PCSK9 inhibitors. PCSK9 inhibitors may be considered in the highest-risk groups, especially FH, but the cost may be prohibitive, and they also may not be available in many low- and middle-income countries (LMICs).

## METABOLIC DYSLIPIDEMIA

The elevated TG/low HDL-c phenotype is the most common dyslipidemia associated with ASCVD. In the setting of obesity and excess caloric intake, particularly from carbohydrates, the liver responds by increasing production of apolipoprotein B and TG containing very low-density lipoprotein (VLDL) particles (8). In the circulation, cholesterol ester is transferred from HDL and LDL to VLDL particles. This creates smaller HDL particles, which are excreted by the kidney, lowering HDL-c levels, and smaller cholesterol-poor LDL particles, which more easily pass into atheroma and are more easily oxidized. Downstream metabolism of VLDL leads to production of atherogenic VLDL particles and increased LDL particle numbers. The net impact of these processes is an increased number of atherogenic apolipoprotein B–containing particles related to measured LDL-c level and decreased HDL capacity for cholesterol efflux from macrophages, all pro-atherogenic changes. As most clinical lipid measurements use calculated LDL-c levels rather than direct measurement, in individuals with metabolic syndrome, T2DM, and hypertriglyceridemia, apolipoprotein B measurement may be preferable. Apolipoprotein B captures the discordance between LDL particle number and the estimated LDL-c from the Friedewald equation and correlates better with ASCVD risk (2).

Beyond the adverse impact on atherogenicity of lipoproteins, elevated TGs are an independent risk factor for future diabetes, with a TG/HDL-c ratio >3 being the simplest biochemical correlate of insulin resistance. These processes can be exacerbated by the presence of common genetic variants that slow TG metabolism.

### Primordial Prevention

In many countries, one third to one half of the adult population has prediabetes or diabetes, with younger individuals at risk because of positive family history, obesity, and metabolic syndrome (high TGs and low HDL-c and elevated blood pressure). The prime driver of the lipid component of this phenotype, excess VLDL production, is excess caloric intake, particularly from added sugars and excess carbohydrates (8, 9). The hormonal, adipokine, and inflammatory milieu associated with obesity creates insulin resistance, which helps drive the atherogenic metabolic processes described earlier.

Public health strategies that encourage appropriate caloric intake for body size and discourage consumption of added sugars will be needed to prevent the obesity epidemic and reduce the prevalence of metabolic dyslipidemia. Encouraging the maintenance of ideal body weight beginning in childhood, particularly given the difficulty in treating obesity, is of paramount importance. While dairy fat contributes to increases in LDL-c, dairy products such as yogurt and cheese are associated with a lower risk of future diabetes. Therefore, encouragement of the use of low-fat dairy products and avoidance of added sugar to them has public health value.

Public health strategies could include greater regulation of the food and beverage industry, including bans on flashy advertisements for food items (especially fried foods, snacks, sweets, and sugar-sweetened beverages), taxation, and stricter control on food preparation in eateries. In this regard, guidelines need to be stricter, as 6–9 tsf of sugar daily is excessive for individuals with overweight, obesity, and metabolic syndrome. Intermittent fasting has emerged as another option to improve insulin sensitivity. Different dietary sources of fat have different impacts on health outcomes—as more is learned, this knowledge can be incorporated into health education and regulation.

In contrast, physical fitness is insulin sensitizing (10). Higher muscle mass relative to fat mass is associated with more efficient metabolism of sugar. This creates a hormonal and adipokine milieu, which reverses the adverse changes associated with obesity and insulin resistance described earlier. The biggest impact on metabolic risk and ASCVD risk reduction is associated with the transition from low to moderate physical fitness levels (10). Therefore, encouragement of moderate levels of physical activity, 30–60 minutes of activity, three to five days per week, can have a beneficial effect on metabolic dyslipidemia and future diabetes. This impact is independent of weight control, with higher levels of fitness conferring greater benefit.

Gene-environment interaction studies suggest that in individuals predisposed to metabolic dyslipidemia, maintenance of normal body weight and increased physical fitness reduce the expression of the adverse metabolic phenotype. Those with genetic predisposition to metabolic dyslipidemia likely benefit the most from behavioral intervention.

## Primary Prevention

Pharmacologic treatment of metabolic dyslipidemia is based on achieving target LDL-c levels as described earlier, with the understanding that more than LDL-c reduction is often needed, given the typical coexistence of other ASCVD risk factors and the need for lifestyle change (3, 4). As discussed earlier, having region- and race/ethnicity-specific risk scores would be helpful. Patients with metabolic dyslipidemia are more likely to have additional ASCVD risk factors compared to those with isolated elevated LDL-c, including diabetes, lowering thresholds for statin initiation. In the setting of elevated TGs such that LDL-c cannot be calculated, non–HDL-c can be used instead by adding 30 mg/dL to LDL-c thresholds. Moderate- to high-intensity statins followed by ezetimibe are the first-choice medications.

Apolipoprotein B levels, as they reflect most accurately the level of atherogenic lipoproteins in the circulation, may prove to be the best marker of ASCVD risk in those with metabolic dyslipidemia (2). As of yet, thresholds for treatment have not been established; hence, making Apo B and direct LDL estimation cheaper and easily available is a public health priority. Measurement of HbA1c should be considered in someone with high TGs and risk for type 2 diabetes.

## Secondary Prevention

Lipid targets in those with metabolic dyslipidemia are the same as those with isolated elevated LDL-c; however, this group is much more likely to have additional risk factors warranting a treatment goal of 55 mg/dL. PCSK9 inhibitors, if available, may be necessary to achieve lower targets (4); longer randomized controlled trials (RCTs) are required to prove survival benefits with their use, as current data are limited to reduction in major vascular events but not mortality even in high-risk ASCVD patients.

While fish oil supplementation to lower TGs and prevent recurrent cardiovascular disease overall is controversial, pharmacologic fish oil preparations, particularly those with highly purified eicosapentaenoic acid (EPA), may be useful in patients with TGs in the 500–1000 mg/dL range and prevalent ASCVD (11). Fish oil lowers TGs but has no impact on LDL-c and may even raise it slightly. The beneficial effect of EPA may be related to beneficial effects on endothelial function, cell membranes, and thrombosis. However, as the benefits are only noted with specific preparations of EPA in high doses and not with others, over-the-counter (OTC) dietary supplements and fish oil preparations should be discouraged.

Though ASCVD prevention is the primary subject of this chapter, those with metabolic dyslipidemia are also at high risk for heart failure, either secondary to myocardial injury from ASCVD or incident heart failure related to risk from hypertension, obesity, and diabetes. Thus, evaluation and control of all risk factors are mandatory in this setting.

## ADDITIONAL CONSIDERATIONS

### Lipoprotein(a)

Lipoprotein(a) is a lipid particle associated with increased cardiovascular risk, though the mechanism is unclear (12). Lipoprotein(a) is not currently part of routine recommended lipid evaluation, but increases risk, probably most in those with elevated LDL-c. For that reason, it should be measured in those with FH, those with prevalent ASCVD, and family members of those with premature ASCVD and no other risk factors. Estimation should become cheaper and easily available, and guidelines should consider making it part of routine lipid estimation, particularly in high-risk groups like Southeast Asians and non-responders to statins.

### Familial Chylomicronemia Syndrome (FCS)

A rare but important cause of severely elevated TGs (>1000 mg/dL) is FCS, an inherited condition associated with pancreatitis but not ASCVD (13). Genetic variants associated with FCS are related to lipoprotein lipase and apolipoprotein C3 function. Current treatment is a very low-fat diet and medium-chain triglyceride (MCT) oil as a substitute for dietary fat. Currently available drug therapy is confined to fibrates, which have limited evidence of clinical benefits; promising experimental treatments are under development.

### Tobacco

Both active smoking and environmental smoke exposure can worsen atherosclerosis or trigger acute ASCVD events; combined with environmental pollution, these are among the strongest risk factors for morbidity and mortality (3). Tobacco use is considered etiologic for abdominal aortic aneurysms. Clean indoor and outdoor air legislation and smoking cessation should be encouraged as public health interventions, as well as primary and secondary prevention strategies.

## Medication Adherence

While evidence-based guidelines hold great promise for reduction of ASCVD, patient adherence to statin medication and the high cost of PCSK9 inhibitors may limit implementation (14). Therefore, public health and provider-based strategies to educate patients regarding the importance of preventive medication and to improve medication access are needed. This includes regulation to keep moderate- and high-intensity statins and ezetimibe affordable, provide coverage for those with the highest-risk conditions such as homozygous FH, and encourage the use of a polypill for those with multiple comorbidities.

## SUMMARY

Management of dyslipidemia to prevent ASCVD requires complementary early, primary, and secondary prevention strategies. It is useful from a public health standpoint to consider separate approaches to the prevention of isolated elevated LDL-c, which requires attention to saturated and trans fats in the diet, and metabolic dyslipidemia, where total caloric intake, added sugars, and exercise are beneficial. Incorporation of heart disease prevention concepts into public education and the workplace environment are needed to lower population-based ASCVD risk Suggestions for future research to improve a public health approach to dyslipidemia are presented in Table 5.9.3. For pharmacologic treatment, LDL-c reduction is the primary target, and statins are the first-choice medications: these are recommended strongly for all with established ASCVD and in high-risk individuals for primary prevention. Genetic information is taking a more important role in diagnosis and treatment; gene-environment interactions provide a rationale for intensification of behavioral intervention in those at risk and provides explanatory information for patients about risk, particularly in those with severe phenotypes such as FH and FCS.

## Table 5.9.3 Issues for Future Research

1. Does routine estimation of ApoB in general population, improve risk assessment? How do we make ApoB estimation a part of the routine lipid assessment by standardizing its measurement and making it easily available?

2. What are the best strategies to improve availability of statins and improve adherence in at-risk individuals, especially in LMICs?

3. What are the feasibility, affordability, and compliance with a polypill, incorporating a statin, in the management of high-risk individuals without established ASCVD?

4. What are the feasibility, safety, and efficacy of a low-carbohydrate diet in the management of individuals with dyslipidemia and prediabetes, diabetes, or metabolic syndrome?

5. Are there regulatory strategies regarding diet and exercise that prevent obesity in populations?

6. Does measurement of lipoprotein(a) as part of lipid profile add to risk stratification?

## REFERENCES

1. Ference BA, Ginsberg HN, Graham I, Ray KK, Packard CJ, Bruckert E, Hegele RA, Krauss RM, Raal FJ, Schunkert H, Watts GF, Borén J, Fazio S, Horton JD, Masana L, Nicholls SJ, Nordestgaard BG, van de Sluis B, Taskinen MR, Tokgözoglu L, Landmesser U, Laufs U, Wiklund O, Stock JK, Chapman MJ, Catapano AL. Low-density lipoproteins cause atherosclerotic cardiovascular disease. 1. Evidence from genetic, epidemiologic, and clinical studies. A consensus statement from the European Atherosclerosis Society Consensus Panel. Eur Heart J. 2017 Aug 21;38(32):2459–2472. doi: 10.1093/eurheartj/ehx144. PMID: 28444290; PMCID: PMC5837225.

2. Sniderman AD, Thanassoulis G, Glavinovic T, Navar AM, Pencina M, Catapano A, Ference BA. Apolipoprotein B particles and cardiovascular disease: A narrative review. JAMA Cardiol. 2019 Dec 1;4(12):1287–1295. doi: 10.1001/jamacardio.2019.3780. PMID: 31642874; PMCID: PMC7369156.

3. Grundy SM, Stone NJ, Bailey AL, Beam C, Birtcher KK, Blumenthal RS, Braun LT, de Ferranti S, Faiella-Tommasino J, Forman DE, Goldberg R, Heidenreich PA, Hlatky MA, Jones DW,

Lloyd-Jones D, Lopez-Pajares N, Ndumele CE, Orringer CE, Peralta CA, Saseen JJ, Smith SC Jr, Sperling L, Virani SS, Yeboah J. 2018 AHA/ACC/AACVPR/AAPA/ABC/ACPM/ADA/AGS/APhA/ASPC/NLA/PCNA Guideline on the management of blood cholesterol: A report of the American College of cardiology/american heart association task force on clinical practice guidelines. J Am Coll Cardiol. 2019 Jun 25;73(24):e285–e350. doi: 10.1016/j.jacc.2018.11.003. Epub 2018 Nov 10. Erratum in: J Am Coll Cardiol. 2019 Jun 25;73(24):3237–3241. PMID: 30423393.

4.  Mach F, Baigent C, Catapano AL, Koskinas KC, Casula M, Badimon L, Chapman MJ, De Backer GG, Delgado V, Ference BA, Graham IM, Halliday A, Landmesser U, Mihaylova B, Pedersen TR, Riccardi G, Richter DJ, Sabatine MS, Taskinen MR, Tokgozoglu L, Wiklund O; ESC Scientific Document Group. 2019 ESC/EAS Guidelines for the management of dyslipidaemias: lipid modification to reduce cardiovascular risk. Eur Heart J. 2020 Jan 1;41(1):111–188. doi: 10.1093/eurheartj/ehz455. PMID: 31504418.

5.  Gidding SS, Champagne MA, de Ferranti SD, Defesche J, Ito MK, Knowles JW, McCrindle B, Raal F, Rader D, Santos RD, Lopes-Virella M, Watts GF, Wierzbicki AS; American Heart Association Atherosclerosis, Hypertension, and Obesity in Young Committee of Council on Cardiovascular Disease in Young, Council on Cardiovascular and Stroke Nursing, Council on Functional Genomics and Translational Biology, and Council on Lifestyle and Cardiometabolic Health. The agenda for familial hypercholesterolemia: A scientific statement from the American Heart Association. Circulation. 2015 Dec 1;132(22):2167–2192. doi: 10.1161/CIR.0000000000000297. Epub 2015 Oct 28. Erratum in: Circulation. 2015 Dec 22;132(25):e397. PMID: 26510694.

6.  Mennella JA, Popkin B, Rowe J, Van Horn L, Whitsel L. Implementing American Heart Association pediatric and adult nutrition guidelines: A scientific statement from the American Heart Association nutrition committee of the council on nutrition, physical activity and metabolism, council on cardiovascular disease in the young, council on arteriosclerosis, thrombosis and vascular biology, council on cardiovascular nursing, council on epidemiology and prevention, and council for high blood pressure research. Circulation. 2009 Mar 3;119(8):1161–1175. doi: 10.1161/CIRCULATIONAHA.109.191856. PMID: 19255356.

7.  Sacks FM, Lichtenstein AH, Wu JHY, Appel LJ, Creager MA, Kris-Etherton PM, Miller M, Rimm EB, Rudel LL, Robinson JG, Stone NJ, Van Horn LV; American Heart Association. Dietary fats and cardiovascular disease: A presidential advisory from the American Heart Association. Circulation. 2017 Jul 18;136(3):e1–e23. doi: 10.1161/CIR.0000000000000510. Epub 2017 Jun 15. Erratum in: Circulation. 2017 Sep 5;136(10):e195. PMID: 28620111.

8.  Ginsberg HN, Huang LS. The insulin resistance syndrome: impact on lipoprotein metabolism and atherothrombosis. J Cardiovasc Risk. 2000 Oct;7(5):325–331. doi: 10.1177/204748730000700505. PMID: 11143762.

9.  Stanhope KL, Schwarz JM, Havel PJ. Adverse metabolic effects of dietary fructose: Results from the recent epidemiological, clinical, and mechanistic studies. Curr Opin Lipidol. 2013 Jun;24(3):198–206. doi: 10.1097/MOL.0b013e3283613bca. PMID: 23594708; PMCID: PMC4251462.

10. Ross R, Blair SN, Arena R, Church TS, Després JP, Franklin BA, Haskell WL, Kaminsky LA, Levine BD, Lavie CJ, Myers J, Niebauer J, Sallis R, Sawada SS, Sui X, Wisløff U; American Heart Association Physical Activity Committee of the Council on Lifestyle and Cardiometabolic Health; Council on Clinical Cardiology; Council on Epidemiology and Prevention; Council on Cardiovascular and Stroke Nursing; Council on Functional Genomics and Translational Biology; Stroke Council. Importance of assessing cardiorespiratory fitness in clinical practice: A case for fitness as a clinical vital sign: A scientific statement from the American Heart Association. Circulation. 2016 Dec 13;134(24):e653–e699. doi: 10.1161/CIR.0000000000000461. Epub 2016 Nov 21. PMID: 27881567.

11. Tummala R, Ghosh RK, Jain V, Devanabanda AR, Bandyopadhyay D, Deedwania P, Aronow WS. Fish oil and cardiometabolic diseases: Recent updates and controversies. Am J Med. 2019 Oct;132(10):1153–1159. doi: 10.1016/j.amjmed.2019.04.027. Epub 2019 May 8. PMID: 31077653

12. Wilson DP, Jacobson TA, Jones PH, Koschinsky ML, McNeal CJ, Nordestgaard BG, Orringer CE. Use of Lipoprotein(a) in clinical practice: A biomarker whose time has come. A scientific statement from the National Lipid Association. J Clin Lipidol. 2019 May-Jun;13(3):374–392. doi: 10.1016/j.jacl.2019.04.010. Epub 2019 May 17. PMID: 31147269.

13. Paquette M, Bernard S, Hegele RA, Baass A. Chylomicronemia: Differences between familial chylomicronemia syndrome and multifactorial chylomicronemia. Atherosclerosis. 2019 Apr;283:137–142. doi: 10.1016/j.atherosclerosis.2018.12.019. Epub 2018 Dec 28. PMID: 30655019.
14. Banach M, Stulc T, Dent R, Toth PP. Statin non-adherence and residual cardiovascular risk: There is need for substantial improvement. Int J Cardiol. 2016 Dec 15;225:184–196. doi: 10.1016/j.ijcard.2016.09.075. Epub 2016 Sep 26. PMID: 27728862.

# 6 Emerging and Life-Course Factors in CVD

*Krithiga Shridhar, Vinita Subramanya, and Poornima Prabhakaran*

## CONTENTS

## INTRODUCTION

Cardiovascular disease (CVD) is the leading cause of mortality worldwide. CVD is one of the more well-studied conditions among chronic diseases in terms of risk factors, disease mechanisms, and treatment and management among men and women. Traditional risk factors such as age, gender, lipid levels, smoking, hypertension, and type 2 diabetes explain the over three-fourths probability of an individual's lifetime CVD risk, and the risk prediction models using these risk factors have clinical utility. This chapter focuses on other important yet often neglected risk factors of CVD.

1  The *Barker hypothesis* of fetal origins of adult disease and the *early life influences* during critical window periods in child development: The role of fetal programming (e.g., low or large birth-weight for gestational age, intrauterine growth) and growth trajectory in early life (e.g., rapid catch-up growth, high childhood body mass index [BMI]) in the incidence of CVD and its risk factors was established a few decades back and is re-emerging with new evidence.

2  *Environmental pollution.* The World Health Organization (WHO, year: 2012–2014) estimates about a quarter of all deaths to be attributable to modifiable environmental risk factors globally (1), with the largest fraction due to CVDs. Air pollution and contamination of water and soil, and thus the food chain with chemical toxins, as well as occupational exposures and environmental noise are the major drivers for this burden. The WHO estimates that around 3.3 million deaths due to CVD are possibly caused by air pollution, and it is found to be greater than from any

DOI: 10.1201/b23266-15

major modifiable CVD risk factors such as smoking, hypertension, hyperlipidemia, or diabetes mellitus. Rapidly accumulating evidence implicates exposure to chemical toxins (e.g., pesticides and heavy metals) in a dose-dependent manner, for the increased risk of CVD risk and mortality. Especially vulnerable are the elderly, obese, pregnant women, and children. The cumulative lifetime risk in children with developing cardiopulmonary systems that are highly susceptible to damage is a greater concern (2). Moreover, maternal exposure to $PM_{2.5}$ and chemical toxins is shown to be negatively correlated with fetal growth indicators, adding interlinks between fetal programming and environmental pollution for CVD risk and mortality, a major public health concern.

Barker's hypothesis, early life influences, and environmental pollution assume a unique perspective in low- and middle-income country (LMIC) settings, where the prevalence of these risk factors as well as the CVD burden are high. For instance, based on the first-ever nationally representative comprehensive Nutrition Survey for ages 0–19 years in India (2016–2018), over a third of Indian children are still stunted (3). Similarly, while the annual median level of $PM_{2.5}$ is <15 µg/m$^3$ in the majority of countries in developed settings, it is over 60–90 µg/m$^3$ in several LMICs, and India is one of the countries with the highest levels of annual air pollution—as high as 92.1 µg/m$^3$ (87.6, 95.7) (4, 5).

## BARKER'S HYPOTHESIS AND DEVELOPMENTAL ORIGINS OF HEALTH AND DISEASE (DOHaD)

A recognition of patterns of mortality in birth cohorts in Europe between 1850 and 1930 (6) commenced a life-course approach that focused on early life influences as potential causal factors for diseases in adulthood. Subsequently, cumulative effects of exposures (7) and early life environmental exposures became the focus of research (8). In the 1970s, Forsdahl demonstrated that environmental conditions and nutritional deficits in early life had an adverse effect on adult coronary heart disease (CHD) risk (9, 10). This led to a resurgence of interest in the fetal origins of disease.

The fetal origins of disease hypothesis, also known as the thrifty phenotype hypothesis, gained traction through the publication of works by David Barker and colleagues in the 1980s (11–14). The theory postulates that fetal undernutrition in mid-to-late gestation leads to programming of metabolic characteristics in the fetus that predisposes it to future disease states in a nutritionally rich environment. Barker and colleagues had noticed that areas in Britain that had the highest infant mortality also had the highest mortality from CHD years later (12). At the time, the most common cause for infant mortality was low birth weight; therefore the hypothesis postulated that low birth weight babies that survived were at a higher risk for CHD later in life. Low birth weight has since been found to be associated with risk factors of CHD such as hypertension, diabetes mellitus, hyperlipidemia, and coagulation factor levels in adulthood (15–19).

Some of the early work assessing the associations of birth weight on CHD and its risk factors were subject to criticisms of inappropriate study design and biased results (20). There was also a lack of consistency of findings with some studies that followed (21–24). This led to the recognition that there were early life influences beyond low birth weight that influenced disease states later in life, such as maternal nutrition, maternal stress, environmental factors, and so forth.

Gluckman and Hanson (25) and Bateson (26) and colleagues (27) separately put forth the idea of developmental plasticity in DOHaD. They hypothesized that there were multiple pathways to initiate disease processes in the prenatal period. Subsequent postnatal stimuli decided the pathway of adaptive or pathological development, depending on if the postnatal environment matched the prenatal one or not, respectively. The postnatal environment was understood to extend to childhood and well into the second decade of life (28). Since its conceptualization, birth weight and supplementary early life exposures have been found to be associated with other health outcomes in adults such as chronic lung disease, certain forms of cancer, psychological outcomes, neurodevelopmental issues, and other characteristics (29). The following section will focus on early life influences and their association with CVD in adults.

## LIFE-COURSE MODELS

A life-course approach in epidemiology refers to understanding exposures and processes at different stages of life, either singly or together, and the way they influence later life disease risk (30). In essence, it is an amalgamation of early life influences and an adult risk model and provides a practical approach to early and primary prevention of disease. Various models are used to explain the life-course approach and are briefly described next.

Critical period model: This model focuses on the occurrence of the exposure at a particular life stage, which exerts its effects through anatomical and physiological changes (25). This usually refers to periods of development that are irreversible (30).

Sensitive period model (30): This model postulates that there are certain periods in development where harmful exposures are able to exert a greater effect compared to other times. Exposures exerting their influence through the critical and sensitive period are modifiable by later life exposures.

Cumulative risk model (30): This model postulates that the effects of exposures accumulate over time. It also provides flexibility for certain periods of susceptibility being greater than others.

Dose-response model (30): In this model, disease risk increases with the duration and number of exposures over the lifetime.

## EARLY LIFE EXPOSURES AND CARDIOVASCULAR DISEASE

### Offspring Factors

#### Birth Weight

Following the recognition of low birth weight (a surrogate marker for intrauterine growth) as a risk factor for adult CHD, subsequent studies found that it was also implicated in the development of hypertension, insulin resistance, and CVD mortality (15). Conversely, high birth weight also has an adverse effect on the adult metabolic profile. A high birth weight also predisposes to long-term cardiovascular risk, including risk for diabetes and metabolic syndrome (31, 32).

#### Growth in Childhood

The interaction between the prenatal and postnatal environment is believed to influence the pathway of choice for adult disease processes (26, 27). One of the postulated mechanisms for adult cardiovascular risk is a rapid rate of postnatal growth, perhaps in a nutritionally enriched environment that follows low birth weight (33–36). The risk for adult CVD is worsened by growth failure in the first year after birth, followed by accelerated growth in subsequent years (37–40). In the period after infancy, higher weight, height, mid upper arm circumference, skinfold thickness, and faster growth were found to be associated with greater CVD risk (41).

Excess weight gain and childhood obesity are associated with the development of diabetes mellitus and higher cardiovascular risk (42–44). Stunting, another measure of growth failure, is commonly seen in developing countries and is secondary to inadequate nutrient intake, malabsorption, and inflammation. Stunting has been found to be associated with hypertension, glucose intolerance, and dyslipidemia (45–47).

### Maternal Factors

Maternal factors have been recognized to contribute to offspring disease risk. Some of the implicated factors are discussed in the following sections.

#### Maternal Diet and Nutrition

An unbalanced diet in different periods of gestation can lead to cardiovascular and nephrological outcomes in offspring. Animal studies have demonstrated a maternal high-fat diet can lead to deleterious effects on offspring growth and predisposes them to obesity and endocrine disorders (48, 49). These findings have been replicated in human studies, and a maternal high-fat diet has been found to be associated with obesity in offspring as well as endothelial dysfunction (49, 50). A maternal high-salt diet, acting through the activation of the renin-angiotensin system, predisposes offspring to hypertension in adulthood (51). In situations where maternal protein intake is limited in pregnancy, supplementation with micronutrients may ameliorate cardiovascular risk. A number of animal studies have demonstrated the protective effects of micronutrients such as folate, vitamin C, vitamin E, and selenium against CVD in offspring whose mothers were fed a protein-restricted diet (52).

#### Breastmilk

Breastmilk is known to provide nutrition as well as immunity to offspring. It is also understood to offer protection from CVD risk factors, such as obesity, by delaying the onset of complementary feeds (53–55). The effects of breastmilk on other cardiovascular risk factors is less clear. There are conflicting results from studies exploring its effects on dyslipidemia (56, 57) and blood pressure (58, 59) later in life.

## Maternal Comorbidities and Behavioral Risk Factors

Maternal obesity in pregnancy is consistently associated with a greater cardiovascular risk in children, from obesity to premature cardiovascular mortality (60–62). Behavioral risk factors, such as maternal smoking during gestation, have been found to result in higher blood pressure levels in offspring (63) and dyslipidemia in offspring. The underlying mechanism is thought to be through shared behavioral risk factors and, to a lesser extent, fetal programming (64, 65). Gestational diabetes exposes the fetus to hyperglycemia in utero, increasing the risk for perinatal mortality. Long-term, there is an increased risk for offspring diabetes, obesity, and CVD. Gestational diabetes results in programming of the fetal hypothalamic pathway and, subsequently, dysregulated lipogenesis (66, 67). Gestational obesity and excess weight gain are implicated in premature mortality from CVD in offspring (68).

## Lifestyle Factors

### Diet

Dietary patterns in childhood determine risk for obesity and, hence, cardiovascular risk. A diet with lower amounts of processed foods is generally protective against CVD risk factor development (69). Other important considerations are calorie intake, salt intake, and adequate fruit and vegetable servings in the diet (69, 70).

### Physical Activity

In conjunction with diet, physical activity levels in childhood are important modifiable factors that determine cardiovascular risk (71). A sedentary lifestyle with greater screen time increases the risk for multiple CVD risk factors (72, 73). Lower CVD risk is associated with moderate-vigorous physical activity levels that are age- and sex-dependent (73). At least one study has also demonstrated a further decrease in cardiovascular risk with athletic training as compared to unstructured physical activity in adolescents (74).

### Others

Adolescents are at the highest risk to initiate smoking and continue with it to adulthood. As in adults, smoking in children has adverse effects on the cardiovascular system with an increase in risk factors, CVD mortality, and all-cause mortality (74, 75).

## Socioeconomic Position

Socioeconomic position in early life is often determined by parental socioeconomic status (SES), household assets, and/or area-level factors. Lower SES in early life is adversely related to CVD (76). Some studies have found a stronger association with hemorrhagic stroke than coronary artery disease. When also accounting for adult SES, studies have found an association with CHD mortality (76, 77). In developing countries, the relationship between SES and CVD is more complex. Studies have found that people with higher SES have a higher risk factor prevalence and those with lower SES have greater mortality from CVD (78–80). Change in SES from childhood to adulthood (in either direction) has also been found to be associated with cardiovascular risk (81), as has persistent low socioeconomic position (82, 83).

## POSTULATED MECHANISMS

There are currently many proposed mechanisms or pathways through which early life exposures are thought to exert their long-term effects.

## Altered Fetal Nutrition

Birth weight is dependent on fetal nutrition, which in turn is dependent on maternal nutrition. Animal studies have demonstrated that inadequate gestational nutrient intake, including protein intake, can lead to low birth weight, higher blood pressure, and higher blood glucose levels (84–88). In human studies too, the effects of altered maternal macronutrient and micronutrient intake results in greater cardiovascular risk in offspring. This is thought to occur due to 'programming' of the fetus in utero to the existing nutrient climate and its subsequent adaptation to the postnatal environment.

## Glucocorticoids

Elevated glucocorticoids, exogenous, maternal, or fetal in origin, or an impaired placental barrier exposes the fetus to higher-than-normal glucocorticoid levels. In animal studies, this results in elevated blood pressure, impaired glucose tolerance, and low birth weight (29). In humans, small-for-gestational-age babies had higher basal cortisol levels in adulthood. The effects of maternal nutrition and glucocorticoids are sometimes hard to separate. Maternal protein restriction causes a fall in 11-β hydroxysteroid dehydrogenase, an enzyme that inactivates glucocorticoids resulting in an increase in glucocorticoid receptor expression in fetal tissues and greater glucocorticoid action, which leads to hypertension in the offspring (89).

## Genetics and Epigenetics

Certain individuals are predisposed to CVD through inheritable traits. Studies, including genome-wide association studies, have found that dyslipidemia (90, 91) and hypertension (92, 93) are associated with common genetic variants. Some of these effects are exerted through epigenetic modifications of the gene expression, wherein there are changes to gene expression without changes to the DNA sequence. Modification such as DNA methylation, histone modifications, and microRNAs have been implicated in disease causation (94). DNA methylation is a process that affects the promoter region of the gene that is rich in cytosine. These regions are methylated in the presence of nutritional deficiencies (e.g., vitamin $B_{12}$, folate, choline, methionine) and can be inherited by subsequent generations. When methylated, gene expression is suppressed and long-term CVD effects are seen. Histones are proteins around which DNA is located. When histones undergo modifications (e.g. methylation, acetylation, phosphorylation), the access of DNA to transcription factors may change, thus impacting gene expression. MicroRNAs are non-coding strands of RNA that are involved in post-transcriptional pathways that affect gene expression. These epigenetic modifications work together to influence cardiovascular risk in adulthood.

## Intergenerational Effects

The transmission of disease risk from the mother to her offspring is known as intergenerational effects. The transmission of these traits across multiple generations refers to transgenerational effects. These effects occur through epigenetic modification and through as yet unidentified factors. Factors that are known to exert intergenerational effects include chemicals and intrauterine malnutrition (95, 96). While most studies have focused on and identified effects through the mother, some exposures are specifically transmitted through the father of the offspring.

## ENVIRONMENTAL POLLUTION FOR CVD RISK AND MORTALITY

Pollution of air and contamination of water and soil by chemical toxins (e.g., heavy metals, pesticides) account for a sizable proportion of health-relevant factors in the environment. The key drivers of environmental pollution are uncontrolled urbanization and industrialization with deforestation and increasing use of toxic chemicals. Nevertheless, household air pollution due to use of coal and solid fuels for heating, lighting, and cooking is still a major concern in a majority of LMIC settings, largely attributed to traditional lifestyles and poverty. Occupational exposures and environmental noise (e.g., traffic, industries) are other relevant, yet often neglected risk factors.

## AMBIENT AIR POLLUTION

Air pollution is the fourth leading risk factor attributed to early deaths worldwide, with 6.7 million deaths in 2019; nearly a half of these deaths is attributed to ischemic heart disease (IHD) and stroke and another one-fifth to diabetes, a risk factor for CVD (4). Ambient fine particulate matter with diameter under 2.5 μm ($PM_{2.5}$), household air pollution, and ozone ($O_3$) are the fairly well-documented components of air pollution (4). The other important components for which evidence to date is emerging but still limited include particulate matter with diameter under 10 μm ($PM_{10}$), black carbon, nitrogen dioxide ($NO_2$) mainly from traffic pollution, sulfur, and diesel exhaust as well as benzene, asbestos, radon, and formaldehyde. The potential biological mechanisms of air pollution for causing CVDs include oxidative stress, systemic inflammation, endothelial dysfunction, abnormal lipid metabolism, disturbance of the autonomic nervous system, arterial vasoconstriction, and abnormal coagulation function. PM may stimulate high cytosolic calcium, with low sarcoplasmic reticulum ion stores causing reduced cardiac contractility and increased hypertrophy. Oxidative stress further may lead to atherosclerosis (accumulation of lipids and fibrous plaque in the arteries) by promoting pro-atherogenic factors (2, 97). Exposure to diesel exhaust was shown to promote platelet activation and thrombus formation. PM may also cause autonomic nervous system dysfunction with sympathetic hyperstimulation over parasympathetic, possibly leading to cardiac arrhythmias and hypertension (2, 97).

Long-term exposure, generally estimated as annual average over a period of time, to elevated levels of air pollution, particularly $PM_{2.5}$, $PM_{10}$, and $NO_2$, are found to be temporally linked (i.e., using cohort study models where exposures precede outcomes) to CVD events such as CHD, acute coronary events, heart failure, atrial fibrillation, cerebrovascular stroke, and mortality in the hazard range of 1.05–1.25 (98). It is interesting to note that short-term exposures in a window period of a few days or months to elevated $PM_{2.5}$ are also strongly associated with hospital admissions, heart rate variability, myocardial infarction (MI), stroke, and heart failure (note: here the exposure is up to seven days) (99). Further, the dose-response curves for air pollution are not very well-defined, yet as emerging evidence points to variations (*see Panel 1*). Countries with international air quality standards have reported increased risk of stroke with small increases in $PM_{2.5}$ (100).

**Panel 1**: Dose-response mechanisms of air pollution for CVD risk and mortality

The fundamental principle of toxicology is that "all things are poison—solely the dose determines that a thing is not a poison (Paracelsus 1493–1541)". The current WHO guidelines for adequate air quality define dose levels for several components of air such as

PM2.5: 10 µg/m3 annual mean; 10 µg/m3 24-hour mean

PM10: 20 µg/m3 annual mean; 50 µg/m3 24-hour mean

$O_3$: 100 µg/m$^3$ 8-hour mean

$NO_2$: 40 µg/m$^3$ annual mean; 200 µg/m$^3$ 1-hour mean

$SO_2$: 20 µg/m$^3$ 24-hour mean; 500 µg/m$^3$ 10-minute mean

Emerging evidence suggests supralinear associations of $PM_{2.5}$ for all-cause and disease-specific mortality, including CVD for concentrations as low as 5 µg/m$^3$ (101).

A large portion of the evidence is from the Western settings, where the exposure levels are low compared to LMIC settings (say, annual median level $PM_{2.5}$: 15.4 µg/m$^3$ [12.8, 17.3] in Europe versus 92.1 µg/m$^3$ [87.6, 95.7] in India). While emphasizing the need for cohort studies from LMICs, a recent systematic review of the status of $PM_{2.5}$ associations for CVDs using data from Brazil, Bulgaria, China, India, and Mexico confirmed positive associations between exposure to $PM_{2.5}$ and cardiometabolic diseases and CVD mortality, with up to 6% increased risk for every 10 µg/m$^3$ increase in $PM_{2.5}$. Further CVD-related hospitalizations and emergency room visits increased up to nearly 20% (98).

## HOUSEHOLD AIR POLLUTION

Household air pollution results from burning of various fuels such as coal, charcoal, wood, agricultural residue, animal dung, kerosene, etc., for heating, lighting, or cooking using open fires or cook stoves with inadequate ventilation. Burning these fuels produces $PM_{2.5}$, black carbon, and carbon monoxide, among others, and this practice is very widespread in sub-Saharan Africa and in certain parts of Asia, including India. While household air pollution has increased in African regions in the last decade between 2010 and 2019, countries in Asia, most notably India (from 73% to 61%) and China (from 54% to 36%), have shown reductions with aggressive campaigns, efforts, and interventions to switch to cleaner fuels. Prospective studies on urban and rural populations in countries such as Bangladesh, Brazil, Chile, China, Colombia, India, Pakistan, Philippines, South Africa, Tanzania, and Zimbabwe have shown associations for individuals living with household air pollution (hazard ratio [HR]:1.08 95% confidence interval [CI]: 0.99, 1.17) compared to individuals in cleaner households) with fatal and non-fatal CVD outcomes (4). The United Nations Sustainable Development Goals (SDG) to reduce premature deaths among people aged 30–69 years from CVD, cancer, diabetes, and chronic lung disease by one third by 2030, aims at a 25% reduction in the use of solid fuels, which is estimated to reduce premature CVD deaths by 1.4% (102).

## CHEMICAL TOXINS IN THE WATER, SOIL, AND FOOD CHAIN

While health effects of air pollution are well characterized, the effects of toxic metals and chemicals in the water and soil, thus affecting the food chain, are still emerging. Pesticides and heavy metals such as arsenic, lead, cadmium, copper, and mercury are the major pollutants studied to date. Although direct exposure of pesticides and heavy metals is greater among agricultural and chemical industry workers, this problem extends to the general population through contamination of food, soil, and water. Toxic chemicals amplify in the food chain, percolate in the environment, and remain in human fatty tissue for a long period following exposure (e.g., organochlorine pesticides), making both short-term and long-term exposures to high and low levels equally harmful.

Insecticides such as organochlorines, organophosphates, carbamates, and pyrethroids, as well as certain fungicides, herbicides, and fumigants, are commonly used as pesticides. These chemicals exhibit toxicity to the cardiovascular system with non-fatal and fatal outcomes in the risk range of 1.1–4.5 times, more so for organochlorines. The acute effects include a lengthened QT interval, sinus tachycardia, and ST segment elevation, while chronic exposure involves the risk for non-fatal MI, peripheral arterial disease, stroke, and CVD mortality. The mechanisms involved in CVD toxicity are inflammation, oxidative stress, and alteration of lipid metabolism leading to increased low-density lipoprotein cholesterol (LDL-C). These toxic chemicals may also act through autonomic and central nervous system dysfunction (e.g., organophosphates), as well as through endocrine dysfunction (e.g., xenoestrogenic activity of organochlorines among women) (103).

Experimental and epidemiological evidence confirms increased risk of CVD, coronary artery disease, and stroke with exposure to heavy metals (e.g., arsenic, lead, cadmium, mercury, and copper). A recent meta-analysis of approximately 350,000 individuals from 37 countries showed that exposure to these toxic metals is associated with an increased risk of CVD incidence (summary RR: 1.15–2.22), having a linear-shaped dose-response curve (104) (*see Panel 2*). Cadmium is the most associated metal and mercury the least with possible J-shaped associations with CVD, IHD, and stroke (104).

**Panel 2**: Dose-response mechanisms of arsenic in water for CVD risk and mortality

WHO guidelines for drinking water quality specifies dose levels targets for toxic chemicals, including pesticides and heavy metals: Aldrin and dieldrin (combined): 0.00003 mg/l (0.03 µg/l)

DDT/metabolites: 0.001 mg/l (1 µg/l); chlorophenoxy herbicides: 0.09 mg/l (90 µg/l)

Chlorpyrifos: 0.03 mg/l (30 µg/l); 2, 4, 6-trichlorophenol: 0.2 mg/l (200 µg/l)

Cadmium: 0.003 mg/l (3 µg/l)

Arsenic: 0.01 mg/l (10 µg/l)

Lead: 0.01 mg/l (10 µg/l)

A review of prospective, retrospective, and ecological studies in arsenic-endemic (e.g., Bangladesh, China, Taiwan, Chile, Mexico) and non-endemic regions (e.g., North American and European countries) has summarized and analyzed systematically significant increased risks of CVD endpoints, including CHD mortality and CVD mortality, as well as combined fatal and nonfatal CVD and carotid atherosclerosis disease, as well as hypertension arising from arsenic concentrations in drinking water between 1 µg/L and 10 µg/L, indicating potential for lowering of the WHO guideline value (105). Earlier investigations confirmed linear dose-response associations for arsenic for CVD risk and mortality across low/moderate to high levels (106).

## OCCUPATIONAL EXPOSURES AND ENVIRONMENTAL NOISE

Occupational exposures to physical (heat, noise, and vibration) and chemical agents (gases, pesticides, and heavy metals) and the associated CVD outcomes historically occupied an important place in the list of put forth by the National Institute of Occupational Safety and Health, 1983 (107). As a consequence of modifications in industrial processes, personal protective guidelines, and preventive approaches, work-related CVD profiles are changing with less acute elevated exposures. These range from organizational policies to protect and minimize occupational exposures, facilitating smoke-free environments, serving healthy food, the promotion and provision of on-site screening, and early detection of chronic diseases. Differences across industries, workplace settings, and types of work create challenges to reaching certain groups and can contribute to disparities, and addressing these can be more challenging in LMIC settings. Occupational exposures are generally higher than the environmental exposures and tend to have a greater impact on health outcomes. For instance, mortality due to stroke is found to be increased up to four times in agricultural workers with long-term exposures to pesticides compared to the workers with less exposures (103). Arrhythmias, heart failure, and mortality due to cardiomyopathy and stroke are also found to be increased by about 1.2–3.5 times with long-term exposures (103).

There is growing, yet limited, evidence linking environmental noise, largely due to traffic and industries, to CVD morbidity and mortality for levels exceeding the guidelines (WHO 50–55 dB during the day and 5–10 dB less during night). A 5 dB noise reduction is estimated to reduce hypertension by 1.4% and IHD by 1.8% (97). Acute exposures, e.g., aircraft noise in the night, also may cause endothelial dysfunction in otherwise healthy individuals, a precursor pathological marker for atherosclerosis. The suggested biological plausibility includes a disrupted autonomic nervous system leading to sympatho-adrenal activation and release of pro-inflammatory mediators. Lipid modification, activation of pro-inflammatory leukocytes, and pro-thrombotic factors, as well as circadian clock disruptions leading to vascular damage, are other mechanisms being explored (97). Recent epidemiological evidence highlights synergistic effects of noise and air pollution on CVD (97).

## RARE ACUTE EXPOSURES AND CVD RISK

Sudden, very high elevated doses of air pollution and toxic chemicals, in addition to acute effects, are reported to have a long-term impact on cardiovascular health. For example, responders of the World Trade Center attacks in the United States (September 2001) reported 1.5–2 times increased risk of CVD in the subsequent 17-year follow-up period compared to responders who joined work at the Trade Center after the attacks. The risk was similar to that observed among firefighters during the attack (108), and it increased in those of young age, female gender, and with exposure to the dust cloud (109).

## ENVIRONMENTAL POLLUTION AND CVD RISK FACTORS

Hypertension, type 2 diabetes mellitus, and dyslipidemia are the modifiable proximal risk factors for CVD. These risk factors are associated with exposure to environmental pollution such as ambient and household air pollution as well as chemical toxins. Hypertension is the leading risk factor for CVD risk, and systematic evidence from developed countries and China indicate associations with both short-term (≤30 days) and long-term exposures (≥30 days) to components of ambient air pollution such as $PM_{2.5}$, $PM_{10}$, $SO_2$, $NO_2$, CO, $O_3$, and hypertension (odds ratio [OR]: 1.05–1.1 per 10 µg/m$^3$) (110). Diastolic and systolic blood pressure increases by 0.15–0.86 mmHg per 10 mg/m$^3$ are also observed (110). While long-term effects were more pronounced in the elderly, short-term exposures affected young adults. In LMIC populations, risk factors like hypertension and type 2 diabetes mellitus increased by odds in the range of 1.14–1.32 per 10 µg/m$^3$ increase of $PM_{2.5}$ (98).

The use of household solid fuel in LMICs, primarily by women, is significantly associated with an increased risk of hypertension, more so in groups controlled for smoking (summary OR: 2.38 versus 1.11 in smoking uncontrolled groups) (111). The suggested biological mechanisms are similar, ranging from stimulation of the sympathetic autonomic nervous system, systemic inflammation by vasoactive molecules, and epigenetic mechanisms such as DNA methylation. Further, air pollution is found to increase the risk of type 2 diabetes in a dose-dependent manner with increasing exposure duration and concentrations of pollutants, particularly among the elderly, obese individuals, and pregnant women. This is possibly due to increased inflammation, oxidative stress, and endoplasmic reticulum stress (112). Lipid dysregulation by up to 4% is observed for the association between $PM_{10}$ and $NO_2$ exposures and increased triglyceride (TG) levels (113).

Although the role of chemical toxins (e.g., pesticides and heavy metals) in water, soil, and the food chain for these risk factors is still emerging, pesticides are found to be associated with the risk of systemic arterial hypertension, type 2 diabetes, hypertensive disorders in pregnancy, and preeclampsia, as well as altered lipid profile (114). While lipid-soluble persistent organic pollutants (POPs, such as polychlorinated dibenzo-p-dioxins, 2-polychlorinated dibenzofurans, and polychlorinated biphenyls [PCBs], 3-brominated flame retardants, and organochlorines) are related to TG and LDL-C, lipid non-soluble POPs (perfluoroalkyl substance) are related to total cholesterol levels (114). Although the exact mechanism of action is unclear, POPs accumulate in adipose tissue and preserved from metabolism, leading to persistent effects. Heavy metals such as arsenic and lead are linked to hypertension. In addition to the suggested mechanisms of action such as chronic inflammation and oxidative stress, these metals also induce immune function impairment and compete with essential nutrients such as iron, calcium, and zinc and cause deficiency (115). The role of these risk factors as a mediator on the environmental pollution adverse CVD effects and different sources of exposures is yet to be studied. For example, recent explorations in endemic regions of India indicate that exposure to arsenic through food items such as rice, wheat, and potatoes is more than through drinking water (116). The temporal effects of environmental pollution on these risk factors in LMIC settings need to be further explored, and a few early longitudinal repeated explorations in India where the environmental pollution levels are one of the highest globally reveal positive associations with $PM_{2.5}$ exposures for systolic blood pressure and incident hypertension that is non-linear (HR: 1.5–1.1 with increasing exposure time) that is more pronounced in obese individuals (5). It is noted that achieving national ambient air quality standards can potentially decrease the prevalence of hypertension by 15% in urban Delhi regions of India (5). Nevertheless, no associations for pesticide exposures for incident type 2 diabetes in the same population despite high exposure levels are found (117).

## EARLY LIFE EXPOSURES TO ENVIRONMENTAL FACTORS AND CVD RISK AND MORTALITY

Every year, >3 million people worldwide die of IHD or stroke attributed to air pollution, more than from other modifiable cardiac disease risks such as obesity, diabetes mellitus, or cigarette smoking. The cardiopulmonary systems of children are rapidly developing and are therefore more vulnerable to injury and inflammation caused by pollutants. The published evidence about the adverse effects of pollution exposure on major CVD risks and cardiovascular phenotypes in pregnant women, neonates, and children is strongly suggestive that the exposure to PM, polycyclic aromatic hydrocarbons (PAHs), or $NO_2$ during pregnancy or in early childhood up to 10–12 years of age impacted hypertension, obesity, dyslipidemia, and glucose metabolism in children during critical windows of growth. For instance, neonatal (from birth to 1 month of life) exposure to $PM_{2.5}$ is associated with increased systolic blood pressure at ages 3–9 years, and insulin resistance increased by 17% for every 2 standard deviations (SDs) of increase in ambient PM and $NO_2$ in 10-year old children. Similarly, with a history of exposure to PAH, the prevalence of obesity was over 20% among 5-year-old children and increased to 33% during follow-ups until age 11 years (2). Evidence indicates that infants (birth to 1 year of life) exposed to high traffic-related pollution in early life may have rapid postnatal weight gain (2). Moreover, maternal exposure to PAH, PM, and $NO_2$ is shown to be negatively correlated with fetal growth indicators, adding interlinks between fetal programming and environmental pollution (118–120).

While environmental pollution contributes to climate change, recent studies have found that climate change has, in turn, some indirect effects on cardiovascular risk. After food insecurity, worsening socioeconomic circumstances, and rising temperatures, maternal nutrition in pregnancy is adversely affected, and this can lead to intrauterine growth restriction. As we've just seen, low birth weight is a consequence of intrauterine growth retardation and has effects on cardiovascular health in later life (88). Additionally, exposure to extreme heat in pregnancy has been found to be associated with preeclampsia and eclampsia, which can lead to premature births and low birth weight offspring (121, 122).

## EXPOSOME AND POLLUTOME (FIGURE 6.1)

In relation to the environmental risk factors and exposures, two recent terminologies include 'exposome' and 'pollutome'. The exposome (proposed by Christopher P. Wild in 2005) is the lifelong contributions of all the environmental risk factors to an individual's pathophysiology. In addition to the environmental factors, lifestyle (i.e., tobacco, alcohol, diet, physical activity), and general environmental factors such as SES, urban environment, pathogens, solar radiation, and climate are included to define an individual's exposome (97). A smaller subset of the exposome is defined as the 'pollutome', which includes "pollutant exposures at a specific period of an individual's life-span, for example, during gestation, infancy, childhood, adulthood, or old age". The pollutome accounts for the sum total of all forms of pollution during the specified period, including occupational exposures, if relevant.

## POLLUTION MITIGATION AND PREVENTION

Pollution mitigation and prevention need intersectoral intervention efforts ranging from awareness and knowledge, to social mobilization to effective policy recommendations, to implementation and impact evaluation. These approaches need to be context- and region-specific; however, lessons from developed regions and other LMICs may be helpful (*see Panel 3*).

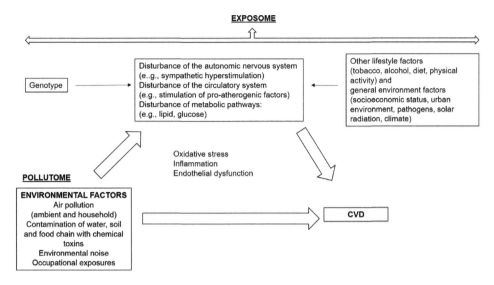

**Figure 6.1** Pollutome and exposome for CVD risk.

**Panel 3**: Household air pollution and toxic chemicals mitigation efforts

Across many LMICs over several decades, programmes have been implemented for reducing household air pollution with variable success rate. Few fairly good examples are improved stove programme (China) and liquefied petroleum gas (LPG) programme- India (123). However, these programmes have not been evaluated adequately for CVD benefits.

### CHINA'S NATIONAL IMPROVED STOVE PROGRAMME

China's National Improved Stove Programme (1982–92) distributed improved cookstoves with chimneys to people in rural areas of China, to reduce smoke from the use of biomass fuel. This programme lowered household air pollution levels with fuel efficiency. However, as the smoke was not actually reduced but only moved to the outside through chimneys, some exposures persisted. Nevertheless, cohort studies in Chinese farmers (1976 to 1992) showed that stove improvement was associated with up to 40% reduction in lung cancer incidence (124) and over 50% reduction in pneumonia deaths (125).

### INDIAN NATIONAL PROGRAMME ON IMPROVED CHULHA AND
### SUBSEQUENT LIQUEFIED PETROLEUM GAS PROGRAMME

The Indian National Programme on Improved Chulha stoves (1984 to 2001), had little effect on fuel efficiency and smoke reduction. This programme has been replaced by liquefied petroleum gas (LPG) programme in 2016, in which families with better socio-economic status give up their LPG subsidy to families below poverty line. The impact of this in terms of CVD and other health outcomes is yet to be studied.

The other prominent examples are Gyapa Stoves Project, Accra, Ghana which improved air quality by 40–45% and Ecuador's electric induction stove programme. Countries with adequate hydropower potential, such as Paraguay and Bhutan, also are trying to implement electric stove projects in their countries (123).

### KURICHI INDUSTRIAL CLUSTER EXPERIENCE, COIMBATORE CITY, TAMILNADU, SOUTH INDIA

Central Pollution Control Board report (2009) implied critical pollution in groundwater in the industrial regions of Coimbatore, a South Indian city. Aggressive monitoring steps were taken by Tamilnadu pollution control Board including reverse-osmosis water treatment plants to treat effluents and rain water harvesting along with water recycling implementation. These efforts led to reduction of pollution levels in the groundwater as comparable to non-industrial regions in 2015 (126).

REFERENCES

1. World Health Organization. Preventing disease through healthy environments: a global assessment of the burden of disease from environmental risks. 2018. Available from: https://www.who.int/publications/i/item/9789241565196

2. Kim JB, Prunicki M, Haddad F, Dant C, Sampath V, Patel R, et al. Cumulative lifetime burden of cardiovascular disease from early exposure to air pollution. J Am Heart Assoc. 2020;9(6):e014944.

3. Ministry of Health and Family Welfare GoI, UNICEF, Population Council. India comprehensive national nutrition survey 2019. Available from: www.popcouncil.org/research/india-comprehensive-national-nutrition-survey

4. Health Effects Institute. State of Global Air. 2020. Available from: www.stateofglobalair.org [accessed 09/06/2022].

5. Prabhakaran D, Mandal S, Krishna B, Magsumbol M, Singh K, Tandon N, et al. Exposure to particulate matter is associated with elevated blood pressure and incident hypertension in urban India. Hypertension (Dallas, Tex: 1979). 2020;76(4):1289–1298.

6. Kermack WO, McKendrick AG, McKinlay PL. Death-rates in Great Britain and Sweden. Some general regularities and their significance. Lancet. 1934:698–703.

7. Ciocco A, Klein H, Palmer CE. Child health and the selective service physical standards. Public Health Rep (1896–1970). 1941:2365–2375.

8. Dubos R, Savage D, Schaedler R. Biological Freudianism: lasting effects of early environmental influences. Pediatrics. 1966;38(5):789–800.

9. Forsdahl A. Are poor living conditions in childhood and adolescence an important risk factor for arteriosclerotic heart disease? J Epidemiol Commun Health. 1977;31(2):91–95.

10. Forsdahl A. Living conditions in childhood and subsequent development of risk factors for arteriosclerotic heart disease. The cardiovascular survey in Finnmark 1974–1975. J Epidemiol Commun Health. 1978;32(1):34–37.

11. Barker DJ, Osmond C, Law C. The intrauterine and early postnatal origins of cardiovascular disease and chronic bronchitis. J Epidemiol Commun Health. 1989;43(3):237–240.

12. Barker DJ, Osmond C. Infant mortality, childhood nutrition, and ischaemic heart disease in England and Wales. Lancet. 1986;327(8489):1077–1081.

13. Barker DJ, Osmond C, Winter P, Margetts B, Simmonds SJ. Weight in infancy and death from ischaemic heart disease. Lancet. 1989;334(8663):577–580.

14. Barker DJ, Forsén T, Uutela A, Osmond C, Eriksson JG. Size at birth and resilience to effects of poor living conditions in adult life: longitudinal study. BMJ (Clinical research ed). 2001;323(7324):1273.

15. Barker D, Bull AR, Osmond C, Simmonds SJ. Fetal and placental size and risk of hypertension in adult life. BMJ. 1990;301(6746):259–262.

16. Barker D, Godfrey K, Osmond C, Bull A. The relation of fetal length, ponderal index and head circumference to blood pressure and the risk of hypertension in adult life. Paediatr Perinat Epidemiol. 1992;6(1):35–44.

17. Hales CN, Barker DJ, Clark PM, Cox LJ, Fall C, Osmond C, et al. Fetal and infant growth and impaired glucose tolerance at age 64. BMJ. 1991;303(6809):1019–1022.

18. Barker D, Martyn C, Osmond C, Hales C, Fall C. Growth in utero and serum cholesterol concentrations in adult life. BMJ. 1993;307(6918):1524–1527.

19. Martyn C, Meade T, Stirling Y, Barker D. Plasma concentrations of fibrinogen and factor VII in adult life and their relation to intra-uterine growth. BrJ Haematol. 1995;89(1):142–146.

20. Huxley R, Neil A, Collins R. Unravelling the fetal origins hypothesis: is there really an inverse association between birthweight and subsequent blood pressure? Lancet. 2002;360(9334):659–665.

21. Stanner SA, Bulmer K, Andres C, Lantseva OE, Borodina V, Poteen V, et al. Does malnutrition in utero determine diabetes and coronary heart disease in adulthood? Results from the Leningrad siege study, a cross sectional study. BMJ (Clinical research ed). 1997;315(7119):1342–1348.

22. Kannisto V, Christensen K, Vaupel JW. No increased mortality in later life for cohorts bom during famine. Am J Epidemiol. 1997;145(11):987–994.

23. Ravelli AC, van der Meulen JH, Michels R, Osmond C, Barker DJ, Hales C, et al. Glucose tolerance in adults after prenatal exposure to famine. Lancet. 1998;351(9097):173–177.

24. Lancet T. An overstretched hypothesis? Elsevier; 2001.

25. Bateson P. Fetal experience and good adult design a. Int J Epidemiol. 2001;30(5):928–934.
26. Bateson P, Barker D, Clutton-Brock T, Deb D, D'Udine B, Foley RA, et al. Developmental plasticity and human health. Nature. 2004;430(6998):419–421.
27. Bateson P, Gluckman P, Hanson M. The biology of developmental plasticity and the Predictive Adaptive Response hypothesis. J Physiol. 2014;592(11):2357–2368.
28. De Boo HA, Harding JE. The developmental origins of adult disease (Barker) hypothesis. Aust N Z J Obstet Gynaecol. 2006;46(1):4–14.
29. Lynch J, Smith GD. A life course approach to chronic disease epidemiology. Annu Rev Public Health. 2005;26:1–35.
30. Gluckman PD, Hanson MA. The developmental origins of health and disease. Early life origins of health and disease. Springer; 2006. pp. 1–7.
31. Stuart A, Amer-Wåhlin I, Persson J, Källen K. Long-term cardiovascular risk in relation to birth weight and exposure to maternal diabetes mellitus. Int J Cardiol. 2013;168(3):2653–2657.
32. Biosca M, Rodríguez G, Ventura P, Samper MP, Labayen I, Collado MP, et al. Central adiposity in children born small and large for gestational age. Nutr Hosp. 2011;26(5):971–976.
33. Jaquet D, Deghmoun S, Chevenne D, Collin D, Czernichow P, Levy-Marchal C. Dynamic change in adiposity from fetal to postnatal life is involved in the metabolic syndrome associated with reduced fetal growth. Diabetologia. 2005;48(5):849–855.
34. Parker L, Lamont D, Unwin N, Pearce M, Bennett S, Dickinson H, et al. A lifecourse study of risk for hyperinsulinaemia, dyslipidaemia and obesity (the central metabolic syndrome) at age 49–51 years. Diabet Med. 2003;20(5):406–415.
35. Ibáñez L, Ong K, Dunger DB, de Zegher F. Early development of adiposity and insulin resistance after catch-up weight gain in small-for-gestational-age children. J Clin Endocrinol Metabol. 2006;91(6):2153–2158.
36. Druet C, Ong KK. Early childhood predictors of adult body composition. Best Pract Res C lin Endocrinol Metab. 2008;22(3):489–502.
37. Eriksson JG, Forsen T, Tuomilehto J, Osmond C, Barker DJ. Early growth and coronary heart disease in later life: longitudinal study. BMJ (Clinical research ed). 2001;322(7292):949–953.
38. Forsen T, Osmond C, Eriksson J, Barker D. Growth of girls who later develop coronary heart disease. Heart. 2004;90(1):20–24.
39. Eriksson J, Forsen T, Tuomilehto J, Osmond C, Barker D. Fetal and childhood growth and hypertension in adult life. Hypertension. 2000;36(5):790–794.
40. Eriksson JG, Forsen T, Tuomilehto J, Osmond C, Barker DJ. Early adiposity rebound in childhood and risk of Type 2 diabetes in adult life. Diabetologia. 2003;46(2):190–194.
41. Joglekar C, Fall C, Deshpande V, Joshi N, Bhalerao A, Solat V, et al. Newborn size, infant and childhood growth, and body composition and cardiovascular disease risk factors at the age of 6 years: the Pune Maternal Nutrition Study. Int J Obesity. 2007;31(10):1534–1544.
42. Juonala M, Magnussen CG, Berenson GS, Venn A, Burns TL, Sabin MA, et al. Childhood adiposity, adult adiposity, and cardiovascular risk factors. New England J Med. 2011;365:1876–1885.
43. Franks PW, Hanson RL, Knowler WC, Sievers ML, Bennett PH, Looker HC. Childhood obesity, other cardiovascular risk factors, and premature death. New England J Med. 2010;362(6):485–493.
44. Gunnell DJ, Frankel SJ, Nanchahal K, Peters TJ, Davey Smith G. Childhood obesity and adult cardiovascular mortality: a 57-y follow-up study based on the Boyd Orr cohort. Am J Clin Nutrit. 1998;67(6):1111–1118.
45. Caulfield LE, Richard SA, Rivera JA, Musgrove P, Black RE. Stunting, wasting, and micronutrient deficiency disorders. Disease Control Priorities in Developing Countries, 2nd edition. Oxford University Press; 2006.
46. Kruger HS, Pretorius R, Schutte AE. Stunting, adiposity, and low-grade inflammation in African adolescents from a township high school. Nutrition. 2010;26(1):90–99.
47. van Rooyen JM, Kruger HS, Huisman HW, Schutte AE, Malan NT, Schutte R. Early cardiovascular changes in 10- to 15-year-old stunted children: the transition and health during urbanization in South Africa in children study. Nutrition. 2005;21(7–8):808–814.
48. Sferruzzi-Perri AN, Vaughan OR, Haro M, Cooper WN, Musial B, Charalambous M, et al. An obesogenic diet during mouse pregnancy modifies maternal nutrient partitioning and the fetal growth trajectory. FASEB J. 2013;27(10):3928–3937.

49. Franco J, Fernandes T, Rocha C, Calvino C, Pazos-Moura C, Lisboa P, et al. Maternal high-fat diet induces obesity and adrenal and thyroid dysfunction in male rat offspring at weaning. J Physiol. 2012;590(21):5503–5518.

50. Retnakaran R, Ye C, Hanley AJ, Connelly PW, Sermer M, Zinman B, et al. Effect of maternal weight, adipokines, glucose intolerance and lipids on infant birth weight among women without gestational diabetes mellitus. CMAJ: Can Med Assoc J = journal de l'Association medicale canadienne. 2012;184(12):1353–1360.

51. Gray C, Al-Dujaili EA, Sparrow AJ, Gardiner SM, Craigon J, Welham SJ, et al. Excess maternal salt intake produces sex-specific hypertension in offspring: putative roles for kidney and gastrointestinal sodium handling. PloS One. 2013;8(8):e72682.

52. Wood-Bradley RJ, Henry SL, Vrselja A, Newman V, Armitage JA. Maternal dietary intake during pregnancy has longstanding consequences for the health of her offspring. Can J Physiol Pharmacol. 2013;91(6):412–420.

53. Reilly JJ, Armstrong J, Dorosty AR, Emmett PM, Ness A, Rogers I, et al. Early life risk factors for obesity in childhood: cohort study. BMJ (Clinical research ed). 2005;330(7504):1357.

54. McCrory C, Layte R. Breastfeeding and risk of overweight and obesity at nine-years of age. Soc Sci Med. 2012;75(2):323–330.

55. Hörnell A, Lagström H, Lande B, Thorsdottir I. Breastfeeding, introduction of other foods and effects on health: a systematic literature review for the 5th Nordic Nutrition Recommendations. Food & Nutrition Research. 2013;57(1):20823.

56. Owen CG, Whincup PH, Odoki K, Gilg JA, Cook DG. Infant feeding and blood cholesterol: a study in adolescents and a systematic review. Pediatrics. 2002;110(3):597–608.

57. Singhal A, Cole TJ, Fewtrell M, Lucas A. Breastmilk feeding and lipoprotein profile in adolescents born preterm: follow-up of a prospective randomised study. Lancet. 2004;363(9421):1571–1578.

58. Kramer MS, Matush L, Vanilovich I, Platt RW, Bogdanovich N, Sevkovskaya Z, et al. Effects of prolonged and exclusive breastfeeding on child height, weight, adiposity, and blood pressure at age 6.5 y: evidence from a large randomized trial. Am J Clin Nutr. 2007;86(6):1717–1721.

59. Kelishadi R, Ardalan G, Gheiratmand R, Majdzadeh R, Delavari A, Heshmat R, et al. Blood pressure and its influencing factors in a national representative sample of Iranian children and adolescents: the CASPIAN Study. Eur J Prevent Cardiol. 2006;13(6):956–963.

60. Haugen M, Brantsæter AL, Winkvist A, Lissner L, Alexander J, Oftedal B, et al. Associations of pre-pregnancy body mass index and gestational weight gain with pregnancy outcome and postpartum weight retention: a prospective observational cohort study. BMC Pregnancy Childbirth. 2014;14(1):1–11.

61. Gruszfeld D, Socha P. Early nutrition and health: short-and long-term outcomes. Evidence-Based Research in Pediatric Nutrition. 108: Karger Publishers; 2013. pp. 32–39.

62. Au CP, Raynes-Greenow CH, Turner RM, Carberry AE, Jeffery H. Fetal and maternal factors associated with neonatal adiposity as measured by air displacement plethysmography: a large cross-sectional study. Early Hum Dev. 2013;89(10):839–843.

63. Brion M-JA, Leary SD, Lawlor DA, Smith GD, Ness AR. Modifiable maternal exposures and offspring blood pressure: a review of epidemiological studies of maternal age, diet, and smoking. Pediatr Res. 2008;63(6):593–598.

64. Mamun AA, O'Callaghan MJ, Williams GM, Najman JM. Maternal smoking during pregnancy predicts adult offspring cardiovascular risk factors—evidence from a community-based large birth cohort study. PloS One. 2012;7(7):e41106.

65. Horta BL, Gigante DP, Nazmi A, Silveira VMF, Oliveira I, Victora CG. Maternal smoking during pregnancy and risk factors for cardiovascular disease in adulthood. Atherosclerosis. 2011;219(2):815–820.

66. Yan J, Yang H. Gestational diabetes mellitus, programing and epigenetics. J Matern Fetal Neonatal Med. 2014;27(12):1266–1269.

67. Cheng X, Chapple SJ, Patel B, Puszyk W, Sugden D, Yin X, et al. Gestational diabetes mellitus impairs Nrf2-mediated adaptive antioxidant defenses and redox signaling in fetal endothelial cells in utero. Diabetes. 2013;62(12):4088–4097.

68. Reynolds RM, Allan KM, Raja EA, Bhattacharya S, McNeill G, Hannaford PC, et al. Maternal obesity during pregnancy and premature mortality from cardiovascular event in adult offspring: follow-up of 1 323 275 person years. BMJ (Clinical Research ed). 2013;347.

69. Golley RK, Smithers LG, Mittinty MN, Emmett P, Northstone K, Lynch JW. Diet quality of UK infants is associated with dietary, adiposity, cardiovascular, and cognitive outcomes measured at 7–8 years of age. J Nutr. 2013;143(10):1611–1617.

70. Patrick H, Hennessy E, McSpadden K, Oh A. Parenting styles and practices in children's obesogenic behaviors: scientific gaps and future research directions. Child Obes. 2013;9(s1):S73–S86.

71. Magnussen CG, Smith KJ, Juonala M. When to prevent cardiovascular disease? As early as possible: lessons from prospective cohorts beginning in childhood. Curr Opin Cardiol. 2013;28(5):561–568.

72. Kelishadi R, Razaghi EM, Gouya MM, Ardalan G, Gheiratmand R, Delavari A, et al. Association of physical activity and the metabolic syndrome in children and adolescents: CASPIAN study. Horm Res. 2007;67(1):46–52.

73. McMurray RG. Insights into physical activity and cardiovascular disease risk in young children: IDEFICS study. BMC Med. 2013;11:173.

74. Subramanian SK, Sharma VK, A V. Comparison of effect of regular unstructured physical training and athletic level training on body composition and cardio respiratory fitness in adolescents. J Clin Diagn Res. 2013;7(9):1878–1882.

75. Whitley E, Lee IM, Sesso HD, Batty GD. Association of cigarette smoking from adolescence to middle-age with later total and cardiovascular disease mortality: theHarvard Alumni Health Study. J Am Coll Cardiol. 2012;60(18):1839–1840.

76. Galobardes B, Smith GD, Lynch JW. Systematic review of the influence of childhood socioeconomic circumstances on risk for cardiovascular disease in adulthood. Ann Epidemiol. 2006;16(2):91–104.

77. Galobardes B, Lynch JW, Davey Smith G. Childhood socioeconomic circumstances and cause-specific mortality in adulthood: systematic review and interpretation. Epidemiol Rev. 2004;26:7–21.

78. Ali MK, Bhaskarapillai B, Shivashankar R, Mohan D, Fatmi ZA, Pradeepa R, et al. Socioeconomic status and cardiovascular risk in urban South Asia: The CARRS Study. Eur J Prev Cardiol. 2016;23(4):408–419.

79. Rosengren A, Smyth A, Rangarajan S, Ramasundarahettige C, Bangdiwala SI, AlHabib KF, et al. Socioeconomic status and risk of cardiovascular disease in 20 low-income, middle-income, and high-income countries: the prospective urban rural epidemiologic (PURE) study. Lancet Glob Health. 2019;7(6):e748–e60.

80. Corsi DJ, Subramanian S. Socioeconomic gradients and distribution of diabetes, hypertension, and obesity in India. JAMA Network Open. 2019;2(4):e190411–e.

81. Glymour MM, Clark CR, Patton KK. Socioeconomic determinants of cardiovascular disease: recent findings and future directions. Curr Epidemiol Rep 2014;1(2):89–97.

82. Power C, Manor O, Matthews S. The duration and timing of exposure: effects of socioeconomic environment on adult health. Am J Public Health. 1999;89(7):1059–1065.

83. McDonough P, Duncan GJ, Williams D, House J. Income dynamics and adult mortality in the United States, 1972 through 1989. Am J Public Health. 1997;87(9):1476–1483.

84. Gardner D, Tingey K, Van Bon B, Ozanne S, Wilson V, Dandrea J, et al. Programming of glucose-insulin metabolism in adult sheep after maternal undernutrition. Am J Physiol Regul Integr Comp Physiol. 2005;289(4):R947–R954.

85. Kind KL, Simonetta G, Clifton PM, Robinson JS, Owens JA. Effect of maternal feed restriction on blood pressure in the adult guinea pig. Experimental physiology. 2002;87(4):469–477.

86. Woodall S, Johnston B, Breier B, Gluckman P. Chronic maternal undernutrition in the rat leads to delayed postnatal growth and elevated blood pressure of offspring. Pediatric Research. 1996;40(3):438–443.

87. Desai M, Crowther NJ, Lucas A, Hales CN. Organ-selective growth in the offspring of protein-restricted mothers. Br J Nutr. 1996;76(4):591–603.

88. Sheffield PE, Landrigan PJ. Global climate change and children's health: threats and strategies for prevention. Environ Health Perspect. 2011;119(3):291–298.

89. Robillard JE, Segar JL. Influence of early life events on health and diseases. Trans Am Clin Climatol Assoc. 2006;117:313.

90. Aulchenko YS, Ripatti S, Lindqvist I, Boomsma D, Heid IM, Pramstaller PP, et al. Loci influencing lipid levels and coronary heart disease risk in 16 European population cohorts. Nat Genet. 2009;41(1):47–55.

91. Kristiansson K, Perola M, Tikkanen E, Kettunen J, Surakka I, Havulinna AS, et al. Genome-wide screen for metabolic syndrome susceptibility Loci reveals strong lipid gene contribution but no evidence for common genetic basis for clustering of metabolic syndrome traits. Circ Cardiovasc Genet. 2012;5(2):242–249.

92. Franceschini N, Reiner AP, Heiss G. Recent findings in the genetics of blood pressure and hypertension traits. Am J Hypertens. 2011;24(4):392–400.

93. Ehret GB. Genome-wide association studies: contribution of genomics to understanding blood pressure and essential hypertension. Curr Hypertens Rep. 2010;12(1):17–25.

94. Santos MS, Joles JA. Early determinants of cardiovascular disease. Best Pract Res Clin Endocrinol Metab. 2012;26(5):581–597.

95. Heindel JJ, Vandenberg LN. Developmental origins of health and disease: a paradigm for understanding disease etiology and prevention. Curr Opin Pediatr. 2015;27(2):248.

96. Almond D, Currie J. Killing me softly: The fetal origins hypothesis. J Econ Perspect. 2011;25(3):153–172.

97. Daiber A, Lelieveld J, Steven S, Oelze M, Kroller-Schon S, Sorensen M, et al. The "exposome" concept—how environmental risk factors influence cardiovascular health. Acta Biochim Pol. 2019;66(3):269–283.

98. Jaganathan S, Jaacks LM, Magsumbol M, Walia GK, Sieber NL, Shivasankar R, et al. Association of long-term exposure to fine particulate matter and cardio-metabolic diseases in low- and middle-income countries: a systematic review. Int J Environ Res Public Health. 2019;16(14).

99. Shah AS, Lee KK, McAllister DA, Hunter A, Nair H, Whiteley W, et al. Short term exposure to air pollution and stroke: systematic review and meta-analysis. Bmj. 2015;350:h1295.

100. Stafoggia M, Cesaroni G, Peters A, Andersen ZJ, Badaloni C, Beelen R, et al. Long-term exposure to ambient air pollution and incidence of cerebrovascular events: results from 11 European cohorts within the ESCAPE project. Environ Health Perspect. 2014;122(9):919–925.

101. Brauer M, Brook JR, Christidis T, Chu Y, Crouse DL, Erickson A, et al. Mortality-air pollution associations in low-exposure environments (MAPLE): Phase 1. Res Rep (Health Effects Institute). 2019(203):1–87.

102. Frieden TR, Cobb LK, Leidig RC, Mehta S, Kass D. Reducing premature mortality from cardiovascular and other non-communicable diseases by one third: achieving sustainable development goal indicator 3.4.1. Glob Heart. 2020;15(1):50.

103. Zago AM, Faria NMX, Favero JL, Meucci RD, Woskie S, Fassa AG. Pesticide exposure and risk of cardiovascular disease: A systematic review. Glob Public Health. 2020:1–23.

104. Chowdhury R, Ramond A, O'Keeffe LM, Shahzad S, Kunutsor SK, Muka T, et al. Environmental toxic metal contaminants and risk of cardiovascular disease: systematic review and meta-analysis. BMJ. 2018;362:k3310.

105. Xu L, Mondal D, Polya DA. Positive association of cardiovascular disease (CVD) with chronic exposure to drinking water arsenic (as) at concentrations below the WHO provisional guideline value: a systematic review and meta-analysis. Int J Environ Res Public Health. 2020;17(7).

106. Moon KA, Oberoi S, Barchowsky A, Chen Y, Guallar E, Nachman KE, et al. A dose-response meta-analysis of chronic arsenic exposure and incident cardiovascular disease. Int J Epidemiol. 2017;46(6):1924–1939.

107. Petronio L. Chemical and physical agents of work-related cardiovascular diseases. Eur Heart J. 1988;9(suppl_L):26–34.

108. Cohen HW, Zeig-Owens R, Joe C, Hall CB, Webber MP, Weiden MD, et al. Long-term cardiovascular disease risk among firefighters after the world trade center disaster. JAMA Netw Open. 2019;2(9):e199775.

109. Sloan NL, Shapiro MZ, Sabra A, Dasaro CR, Crane MA, Harrison DJ, et al. Cardiovascular disease in the world trade center health program general responder cohort. Am J Ind Med. 2021;64(2):97–107.

110. Yang BY, Qian Z, Howard SW, Vaughn MG, Fan SJ, Liu KK, et al. Global association between ambient air pollution and blood pressure: a systematic review and meta-analysis. Environ Pollut. 2018;235:576–588.

111. Li L, Yang A, He X, Liu J, Ma Y, Niu J, et al. Indoor air pollution from solid fuels and hypertension: a systematic review and meta-analysis. Environ Pollut. 2020;259:113914.

112. Li Y, Xu L, Shan Z, Teng W, Han C. Association between air pollution and type 2 diabetes: an updated review of the literature. Ther Adv Endocrinol Metab. 2019;10:2042018819897046.

113. Gaio V, Roquette R, Dias CM, Nunes B. Ambient air pollution and lipid profile: Systematic review and meta-analysis. Environ Pollut. 2019;254(Pt B):113036.

114. Lind PM, Lind L. Are persistent organic pollutants linked to lipid abnormalities, atherosclerosis and cardiovascular disease? A review. J Lipid Atheroscler. 2020;9(3):334–348.

115. Yang AM, Lo K, Zheng TZ, Yang JL, Bai YN, Feng YQ, et al. Environmental heavy metals and cardiovascular diseases: status and future direction. Chronic Dis Transl Med. 2020;6(4):251–259.

116. Mondal D, Rahman MM, Suman S, Sharma P, Siddique AB, Rahman MA, et al. Arsenic exposure from food exceeds that from drinking water in endemic area of Bihar, India. Sci Total Environ. 2021;754:142082.

117. Jaacks LM, Yadav S, Panuwet P, Kumar S, Rajacharya GH, Johnson C, et al. Metabolite of the pesticide DDT and incident type 2 diabetes in urban India. Environ Int. 2019;133(Pt A):105089.

118. Zhao Y, Song Q, Ge W, Jin Y, Chen S, Zhao Y, et al. Associations between in utero exposure to polybrominated diphenyl ethers, pathophysiological state of fetal growth and placental DNA methylation changes. Environ Int. 2019;133(Pt B):105255.

119. van den Hooven EH, Pierik FH, de Kluizenaar Y, Willemsen SP, Hofman A, van Ratingen SW, et al. Air pollution exposure during pregnancy, ultrasound measures of fetal growth, and adverse birth outcomes: a prospective cohort study. Environ Health Perspect. 2012;120(1):150–156.

120. Iñiguez C, Esplugues A, Sunyer J, Basterrechea M, Fernández-Somoano A, Costa O, et al. Prenatal exposure to NO2 and ultrasound measures of fetal growth in the Spanish INMA cohort. Environ Health Perspect. 2016;124(2):235–242.

121. Subramaniam V. Seasonal variation in the incidence of preeclampsia and eclampsia in tropical climatic conditions. BMC Womens Health. 2007;7:18.

122. Deschenes O, Greenstone M, Guryan J. Climate change and birth weight. Am Econ Rev. 2009;99(2):211–217.

123. Landrigan PJ, Fuller R, Acosta NJR, Adeyi O, Arnold R, Basu NN, et al. The Lancet Commission on pollution and health. Lancet. 2018;391(10119):462–512.

124. Hosgood HD, 3rd, Chapman R, Shen M, Blair A, Chen E, Zheng T, et al. Portable stove use is associated with lower lung cancer mortality risk in lifetime smoky coal users. Br J Cancer. 2008;99(11):1934–1939.

125. Shen M, Chapman RS, Vermeulen R, Tian L, Zheng T, Chen BE, et al. Coal use, stove improvement, and adult pneumonia mortality in Xuanwei, China: a retrospective cohort study. Environ Health Perspect. 2009;117(2):261–266.

126. Mohankumar K, Hariharan V, Rao NP. Heavy metal contamination in groundwater around industrial estate vs residential areas in Coimbatore, India. J Clin Diagnostic Res: JCDR. 2016;10(4):BC05–BC07.

# 7 Social Determinants of Cardiovascular Diseases

*Panniyammakal Jeemon and K. Srinath Reddy*

## CONTENTS

## INTRODUCTION

Globally, cardiovascular disease (CVD) is the leading cause of death and morbidity.[1,2] In 2017, close to 18 million deaths were attributed to CVD globally.[1] Further, 486 million CVD cases were estimated to be prevalent in 2017.[2,3] Together the mortality and morbidity correspond to 330 million years of life lost and another 35.6 million years lived with disability.[1,4] The steep rise in the epidemic of CVD burden is reflected in the 21% increase in number of deaths in 2017 as compared with the deaths in 2007.[1,3] Ischemic heart disease (IHD) and stroke are the main constituents of CVD.[5] Worldwide, close to 9 and 6 million deaths are attributable to IHD and stroke, respectively.[5] The mean lifetime risk of stroke is estimated to be around 25% globally.[6]

Low- and middle-income countries (LMICs) bear disproportionately higher burdens due to CVD. For example, nearly 80% of global CVD deaths occur in LMICs.[5] Traditional cardiovascular risk factors explain a large proportion of the burden attributable to CVD. However, many of them are mediated by social determinants of health. The World Health Organization (WHO) defines the social determinants of health quite broadly as "the circumstances in which people are born, grow, live, work, and age, and the systems put in place to deal with illness.[7]" It is based on the understanding that health and illness often cluster at the intersections of social, economic, environmental, and interpersonal forces. CVD is not an exception to this rule, and it is influenced by social determinants. However, the social determinants of CVD are often an overlooked component in many parts of the world.

In this chapter, we aim to increase awareness of the influence of social factors on the prevalence, incidence, treatment, and outcomes of CVD among students interested in global health. We summarize the current state of knowledge about the social factors associated with CVD globally. Additionally, we suggest future directions in research, particularly research on effective interventions to alleviate the potential adverse social influences.

## MEASURING SOCIAL DETERMINANTS OF HEALTH

Social determinants of health are a spectrum of social, economic, political, and environmental variables. The indicators of socioeconomic position are often interrelated with each other, and none of them individually measure the influence of all the variables. However, indicators such as wealth, income, education, employment, occupation, race, ethnicity, cast, social support, social network, culture, and residential environment collectively reflect the socioeconomic position of an individual. Nobel Laureate Joseph Stiglitz headed the Commission on the Measurement of Economic Performance and Social Progress, describes and emphasizes the multidimensional nature of socioeconomic position.[8] A conceptual framework (Figure 7.1) developed by the WHO on social determinants of health describes the sociopolitical context that defines the structural mechanisms to generate social stratification, class divisions, and socioeconomic position, in order to account for them in the design of public health policy.[9] Further, it explains that the health system as a social determinant of health plays an important role in mediating the different outcomes of diseases that generate health inequities.[9]

The left-to-right arrows indicate how the hierarchy of structural and intermediary determinants contribute to shape the state of health and well-being of the populations. Right-to-left arrows indicate how intersectoral policies may proceed from a population basis, affecting the public health and societal sectors.

DOI: 10.1201/b23266-16

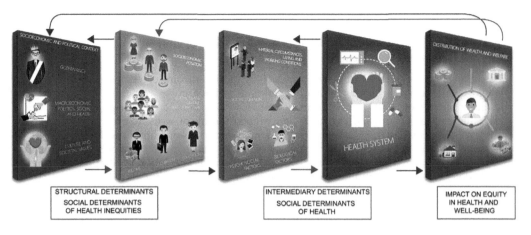

Conceptual framework of social determinants of child health. Source: adapted from Solar & Irwin (2010)

**Figure 7.1**   Social determinants and public health policy.

*Source*: https://doi.org/10.1371/journal.pone.0190960.g002

## IMPORTANCE OF STUDYING SOCIAL DETERMINANTS OF CARDIOVASCULAR DISEASE

Undoubtedly, the social environment shapes human health. It produces strong relationships between social factors, disease risk, and survival. Globally, social inequalities in risk factors account for more than half of inequalities in CVDs.[10] The health policy and practice to address the rising burden of CVD and their disproportionate increase in LMICs need to recognize that optimal cardiovascular health is a result of complex and dynamic processes, whose interactions are shaped by social, political, economic, and organizational factors. Further, the integration of available knowledge on the complexities in promoting ideal cardiovascular health is essential in policy making.

## MECHANISMS MEDIATING THE RELATIONSHIP BETWEEN SOCIOECONOMIC DISADVANTAGE AND ADVERSE HEALTH OUTCOMES

Socially induced stress is sufficient to negatively impact health and shorten life expectancy in human beings. Belonging to a disadvantaged social group also may involve, through discrimination, psychosocial effects on health and well-being. A recent review in *Science* clearly demonstrates strong evolutionary roots in the relationship between social environment and health disparities.[11] Evolutionary biologists demonstrate strong parallels between the consequences of social adversity in human populations and in other social mammals. They reveal that social integration, social support, and social status independently predict life span in at least four different mammalian orders.[11] Importantly, the effect sizes that relate social status and social integration to natural life span in other mammals aligned with those estimated for social environmental effects in humans.[11] The interaction of educational status and genetic markers suggests that educational attainment often acts as a surrogate for other unmeasured innate and environmental exposures and behaviors modifying the genetic effect on cardiovascular risk factors such as blood pressure.[12]

## ASSOCIATION OF SOCIOECONOMIC POSITION WITH CARDIOVASCULAR DISEASE

Education, income, and occupation are the three main measures of socioeconomic position that have been studied extensively in the context of cardiovascular health. However, a data-mining approach, followed by a network analysis of the interrelationship between key terms, identified several themes and variables in studies related to social determinants of CVD globally.[9] They are largely grouped into the following three domains:

(1) *Political context of health inequities* that included global governance, macroeconomic policies, social policies (as a labour market, housing or land) and any other public policies (education, health and social protection), also culture and social values, (2) *Structural determinants of*

*health inequities* such the socioeconomic position and social class (education, occupation and income) and (3) *Intermediary determinants of health*, material circumstances (living and working conditions, food availability), behaviours, biological, social-environmental and psychological factors as well as health system.[9]

Lower levels of socioeconomic position, especially in high-income countries, is associated with greater prevalence of risk factors, higher incidence of cardiovascular conditions, and greater rates of mortality from CVD.[7,13,14] A recent systematic review indicates that social and economic disadvantages are associated with health inequalities in terms of access to care, increased risk of disease, and early death in the Organisation for Economic Co-operation and Development (OECD) countries.[15] Low household income was associated with greater risk of heart failure and myocardial infarction in a large study of over 300,000 patients with atrial fibrillation.[16] Further, socially determined vulnerabilities increase the risk for incident heart failure hospitalization in the reasons for geographical and racial differences in stroke (REGARDS) cohort.[17] Similarly, an incremental increase in the number of social determinants of health was associated with a higher risk of incident stroke in the REGARDS cohort.[18] Accumulated income, a measure of both duration and extent of low income, is considered the driving force behind educational differences in premature CVD mortality.[19] In the life-course analysis on accumulated income and incident acute myocardial infarction in a Danish cohort study, the inverse social gradient was steeper in women as compared to men.[20] Food, housing, and financial insecurity are also strongly associated with CVD outcomes.[21] Food-insecure individuals in the National Health and Nutrition Examination Survey reported higher CVD mortality in a 10-year follow-up study conducted in the United States of America.[22] A recent systematic review highlights housing as one of the prominent social determinants of cardiovascular health and well-being, with higher risk in the homeless and individuals with housing insecurity.[23]

In a prospective study conducted in China, low education level was independently associated with increased risk of mortality, recurrent stroke, and cardiovascular events in patients with acute ischemic stroke.[24] In a nationally representative study conducted in South Korean adults, unit increase in social risk was associated with a higher risk of stroke diagnosis even after controlling for other risk factors.[25] Additionally, in a recent systematic review, metabolic syndrome components were much less frequent among individuals with a higher educational level and income level.[26] In a representative survey conducted among older adults (>60 years) in Columbia (an upper middle-income country from the Latin American region), an inverse relationship between socioeconomic status and risk of hypertension was evident.[27] There are, however, recent examples of reduction in social inequities in terms of CVD and mortality outcomes in high-income countries. For example, the social gradient in myocardial infarction and mortality outcomes almost disappeared in Germany based on a recent study conducted in the claims database.[28]

An inverse association between childhood social circumstances and adult CVD risk is also documented in studies conducted mostly in high-income countries.[29] However, the association between poor childhood socioeconomic conditions and CVD outcomes are often mediated through adulthood risk factors.[30,31] The mechanisms and biological sequelae of interactions among early life socioeconomic environments and risk factor trajectories indicate a life-course process linking early life socioeconomic position or class to CVD conditions and mortality. Prenatal deprivation, low birth weight, and intrauterine growth retardation are also linked to cardiovascular conditions and outcomes in adults.[13] These are discussed in the chapter "Emerging and Life-Course Factors in CVD".

Due to the complex relationship between socioeconomic position and CVD, the cardiovascular risk prediction in different socioeconomic groups often results in relatively less valid results. For example, the Framingham Risk Score overestimates the risk of coronary heart disease in individuals from high socioeconomic levels and underestimates the risk in low-socioeconomic status individuals.[32,33] Further, it has been shown that adding socioeconomic indicators to the Framingham Risk Score improves the overall risk classification.[34] An improvement in risk classification may prevent potential under treatment in the socially deprived groups.

The link between social support (the subjective feeling that a person is cared for and loved, esteemed, and a member of a network of mutual obligations) and CVD is reasonably well-established. Several studies established the link between poor social support and incident CVD and mortality associated with cardiovascular conditions.[35–38] The pre-diagnosis social support was inversely associated with post-diagnosis survival among heart failure patients in the

Cardiovascular Health Study conducted in the United States of America.[37] A smaller social network was positively associated with higher prevalence of metabolic syndrome in a study conducted in the Cardiovascular and Metabolic Diseases Etiology Research Center (CMERC) Cohort.[39] However, intervention in general directed at improving social support did not improve cardiovascular outcomes.[40] A recent scoping review suggests that caregiver-oriented strategies may offer a promising avenue for enhancing social support and improving CVD outcomes.[41] Social networks focus on a group of individuals and are characterized by their size, density, and characteristics of the connection. Although several studies postulate theories linking social networks and CVD,[42,43] the available data are limited to make valid conclusions.

Residential environments, often referred to as neighborhoods, are linked to CVD outcomes. For example, in the Atherosclerosis Risk in Communities (ARIC) study, neighborhood socioeconomic disadvantage was associated with higher risk of incident coronary heart disease.[44] In the Cardiovascular Health Study, higher risk of incident stroke was observed in the most disadvantaged neighborhoods among whites.[45] Further, higher mortality one year after incident stroke was observed in individuals living in the socioeconomically disadvantaged neighborhoods.[46] However, this relationship was not observed among blacks. Better walkability and low witnessed violence were associated with better carotid artery intima-media thickness in adults in the Brazilian Longitudinal Study of Adult Health.[47]

## ASSOCIATION OF SOCIOECONOMIC POSITION WITH CARDIOVASCULAR DISEASE IN LOW- AND MIDDLE-INCOME COUNTRIES

Research led by authors from LMICs on socioeconomic position and CVD are limited.[48] However, the highest risks of dying from most of the non-communicable diseases are observed in LMICs.[49] A systematic review shows that low socioeconomic status or living in LMICs increases the risk of developing CVD.[50] Further, most common non-communicable disease conditions, including CVD, impose catastrophic health spending,[51] increase inequality, and push families into the vicious cycle of poverty and chronic conditions in LMICs. A recent systematic review focused on LMIC settings[52] suggests that lower-socioeconomic groups are more likely to drink alcohol, use tobacco, and consume insufficient fruit and vegetables than more advantaged groups. Lack of data from the majority of LMICs on the association between socioeconomic status and alcohol use is noted in another systematic review.[53] The relatively high rates of risk factors in the lower-socioeconomic group may further increase the risk of CVD events and mortality in the disadvantaged group and widen the inequality further. In another systematic review, the risk of getting type 2 diabetes was associated with low socioeconomic position in high-, middle- and low-income countries and overall.[54] In a representative survey of adult women in Sudan, the socioeconomic gradient in hypertension was not observed in the urban areas, while hypertension risk was higher in individuals with high education and wealth in the rural areas.[55] The financial protection for health care costs for people with CVD is inadequate in LMICs.[56] Hence, a high proportion of women forgo care due to cost, which has serious implications for future morbidity and mortality.[56]

Limited and conflicting data are available from India on social determinants of CVD. However, the conflicting findings are largely due to the data presentation and analysis. There were early indications of the reversal of social gradients in some of the CVD risk factors and outcomes (inverse association between socioeconomic position and CVD) in studies conducted in India.[57,58] Detection or diagnosis of cardiovascular risk factors such as diabetes were poor in the low education group in India.[59] Hence, self-reported prevalence estimates are not useful in comparing the data across socioeconomic groups in India. Tobacco and alcohol use and low intake of fruits and vegetables were more common in lower-socioeconomic positions in a study conducted in the rural regions of India.[60] Although behavioral risk factors such as alcohol and tobacco use were higher in the low-education group in a study conducted in Himachal Pradesh, the obesity, diabetes, and hypertension rates were higher in the high-education group.[61] Similarly, a large study on socioeconomic gradients and distribution of diabetes, hypertension, and obesity in India suggests that a major proportion of the burden of these conditions was among high-socioeconomic groups.[62] However, the inaccurate socioeconomic status definition that the authors used in this large study from India classified 65–80% of Indians in the high-socioeconomic group.[63] Further, even individuals who have studied only up to primary school (fifth-grade equivalent) were counterintuitively described as being a higher socioeconomic group in the education measure.[63] It is therefore important to follow standard definitions for socioeconomic position, educational status, and income groups for better comparison across studies conducted in LMIC settings.

## RESEARCH GAPS

A comprehensive set of actions across social, health, economic, and environmental sectors that could potentially reduce the burden of CVD and global health inequalities is available.[64] Despite experiencing a disproportionately higher burden of CVD, intervention studies aligned to the WHO "best buys" are limited in LMICs.[65] In order to tackle the socioeconomic inequalities in terms of access to resources for prevention and treatment, improved international regulations across jurisdictions that eliminate the legal and practical barriers in the implementation of CVD control initiatives in LMIC are essential.[66]

In order to unpack the complexities associated with social determinants and CVD in LMIC settings, we propose the following research initiatives; (1) develop standardized measures of actionable social determinants of health, stratify the population according to the key socioeconomic variables, and study the secular trend in CVD risk factor progress and development of incident conditions; (2) explore in detail the intergenerational transmission of social disadvantage and its likely impact on CVD; (3) understand the predictors of interindividual and intersocietal differences in response to social adversity and CVD; (4) study the psycho-social, behavioral, and biological mechanisms associated with development of adverse CVD outcomes in socially disadvantaged groups; and (5) develop and test socially acceptable, culturally relevant, and resource-sensitive interventions for prevention and control of CVD in socially disadvantaged groups.

## REFERENCES

1. Collaborators GBDCoD. Global, regional, and national age-sex-specific mortality for 282 causes of death in 195 countries and territories, 1980–2017: a systematic analysis for the Global Burden of Disease Study 2017. *Lancet* 2018;392(10159):1736–1788. doi: 10.1016/S0140-6736(18)32203-7
2. Virani SS, Alonso A, Benjamin EJ, et al. Heart disease and stroke statistics-2020 update: A report from the American heart association. *Circulation* 2020;141(9):e139–e596. doi: 10.1161/CIR.0000000000000757
3. Global Burden of Disease Study 2017 (GBD 2017). Seattle, WA: Institute for Health Metrics and Evaluation, University of Washington; 2018. http://ghdx.healthdata.org/gbd-results-tool.
4. DALYs GBD, Collaborators H. Global, regional, and national disability-adjusted life-years (DALYs) for 359 diseases and injuries and healthy life expectancy (HALE) for 195 countries and territories, 1990–2017: a systematic analysis for the global burden of disease study 2017. *Lancet* 2018;392(10159):1859–1922. doi: 10.1016/S0140-6736(18)32335-3
5. Roth GA, Johnson C, Abajobir A, et al. Global, regional, and national burden of cardiovascular diseases for 10 causes, 1990 to 2015. *J Am Coll Cardiol* 2017;70(1):1–25. doi: 10.1016/j.jacc.2017.04.052
6. Collaborators GBDLRoS, Feigin VL, Nguyen G, et al. Global, regional, and country-specific lifetime risks of stroke, 1990 and 2016. *N Engl J Med* 2018;379(25):2429–2437. doi: 10.1056/NEJMoa1804492
7. Marmot M, Friel S, Bell R, et al. Closing the gap in a generation: health equity through action on the social determinants of health. *Lancet* 2008;372(9650):1661–1669. doi: 10.1016/S0140-6736(08)61690-6
8. Stiglitz JE, Sen A, Fitoussi J-P. Mismeasuring our lives: why GDP doesn't add up. The report by the commission on the measurement of economic performance and social progress. New York, NY: The New Press; 2010.
9. Martinez-Garcia M, Salinas-Ortega M, Estrada-Arriaga I, et al. A systematic approach to analyze the social determinants of cardiovascular disease. *PLoS One* 2018;13(1):e0190960. doi: 10.1371/journal.pone.0190960
10. Di Cesare M, Khang YH, Asaria P, et al. Inequalities in non-communicable diseases and effective responses. *Lancet* 2013;381(9866):585–597. doi: 10.1016/S0140-6736(12)61851-0
11. Snyder-Mackler N, Burger JR, Gaydosh L, et al. Social determinants of health and survival in humans and other animals. *Science* 2020;368(6493) doi: 10.1126/science.aax9553
12. Basson J, Sung YJ, Schwander K, et al. Gene-education interactions identify novel blood pressure loci in the Framingham Heart Study. *Am J Hypertens* 2014;27(3):431–444. doi: 10.1093/ajh/hpt283

13. Havranek EP, Mujahid MS, Barr DA, et al. Social determinants of risk and outcomes for cardiovascular disease: A scientific statement from the american heart association. *Circulation* 2015;132(9):873–898. doi: 10.1161/CIR.0000000000000228

14. Petrelli A, Di Napoli A, Sebastiani G, et al. Italian Atlas of mortality inequalities by education level. *Epidemiol Prev* 2019;43(1S1):1–120. doi: 10.19191/EP19.1.S1.002

15. Lago-Penas S, Rivera B, Cantarero D, et al. The impact of socioeconomic position on non-communicable diseases: what do we know about? *Perspect Public Health* 2020:1757913920914952. doi: 10.1177/1757913920914952

16. LaRosa AR, Claxton J, O'Neal WT, et al. Association of household income and adverse outcomes in patients with atrial fibrillation. *Heart* 2020 doi: 10.1136/heartjnl-2019-316065

17. Pinheiro LC, Reshetnyak E, Sterling MR, et al. Multiple vulnerabilities to health disparities and incident heart failure hospitalization in the REGARDS study. *Circ Cardiovasc Qual Outcomes* 2020:CIRCOUTCOMES119006438. doi: 10.1161/CIRCOUTCOMES.119.006438

18. Reshetnyak E, Ntamatungiro M, Pinheiro LC, et al. Impact of multiple social determinants of health on incident stroke. *Stroke* 2020;51(8):2445–2453. doi: 10.1161/STROKEAHA.120.028530

19. Ariansen I, Strand BH, Kjollesdal MKR, et al. The educational gradient in premature cardiovascular mortality: Examining mediation by risk factors in cohorts born in the 1930s, 1940s and 1950s. *Eur J Prev Cardiol* 2019;26(10):1096–1103. doi: 10.1177/2047487319826274

20. Kriegbaum M, Hougaard CO, Andersen I, et al. Life course analysis on income and incident AMI: a Danish register-based cohort study. *J Epidemiol Community Health* 2019;73(9):810–816. doi: 10.1136/jech-2018–212043

21. Parekh T, Desai R, Pemmasani S, et al. Impact of social determinants of health on cardiovascular disease *JACC* 2020;75(11):1989.

22. Banerjee S, Radak T, Khubchandani J, et al. Food Insecurity and mortality in american adults: results from the NHANES-linked mortality study. *Health Promot Pract* 2020:1524839920945927. doi: 10.1177/1524839920945927

23. Sims M, Kershaw KN, Breathett K, et al. Importance of housing and cardiovascular health and well-being: a scientific statement from the american heart association. *Circ Cardiovasc Qual Outcomes* 2020:HCQ0000000000000089. doi: 10.1161/HCQ.0000000000000089

24. Che B, Shen S, Zhu Z, et al. Education level and long-term mortality, recurrent stroke, and cardiovascular events in patients with Ischemic stroke. *J Am Heart Assoc* 2020:e016671. doi: 10.1161/JAHA.120.016671

25. Lee HH, Kang AW, Lee H, et al. Cumulative social risk and cardiovascular disease among adults in South Korea: a cross-sectional analysis of a nationally representative sample. *Prev Chronic Dis* 2020;17:E39. doi: 10.5888/pcd17.190382

26. Blanquet M, Legrand A, Pelissier A, et al. Socio-economics status and metabolic syndrome: a meta-analysis. *Diabetes Metab Syndr* 2019;13(3):1805–1812. doi: 10.1016/j.dsx.2019.04.003

27. Hessel P, Rodriguez-Lesmes P, Torres D. Socio-economic inequalities in high blood pressure and additional risk factors for cardiovascular disease among older individuals in Colombia: results from a nationally representative study. *PLoS One* 2020;15(6):e0234326. doi: 10.1371/journal.pone.0234326

28. Geyer S, Tetzlaff J, Eberhard S, et al. Health inequalities in terms of myocardial infarction and all-cause mortality: a study with German claims data covering 2006 to 2015. *Int J Public Health* 2019;64(3):387–937. doi: 10.1007/s00038-019-01224-1

29. Galobardes B, Smith GD, Lynch JW. Systematic review of the influence of childhood socioeconomic circumstances on risk for cardiovascular disease in adulthood. *Ann Epidemiol* 2006;16(2):91–104. doi: 10.1016/j.annepidem.2005.06.053

30. Kamphuis CB, Turrell G, Giskes K, et al. Socioeconomic inequalities in cardiovascular mortality and the role of childhood socioeconomic conditions and adulthood risk factors: a prospective cohort study with 17-years of follow up. *BMC Public Health* 2012;12:1045. doi: 10.1186/1471-2458-12-1045

31. Kamphuis CB, Turrell G, Giskes K, et al. Life course socioeconomic conditions, adulthood risk factors and cardiovascular mortality among men and women: a 17-year follow up of the GLOBE study. *Int J Cardiol* 2013;168(3):2207–2213. doi: 10.1016/j.ijcard.2013.01.219

32. Brindle PM, McConnachie A, Upton MN, et al. The accuracy of the Framingham risk-score in different socioeconomic groups: a prospective study. *Br J Gen Pract* 2005;55(520):838–845.

33. Tunstall-Pedoe H, Woodward M, estimation Sgor. By neglecting deprivation, cardiovascular risk scoring will exacerbate social gradients in disease. *Heart* 2006;92(3):307–310. doi: 10.1136/hrt.2005.077289

34. Fiscella K, Tancredi D, Franks P. Adding socioeconomic status to Framingham scoring to reduce disparities in coronary risk assessment. *Am Heart J* 2009;157(6):988–994. doi: 10.1016/j.ahj.2009.03.019

35. Williams RB, Barefoot JC, Califf RM, et al. Prognostic importance of social and economic resources among medically treated patients with angiographically documented coronary artery disease. *JAMA* 1992;267(4):520–524.

36. Berkman LF, Leo-Summers L, Horwitz RI. Emotional support and survival after myocardial infarction. A prospective, population-based study of the elderly. *Ann Intern Med* 1992;117(12):1003–1009. doi: 10.7326/0003-4819-117-12-1003

37. Kaiser P, Allen N, Delaney JAC, et al. The association of prediagnosis social support with survival after heart failure in the Cardiovascular Health Study. *Ann Epidemiol* 2020;42:73–77. doi: 10.1016/j.annepidem.2019.12.013

38. Green YS, Hajduk AM, Song X, et al. Usefulness of social support in older adults after hospitalization for acute myocardial infarction (from the SILVER-AMI study). *Am J Cardiol* 2020;125(3):313–319. doi: 10.1016/j.amjcard.2019.10.038

39. Kim K, Jung SJ, Baek JM, et al. Associations between social network properties and metabolic syndrome and the mediating effect of physical activity: findings from the Cardiovascular and Metabolic Diseases Etiology Research Center (CMERC) Cohort. *BMJ Open Diabetes Res Care* 2020;8(1) doi: 10.1136/bmjdrc-2020-001272

40. Berkman LF, Blumenthal J, Burg M, et al. Effects of treating depression and low perceived social support on clinical events after myocardial infarction: the Enhancing Recovery in Coronary Heart Disease Patients (ENRICHD) randomized trial. *JAMA* 2003;289(23):3106–3116. doi: 10.1001/jama.289.23.3106

41. Clayton C, Motley C, Sakakibara B. Enhancing social support among people with cardiovascular disease: a systematic scoping review. *Curr Cardiol Rep* 2019;21(10):123. doi: 10.1007/s11886-019-1216-7

42. Joo WT, Lee CJ, Oh J, et al. The association between social network betweenness and coronary calcium: a baseline study of patients with a high risk of cardiovascular disease. *J Atheroscler Thromb* 2018;25(2):131–141. doi: 10.5551/jat.40469

43. Valtorta NK, Kanaan M, Gilbody S, et al. Loneliness and social isolation as risk factors for coronary heart disease and stroke: systematic review and meta-analysis of longitudinal observational studies. *Heart* 2016;102(13):1009–1016. doi: 10.1136/heartjnl-2015-308790

44. Diez Roux AV, Merkin SS, Arnett D, et al. Neighborhood of residence and incidence of coronary heart disease. *N Engl J Med* 2001;345(2):99–106. doi: 10.1056/NEJM200107123450205

45. Brown AF, Liang LJ, Vassar SD, et al. Neighborhood disadvantage and ischemic stroke: the Cardiovascular Health Study (CHS). *Stroke* 2011;42(12):3363–3368. doi: 10.1161/STROKEAHA.111.622134

46. Brown AF, Liang LJ, Vassar SD, et al. Neighborhood socioeconomic disadvantage and mortality after stroke. *Neurology* 2013;80(6):520–527. doi: 10.1212/WNL.0b013e31828154ae

47. Willets C, Santos IS, Lotufo PA, et al. Association between perceived neighborhood characteristics and carotid artery intima-media thickness: cross-sectional results from the ELSA-brasil study. *Glob Heart* 2019;14(4):379–385. doi: 10.1016/j.gheart.2019.09.002

48. Allen LN, Fox N, Ambrose A. Quantifying research output on poverty and noncommunicable disease behavioural risk factors in low-income and lower middle-income countries: a bibliometric analysis. *BMJ Open* 2017;7(11):e014715. doi: 10.1136/bmjopen-2016–014715

49. NCDC collaborators. NCD Countdown 2030: worldwide trends in non-communicable disease mortality and progress towards sustainable development goal target 3.4. *Lancet* 2018;392(10152):1072–1088. doi: 10.1016/S0140-6736(18)31992-5

50. Sommer I, Griebler U, Mahlknecht P, et al. Socioeconomic inequalities in non-communicable diseases and their risk factors: an overview of systematic reviews. *BMC Public Health* 2015;15:914. doi: 10.1186/s12889-015-2227-y

51. Jaspers L, Colpani V, Chaker L, et al. The global impact of non-communicable diseases on households and impoverishment: a systematic review. *Eur J Epidemiol* 2015;30(3):163–188. doi: 10.1007/s10654-014-9983-3

52. Allen L, Williams J, Townsend N, et al. Socioeconomic status and non-communicable disease behavioural risk factors in low-income and lower-middle-income countries: a systematic review. *Lancet Glob Health* 2017;5(3):e277-e89. doi: 10.1016/S2214-109X(17)30058-X

53. Allen LN, Townsend N, Williams J, et al. Socioeconomic status and alcohol use in low- and lower-middle income countries: A systematic review. *Alcohol* 2018;70:23–31. doi: 10.1016/j.alcohol.2017.12.002

54. Agardh E, Allebeck P, Hallqvist J, et al. Type 2 diabetes incidence and socio-economic position: a systematic review and meta-analysis. *Int J Epidemiol* 2011;40(3):804–818. doi: 10.1093/ije/dyr029

55. Osman S, Costanian C, Annan NB, et al. Urbanization and socioeconomic disparities in hypertension among older adult women in Sudan. *Ann Glob Health* 2019;85(1). doi: 10.5334/aogh.2404

56. Murphy A, Palafox B, Walli-Attaei M, et al. The household economic burden of non-communicable diseases in 18 countries. *BMJ Glob Health* 2020;5(2):e002040. doi: 10.1136/bmjgh-2019-002040

57. Jeemon P, Reddy KS. Social determinants of cardiovascular disease outcomes in Indians. *Indian J Med Res* 2010;132:617–622. doi: 10.4103/0971-5916.73415

58. Reddy KS, Prabhakaran D, Jeemon P, et al. Educational status and cardiovascular risk profile in Indians. *Proc Natl Acad Sci U S A* 2007;104(41):16263–16268. doi: 10.1073/pnas.0700933104

59. Claypool KT, Chung MK, Deonarine A, et al. Characteristics of undiagnosed diabetes in men and women under the age of 50 years in the Indian subcontinent: the National Family Health Survey (NFHS-4)/demographic health survey 2015–2016. *BMJ Open Diabetes Res Care* 2020;8(1) doi: 10.1136/bmjdrc-2019-000965

60. Kinra S, Bowen LJ, Lyngdoh T, et al. Sociodemographic patterning of non-communicable disease risk factors in rural India: a cross sectional study. *BMJ* 2010;341:c4974. doi: 10.1136/bmj.c4974

61. Agarwal A, Jindal D, Ajay VS, et al. Association between socioeconomic position and cardiovascular disease risk factors in rural north India: The Solan Surveillance Study. *PLoS One* 2019;14(7):e0217834. doi: 10.1371/journal.pone.0217834

62. Corsi DJ, Subramanian SV. Socioeconomic gradients and distribution of diabetes, hypertension, and obesity in India. *JAMA Netw Open* 2019;2(4):e190411. doi: 10.1001/jamanetworkopen.2019.0411

63. Patel SA, Cunningham SA, Tandon N, et al. Chronic diseases in India-ubiquitous across the socioeconomic spectrum. *JAMA Netw Open* 2019;2(4):e190404. doi: 10.1001/jamanetworkopen.2019.0404

64. Ezzati M, Pearson-Stuttard J, Bennett JE, et al. Acting on non-communicable diseases in low- and middle-income tropical countries. *Nature* 2018;559(7715):507–516. doi: 10.1038/s41586-018-0306-9

65. Allen LN, Pullar J, Wickramasinghe KK, et al. Evaluation of research on interventions aligned to WHO 'Best Buys' for NCDs in low-income and lower-middle-income countries: a systematic review from 1990 to 2015. *BMJ Glob Health* 2018;3(1):e000535. doi: 10.1136/bmjgh-2017-000535

66. Niessen LW, Mohan D, Akuoku JK, et al. Tackling socioeconomic inequalities and non-communicable diseases in low-income and middle-income countries under the Sustainable Development agenda. *Lancet* 2018;391(10134):2036–2046. doi: 10.1016/S0140-6736(18)30482-3

# 8 How Do We Frame Public Health Policies?

*Anand Krishnan, Tilahun Haregu, and Brian Oldenburg*

## CONTENTS

## INTRODUCTION

Public policy is the process by which governments and their stakeholders translate their political vision into programs and actions to deliver 'outcomes' or the changes that they desire in the world. Policy development is a key function of all government systems. Policies and procedures provide the framework within which the government operates and allow other stakeholders to operate. They define what they do (their priorities) and how to do it. Having clear policies offers clarity and helps different wings of the government and other stakeholders to operate more harmoniously and effectively. Developing and implementing policy is a process of continuous improvement. Policymaking is neither objective nor neutral; it is an inherently political process.

## WHAT IS HEALTH POLICY?

Health policy refers to decisions, plans, and actions that are undertaken to achieve specific health care goals within a society. An explicit health policy defines a vision for the future, which in turn helps to establish targets and points of reference for the short- and medium-term outcomes. It outlines priorities and identifies different stakeholders and their expected roles and usually reflects a consensus or a majority opinion of the people.[1] While there may be an overarching health policy at the national or sub-national level, there could be policies which address specific areas of health as well—for example, mental health policy, emergency care policy, vaccination policy, or tobacco control policy. A number of different factors affect policymaking at an individual level—for example, a policymaker's own experience, expertise, and judgement—and at an institutional level—for example, in terms of institutional capacity and objective.

## HEALTH POLICY DEVELOPMENT PROCESS

Health policymaking involves[2] an exhausting and time-consuming 'policy cycle'. The basic stages of the policy cycle are as follows: a problem is identified, a policy response is formulated, the policy is adopted and implemented, and finally the policy is evaluated as to whether the original problem has been solved and, if not, why and what is an alternative course of action, thus, returning policymakers to the very first step: the identification of a problem. It should be remembered

DOI: 10.1201/b23266-17

## Table 8.1 Stages in Policy Development and Their Descriptions

| Stages in Policy Development | Objectives | Issues to Be Addressed | Expected Outcome | Lead Actors |
|---|---|---|---|---|
| Scoping for policy change | To convince the 'powers' about the need for a review of the policy, its proposed direction of change, and the process to be followed. | • Is a policy change required or is the problem better addressed through other means? <br> • Why is policy change needed, what is needed, and what is the process to be followed for its development? | Discussion note or policy brief | Concerned ministry cell or division |
| Preparing a draft policy document | To bring clarity on the policy gap, review the different options, and get stakeholder feedback in preparing the draft policy. | • What are the policy objectives and strategic options and their pros and cons? <br> • Who are the affected stakeholders? <br> • What baseline information is needed for later evaluation of the policy? | Discussion papers Background papers Draft policy document | Core policy team, preferably interministerial |
| Public and stakeholders' feedback | To solicit feedback by putting the draft policy document in the public domain and revising the document based on the feedback. | • What are the comments of different stakeholders? <br> • What is the process of public consultation and its timeframe to ensure transparency? | Revised document for submission | Core policy team |
| Policy adoption | Finalize and adopt the policy by the executive or legislative bodies. | • What will be its implementation strategy, including financial and staffing implications, responsibilities, and monitoring process, including key deliverables? | Approved final policy document | Executive or legislative bodies |
| Policy implementation | To implement the adopted policy | • What needs to be done to implement the policy? <br> • How well is it being implemented based on the reports on performance measures? | Routine report | Executive wings of the government and other stakeholders |
| Policy evaluation | This stage closes the policy cycle and involves the monitoring and review of the policy based on a pre-decided framework. | • How much did we achieve what we set out to achieve by the policy change? <br> • What were the facilitatory and impedimentary factors in the achievement? | Evaluation report | Think tanks |

that there is an inherent inertia to not change a policy. This is because once a country has set on a certain policy path, it is difficult to change this path because actors and policies have become institutionalized, and a change necessitates great efforts and costs by actors who desire change (theory of path dependence).[3] Therefore, the onus is on the advocates of change to convince that there is a need to change the policy. In most situations and countries, the process of policy change or development is well established. The stages in policy development are described in Table 8.1.[4]

### Stage 1: Issue Identification and Scoping for Health Policy

The first question to ask in the health policy development process is whether the health issue requires a new policy or is better addressed through other means. There are three possible scenarios: one where no existing policy covers the area of interest (new policy), second a major change is required (policy reform), or third a minor change or tweak is required (policy refinement). For the rest of the chapter, all three options will be treated similarly as policy change. If a policy change is required, a discussion note or brief should be prepared that clearly articulates its need and the process to be followed for its development. The main purpose at this stage is to convince the 'powers' for a need to have a relook at the policy and the proposed direction of change.

## Stage 2: Preparing a Draft Health Policy

Once they are convinced, a core team with competency in necessary areas should be set up to navigate the entire process of policy development. The aim of this stage is to have clarity on issues that will be affected by the policy change, as well as review the different options available to address the policy gap. Consultation with all stakeholders or interest groups at this stage is critical, as this is when key issues and objectives are clarified, strategies are developed, and the feasibility of options tested. The consultation process should document the perspectives of those affected by the policy and ensure the stakeholders and public have effective and appropriate input into developing policies. Based on these inputs, a draft document is prepared for internal consultation. A workshop may be held with relevant staff and senior management to provide feedback on the draft discussion paper. The team revises the draft document and prepares a final draft policy document. A baseline of information against which to measure performance of the final policy should be established.

## Stage 3: Public Feedback on Draft Health Policy Document

After approval from the requisite authority, the draft health policy document is released in the public domain for comments and suggestions from everyone within a given timeframe. This process of public consultation could be in the form of online feedback as well as publicized public consultations/open houses/public hearings. The team then revises the policy based on the outcomes of public consultation on the discussion paper.

## Stage 4: Health Policy Adoption

The revised policy document is put up to the final authority for approval. This could include executive or legislative bodies and could include open or closed debates/discussions on the policy. The final policy should include an implementation plan that identifies performance measures, key deliverables, and responsibilities for implementation, including financial and staffing implications.

## Stage 5: Health Policy Implementation

Once approved, the responsibility shifts to the implementation nodal point—which would be the ministry of health in this case. It is often noted that there is a large interval between policy adoption and its implementation, either because the processes have not been well defined or because the political landscape has changed in the interim. Implementation will benefit from clarifying the reporting arrangements and performance measures against which the policy will be monitored.

## Stage 6: Health Policy Evaluation

The final stage involves the monitoring and review of the policy. This stage closes the policy cycle and involves understanding how well the policy change achieved its objective, as outlined in the first stage, and what policy options worked or did not work and why. Was it a design issue or more of an implementation issue or that the circumstances changed? Addressing these may require policy refinement or a new policy.

These stages are an ideal model. However, the policy development process is often not linear. These six stages include multiple sub-steps. The actual policy processes vary depending on the scope and complexity of the issue, changes in circumstances and priorities over the cycle period, and consultations.

## FRAMING OF HEALTH POLICIES

While framing a policy could mean development of a policy, framing in the policy context could also mean political framing of the policy. As already said, policy development is an inherently political process. The term 'frame' can be used to describe a variety of ideas, packaged as values, social problems, metaphors, or arguments.[5] The framing of ideas in a particular way evokes deeply held values that shift the terrain of the debate along an ideological path, transforming it into a social issue with an implicit set of solutions resulting in forming coalitions of interest.

- ■ Frames: Conceptual structures with mostly subconscious reference points that determine how knowledge is constructed, shaping our ideas, and the way we reason and act.

■ Framing: Strategic efforts by groups to shape shared understandings of the world and that provide legitimacy and motivate certain actions.

## FRAMING OF A GLOBAL HEALTH AGENDA: A CASE STUDY OF HIV

The process of prioritizing health issues at the global level is complex and deeply political. However, global experience with HIV/AIDS can give us valuable lessons on how to successfully get a public health problem into global development agenda.

I. Framing: The HIV epidemic was framed both as a humanitarian crisis and a threat to economic development and security. The fear of disease, but also of violence and instability, was fundamental to the health security framing for HIV/AIDS. Experience with HIV suggests that it is the novelty and lethality of pathogens that disrupt societies and threaten political power, rather than disease prevalence per se.

II. Simple policy/program options: In addition, for HIV there was one main issue of access to antiretroviral therapy (ART) that the movement could coalesce around. Access to AIDS treatment was framed as a matter of economic justice.

III. Global stewardship: The creation of UNAIDS as a joint and co-sponsored program, bringing together the 11 main UN agencies involved into a coordinated response, was further recognition that a medical response on its own would be entirely insufficient and that HIV was a health and development issue.

IV. Adequate funding: This resulted in many national AIDS programs being housed in the 'heads of the state' office—often encouraged by external funding as well as higher funding from the national governments. The establishment of the Global Funds for AIDS, Tuberculosis and Malaria (GFATM) ensured adequate funding for national HIV/AIDS programs in poor countries and is one of the major reasons for its global success.

## FRAMING OF NONCOMMUNICABLE DISEASES IN THE GLOBAL AGENDA

The way AIDS was framed in this process may have lessons for how noncommunicable disease (NCD) actors can implement the 'whole of government'.[6,7] However, NCDs are currently not perceived as novel threats and are often incorrectly considered diseases only of the elderly or of the wealthy. Despite being the leading cause of morbidity and mortality worldwide, NCDs have not received the same political or financial attention from the global health community as other conditions, such as HIV/AIDS. We can use the previous framework to analyze the NCD policy framing.

### Framing

NCDs have been variously framed as a medical and clinical problem; an obstacle to economic growth; an equity and human rights issue; a development issue central to achieving the Sustainable Development Goals (SDGs); an externality of transnational corporate practice; and a multisectoral issue, requiring a 'whole-of-government', 'whole-of-society' approach.[8,9,10] The multiplicity of framings reflects the heterogeneous nature of NCDs as a concept, as well as the fragmentation and range of issues involved in the response. Other reasons cited for ineffective framing of NCDs include vested commercial interests and a lack of a 'fear factor'. The framing of NCDs as a 'health' problem of four risk factors and four diseases did not resonate with the larger policy community, but the economic and development argument enabled some traction to be gained. Some recommend that NCDs be framed as an issue of global health security, as health systems will collapse in developing countries due to the burden that will have global implications. Some also advocate linking NCDs to major social movements, such as climate action, by building new alliances.

### Simple Policy Options

The technocratic solutions offered for NCDs was the World Health Organizations (WHO's) Best Buys, but their applicability globally, especially in low- and middle-income countries, is questionable. More recently, treatment of NCDs has been framed as a part of the Universal Health Coverage (UHC). While WHO has also listed policy interventions (fiscal, legislative, structural, or informational instruments) for tobacco, alcohol, diet, and physical activity, these have not been promoted effectively into an attractive package. Overall, there is the need for the NCD community to divide the issue into two components—prevention of NCDs and treatment and care of people

## BOX 8.1 CASE STUDIES ON FRAMING OF NCDS

1. <u>Taxation on Sugar-Sweetened Beverages:</u> Framing the tax on sugar-sweetened beverages (SSBs) as a way to reduce the prevalence of NCDs is popular among the public, especially where awareness of NCDs is high and the issue of NCDs is most pressing. Additional factors that helped governments frame the need for an SSB tax included availability of evidence demonstrating the prevalence of NCDs and child obesity in the area, academics and professional associations supporting the tax, the growing international precedent of SSB taxes being implemented in other countries, and existence of recommendations from credible international organizations such as the World Health Organization (WHO). Earmarking the tax for a social or public good (child education or fighting childhood obesity) is a successful way to frame the tax, which helps to increase both public and political support for it.

2. <u>Tobacco Control:</u> The WHO's Framework Convention on Tobacco Control (FCTC) provides an excellent platform for countries to build on. Studying the considerable variation in its implementation among European countries, it was seen that in countries where the health civil society had relative policy dominance, tobacco consumption was predominantly framed as a health issue, nongovernmental organization (NGO) communities were well developed, the industry was largely absent in terms of production and manufacture, the health ministries played central roles in the policymaking process, and FCTC provisions were strictly interpreted. In countries where the tobacco industry had relative policy dominance, tobacco was framed as a private problem, NGO communities were absent or weak, the industry was well represented, the health ministries played subordinate roles in the policymaking process, and FCTC provisions were implemented only partially.[13]

with NCDs. These require different policy responses at the global and national level to 'ensure healthy lives and promote well-being for all at all ages'.

### Global Stewardship

While like in the case of HIV/AIDS, a United Nations high-level meeting on NCDs was convened in 2011, it was not followed by a similar WHO signature initiative on NCDs. Richard Horton, in a *Lancet* editorial, has critiqued WHO's director-general, Tedros Adhanom Ghebreyesus, for not mentioning NCDs among the four urgent issues: health emergencies; universal health coverage; women's, children's, and adolescents' health; and climate change.[10] The institutional constraints of the WHO resulted in missing many policy windows. The SDGs offer the NCD community an opportunity, as they not only include NCD-specific targets but also wide-ranging factors relevant to addressing this health challenge. The complex and intersectoral actions, civil society mobilization, and a coalition beyond the health sector require leadership which is still missing.

### Adequate Funding

A review of global development assistance for health revealed that in 2007, 3% ($503 million out of $22 billion) was dedicated to NCDs. In terms of burden of disease, donors provided about $0.78/DALY attributable to NCDs in developing countries as compared to $23.9/DALY attributable to HIV, tuberculosis, and malaria.[11] The potential conflicts of interest among the many parties involved in the multibillion-dollar industry and nontransparent tracking of international program funding and finances have undermined the global efforts for sourcing funds required to combat NCDs.[12]

We look at two case studies (Box 8.1) to understand the framing of issues as relevant in the NCDs context.

### CASE STUDY: HIV-NCD INTEGRATION: IMPLICATIONS FOR POLICY FRAMING[14,15,16]

HIV infection being a chronic disease with behavioral risk factors provides an excellent template to adapt for NCD management and prevention policies. In addition to their epidemiological overlap, HIV/AIDS and NCD epidemics have many important similarities in their etiology,

## Table 8.2 Policy Framing Related to HIV/AIDS in Four Countries: A Case Study

| Country | Policy Structures for NCDs |
|---------|---------------------------|
| South Africa | National Health Commission chaired by the presidency and involving all relevant government sectors and others. In addition, it had established an advisory committee. It also had an interministerial committee on the prevention of substance abuse. |
| Sri Lanka | National Health Council for promoting collaboration and National NCD steering committee for monitoring policy implementation. |
| Malaysia | Cabinet Committee for Health Promoting Environment chaired by the deputy prime minister and involving the major ministries. |
| Ethiopia | National Technical working group drafted the strategic framework for the prevention and control of NCDs. A national-level NCD consortium was also established. |

pathogenesis, and management. In this regard, one key aspect of policy framing is to develop and implement an integrated chronic disease prevention and control policy that can address both infectious diseases and NCDs. This case study presents the case for South Africa, Ethiopia, Malaysia, and Sri Lanka in the 10-year period between 2006 and 2015[17] (Table 8.2).

Policy-related processes in the national response to HIV/AIDS in the case countries were categorized into four major processes. The first one was *political leadership*. This involved the highest political bodies of a country (cabinet/members/ministers/presidents, etc.). The second process was a *policymaking process* which encompasses drafting (and approving) the policy and oversight of its implementation. The third process was a *policy advisory role* that addresses policy and technical issues. The final process is *program governance* which was spearheaded by national (HIV/AIDS) secretariat/working group/taskforce (members). From the NCD perspective, all four case countries had a responsible body in the ministry of health. NCD-specific policy processes and governance structures varied widely across the case countries.

Both HIV/AIDS and NCDs were included in the sector-wide policies for health in all the case countries. All the four countries had stand-alone policy/strategy frameworks for both HIV/AIDS and NCDs. The four countries also had HIV policies specific to some population groups and specific technical areas. South Africa and Sri Lanka had operational policy documents on the four major NCDs and the four common NCD risk factors. However, there were concerns in the alignment of HIV/AIDS and NCD-specific policies/strategies with the sector-wide policies/strategies. The alignment of NCD-specific policies with disease/risk factor–specific policies was also another area of concern in the integrated response to NCDs. In this regard, evidence-informed policy framing for HIV/NCD integration would be important in to address these challenges.[18,19]

### ROLE OF SCIENTIFIC EVIDENCE IN HEALTH POLICY DEVELOPMENT

There cannot be any doubt that the policy development should be led by evidence. Scientists usually portray 'evidence' as an apolitical, neutral, and objective policy tool.[20,21] There are three main issues surrounding the use of evidence-based policy development.[22] First, policy should be informed by a wide breadth of evidence, not simply hard research. Second, evidence has the potential to influence the policymaking process at each stage mentioned earlier. However, different evidence and different mechanisms may be required at each of the policy stages. Finally, several constraints limit the extent to which evidence can affect policy. The three obstacles to promoting evidence-based policy development globally have been described as too little primary research that specifically examines the value of interventions among poor communities, assumption that policymaking is a linear process, and finally being unable to understand the 'black box' of implementation.[23] Peter John characterizes policymaking as a slippery interaction between 'four I's': institutions, interests, incidents, and ideas.[24] The five "S" factors which limit evidence-based decision making are speed or time pressure, superficiality of knowledge of policymakers, spin or the perception game, secrecy of evidence and interests, and finally scientific ignorance.

### HEALTH POLICY DEVELOPMENT IN LOW- AND MIDDLE-INCOME COUNTRIES

The process of health policy development in an LMIC country context presents a considerable challenge. Due to the considerable diversity of cultural, economic, and political contexts, global evidence may not be entirely applicable and local evidence may not be available. The other biggest challenges to policy development in the LMIC context is that it is based on a top-down approach of a small group of experts, without considering the wider stakeholders in the policy process. The policy processes tend to be centralized and often less open in LMICs, especially in terms of policy formulation. These countries often have a more troubled political context characterized by limited political freedoms or restricted democratic spaces. There may be less public representation, weak structures for aggregating and arbitrating interests in society, and weak systems of accountability. LMICs tend to be more politically volatile, which tends to have a negative impact on the use of evidence in policy processes. Academic and media freedom and the role of civil society in articulation of public interests are critical for evidence-based policy. In addition, there can be problems with accountability, participation, corruption, and the lack of incentives and capacity to draw in evidence in policy implementation.

## ROLE OF CIVIL SOCIETY IN HEALTH POLICY FRAMING

The increasingly accepted understanding of the term civil society organizations (CSOs) is that of nonstate, not-for-profit voluntary organizations formed by people in that social sphere. Civil society can, with its low cost of entry, bring innovative solutions to address new tasks quickly that could eventually be adopted by public and private organizations.[25] Civil society can therefore compensate for policy failures through quick responses and incubation of alternative organizational models. CSOs often play a key role in advocacy, trying to drive social change through direct campaigns on topics such as disease awareness or public health issues such as smoking and domestic violence. In health policy development, civil society can bring expertise, ideas, and diverse perspectives. A policy that is pushed through in the face of opposition from affected civil society groups might be perfectly legitimate, but it will also be contentious and face difficulties.[26]

Power and trust equations between government and civil society are often uncomfortable. The advocacy of new ideas, efforts to shape the political agenda, and connection with less powerful and more vulnerable groups in society, thus empowering them, make the incumbent powers uncomfortable. If governments want to work with civil society, they must learn to cope with criticism. Nonetheless, better partnership is possible. The benefits to policymakers of civil society participation in policymaking are better information, better legitimacy, and diverse ideas.

However, for CSOs to bring any kind of information and ideas into policymaking, suitable mechanisms need to exist. The engagement of civil society with health policy and health is substantially dependent on the legal and political framework of the country. There are many consultation mechanisms to involve civil society, including consultative forums and publication of government proposals for comment. Also, narrow and specific forums where CSOs can exchange ideas with policymakers on specific topics such as food regulation are also highly effective. One also needs to acknowledge the limitations of working with CSOs. Some organizations representing citizens and patients have been criticized for opacity regarding their funding sources and lines of accountability, raising suspicions that vested interests are using CSOs as a vehicle to undermine certain policies, such as tobacco control. It is worth remembering that the benefits of civil society engagement come partly from its independence from the state. A credible civil society is necessary if its endorsement is to make policy more credible.

## POLICY IMPLEMENTATION AND ITS CHALLENGES

There is an increasing awareness that policies do not 'succeed or fail' on their own merits; rather, their progress is dependent upon the process of implementation.[27] As already said, the policy development process is nonlinear and messy. However, the implementation is unarguably much harder. The governments are increasingly recognizing that more needs to be done to try to manage the implementation process so as to ensure intentions are turned into results. Four broad contributors to policy failure can be identified: overly optimistic expectations, implementation through fragmented governance, inadequate collaborative policymaking, and the vagaries of the political cycle.

## SUMMARY

Health policy defines a vision for the future which in turn helps to establish targets and points of reference for the short- and medium-term outcomes. Policymaking is an inherently political process, and there will always be an inherent inertia to not change a policy. Health policymaking goes through a time-consuming 'policy cycle' of identification of a problem, formulation of a policy response, adoption of the policy, its implementation, and finally its evaluation. While policy should be based on evidence, political 'framing' of an issue is often considered as a way to get it into the agenda of the government. The successful framing of the HIV agenda in the global development agenda and the failure of NCDs to tap global resources are good examples to learn from. CSOs have an important role to play in all stages of policy development. The ultimate test of a policy change is its impact on the ground level, which is often much later due to implementation challenges.

## REFERENCES

1  World Health organization. Health Policy. www.who.int/topics/health_policy/en/ accessed on 20th August 2020.

2  Eastern Metropolitan Regional Council. EMRC policy development guidelines. 71240. ASCOT WA 6104.

3  Cerna L. The nature of policy change and implementation: a review of different theoretical approaches. Paris: Organization for Economic Co-operation and Development, 2013.

4  European Commission. Quality of public administration. A toolbox for practitioners. Luxembourg: European Commission, 2017. doi:10.2767/879305

5  Koon AD, Hawkins B, Mayhew SH. Framing and the health policy process: a scoping review. Health Policy Plan. 2016 Jul;31(6):801–816. doi: 10.1093/heapol/czv128

6  Palma AM, Rabkin M, Nuwagaba-Biribonwoha H, Bongomin P, Lukhele N, Dlamini X, et al. Can the success of HIV scale-up advance the global chronic NCD agenda? Glob Heart [Internet]. 2016 Dec 1 [cited 2018 Aug 13];11(4):403–408. Available from: www.sciencedirect.com/science/article/pii/S2211816016307487

7  Labonté R, Gagnon ML. Framing health and foreign policy: lessons for global health diplomacy. Global Health. 2010;6:1–19.

8  Adjaye-Gbewonyo K, Vaughan M. Reframing NCDs? An analysis of current debates, Global Health Action. 2019;12(1):1641043. doi: 10.1080/16549716.2019.1641043

9  Heller O, Somerville C, Suggs LS, et al. The process of prioritization of non-communicable diseases in the global health policy arena. Health Policy Plan. 2019;34(5):370–383.

10  Horton R. Offline: NCDs-why are we failing? Lancet. 2017;390(10092):346. doi:10.1016/S0140-6736(17)31919-0

11  Nugent RA, Feigl AB. Where have all the donors gone? Scarce donor funding for non-communicable diseases (Working Paper 228). Washington: Center for Global Development, 2010.

12  Banerjee A. Tracking global funding for the prevention and control of noncommunicable diseases. Bull World Health Organ. 2012 Jul 1;90(7):479–479A. doi: 10.2471/BLT.12.108795. PMID: 22807589; PMCID: PMC3397713.

13  Kuijpers TG, Kunst AE, Willemsen MC. Who calls the shots in tobacco control policy? Policy monopolies of pro and anti-tobacco interest groups across six European countries. BMC Public Health. 2019;19(1):800.

14  Haregu TN, Setswe G, Elliott J, Oldenburg B. National responses to HIV/AIDS and non-communicable diseases in developing countries: analysis of strategic parallels and differences. J Public Health Res. 2014;3(1):99.

15  Haregu TN, Setswe G, Elliott J, Oldenburg B. Developing an action model for integration of health system response to HIV/AIDS and noncommunicable diseases (NCDs) in developing countries. Glob J Health Sci. 2013;6(1):9–22.

16  Njuguna B, Vorkoper S, Patel P, Reid MJA, Vedanthan R, Pfaff C, et al. Models of integration of HIV and noncommunicable disease care in sub-Saharan Africa: lessons learned and evidence gaps. Aids. 2018;32 Suppl 1(Suppl 1):S33–S42.

17  Haregu TN, Setswe G, Elliott J, Oldenburg B. National responses to HIV/AIDS and Non-communicable diseases in developing countries: analysis of strategic parallels and differences. J Public Health Res. 2014;3(1):99.

18  Haregu TN, Setswe G, Elliott J, Oldenburg B. Developing an action model for integration of health system response to HIV/AIDS and noncommunicable diseases (NCDs) in developing countries. Glob J Health Sci. 2013;6(1):9–22.

19  Njuguna B, Vorkoper S, Patel P, Reid MJA, Vedanthan R, Pfaff C, et al. Models of integration of HIV and noncommunicable disease care in sub-Saharan Africa: lessons learned and evidence gaps. Aids. 2018;32 Suppl 1(Suppl 1):S33–S42.

20  Cairney P, Oliver K. Evidence-based policymaking is not like evidence-based medicine, so how far should you go to bridge the divide between evidence and policy? Health Res Policy Syst. 2017;15(1):35.

21 Sutcliffe S, Court J. What is it? How does it work? What relevance for developing countries? London: Overseas Development Institute, November 2005.

22 Gómez-Olivé FX, Ali SA, Made F, Kyobutungi C, Nonterah E, Micklesfield L, et al. Regional and sex differences in the prevalence and awareness of hypertension: an H3Africa AWI-gen study across 6 sites in sub-Saharan Africa. Global Heart. 2017;12(2):81–90.

23 Yamey G, Feachem R. Evidence-based policymaking in global health—the payoffs and pitfalls. BMJ Evidence-Based Medicine. 2011;16:97–99.

24 John P. Analyzing public policy. London: Continuum International Publishing Group, 2000.

25 Kuruvilla S. CSO participation in health, research and policy: A review of models, mechanisms and measures. Working Paper 251. Overseas Development Institute London, August 2005.

26 Court J, Mendizabal E, Osborne D, Young J. Policy engagement how civil society can be more effective. Overseas Development Institute London, 2006.

27 Hudson B, Hunter D, Peckham S. Policy failure and the policy-implementation gap: can policy support programs help? Policy Design Practice. 2019;2(1):1–14.

# 9 Public Health Policies for Prevention and Control of Cardiovascular Diseases

*Sailesh Mohan*

## CONTENTS

## INTRODUCTION

Worldwide, cardiovascular diseases (CVDs) are the leading cause of mortality, with two-thirds of all CVD deaths occurring currently in low- and middle-income countries (LMICs). This is highly disconcerting from a health as well as societal perspective and can be attributed to varied health transitions underway in most LMICs, resulting in increased longevity and exposure to CVD risk factors such as tobacco use, unhealthy diets, physical inactivity, and high blood pressure. The increasing trends in CVDs are expected to continue for the foreseeable future in the absence of appropriate and effective public health action to stem the rise.[1,2]

This chapter examines the decline of CVDs in many high-income countries (HICs), the rationale for implementing evidence-based public health policies, and how LMICs can leverage lessons from the declines in CVD observed in HICs and implement public health policies to reduce the rising CVD burden.

## THE DECLINE OF CVDs IN HICs

The last half of the 20th century saw an acceleration of research into the causes of CVDs. The premature death of US President Roosevelt due to hypertensive heart disease (a blood pressure of 300/190 mmHg) and stroke in 1945 and the rising national disease burden in the 1940s, when CVD had become the number one cause of mortality among Americans, accounting for one in two deaths, catalyzed the development of the landmark epidemiological study, The Framingham Heart Study (FHS), in 1948 to understand the major modifiable risk factors contributing to CVDs.[3,4] The FHS helped in identifying these risk factors such as high blood pressure, high cholesterol, smoking, and diabetes, as well as contributing to altering various fallacies of physicians at that time. This included the belief that high blood pressure is important to force blood through stiffened arteries and a normal attribute associated with aging and that diastolic blood pressure was of prime importance. Systolic blood pressure was considered innocuous, particularly in the elderly. The FHS also generated evidence on smoking as a risk factor for heart attacks.[3,4] Importantly, it also helped shift the focus from treatment of individuals with CVD to prevention of the disease in those at risk and enabled the targeting of preventive interventions. The development of "risk profiles" or "risk scores" enabled physicians to calculate an individual's risk of developing the CVD. The first one was published in 1976 by Kannel and colleagues, while the widely regarded and used Framingham Risk Score was published in 1998 by Wilson and colleagues.[5,6]

Based on the scientific evidence generated through FHS and other similar global studies and the implementation of evidence-based public health policies, especially for tobacco control and improved treatments, a remarkable decline in mortality due to CVDs was observed in the United States since the 1970s. Similar declines were observed in other HICs as well, such as Australia, Western Europe, and the UK. For example, there was a 70% decline in CVD mortality rates in the Netherlands, whereas in the UK and Ireland from 1980 to 2009 a 60% decline was reported.[7] Annual age-adjusted CVD mortality rates have continued to decline in the United States, falling by 22% from 1990 to 2013.[4]

Finland, which had one of the highest rates of CVD in the world in the 1970s, provides one of the best exemplars of effective translation of available evidence into policies to modify CVD risks at the population level. A community-based prevention project involving multiple sectors resulted in lowering CVD in the demonstration area (North Karelia). This was later expanded nationwide

DOI: 10.1201/b23266-18

to modify the main CVD risk factors (cholesterol, blood pressure, smoking, diet) at the population level, utilizing community health education and empowerment; improving health service delivery; initiating prevention in multiple settings (such as schools and workplaces); collaboration with media, civil society organizations, and the private sector; implementation of public health regulations (food labeling); and international collaboration. Notably, there were remarkable decreases in mortality from CVD (>70%) from 1972 to 2014, leading to increased life expectancy and better quality of life.[8] In Mauritius, the government's policy to substitute the main cooking oil from high saturated fat palm oil to unsaturated soybean oil led to a 15% decline in population cholesterol levels.[9] Similarly in Poland, removal of subsidies for animal-based dairy products (butter, lard) and a liberal import policy on vegetable oils, fruits, and vegetables led to marked substitution of saturated fats by unsaturated fats and subsequent decrease in CVD mortality.[10] Fiscal policies have been documented to be impactful in driving reductions in population tobacco use in most countries and are being increasingly used for other risks such as excess alcohol intake and unhealthy foods and beverages.

## RATIONALE FOR IMPLEMENTING EVIDENCE-BASED PUBLIC HEALTH POLICIES

Population-wide risk factor modification (such as modest reductions in tobacco use/salt intake/fat intake/sugar intake and increase in physical activity/fruit and vegetable intake) could prevent a large proportion of disease events in the whole population, given that most disease events occur at modest elevations of multiple risk factors rather than at marked elevations of a single risk factor. For example, a population-wide decrease of just 2 mmHg systolic blood pressure, such as that easily achievable by modest salt reduction, would be estimated to lower total mortality as well mortality from stroke and coronary heart disease, with further decreases in blood pressure yielding higher reductions (Figure 9.1).[11] Another estimate indicated that a 2 mmHg diastolic blood pressure reduction in the population would be estimated to lower the prevalence of hypertension by 17%, coronary heart disease by 6%, and the risk of stroke by 15%, with many of the benefits occurring among patients with normal blood pressure.[12] These experiences underline the favorable impact of healthy public policies on CVD prevention and control.

Even though clinical approaches to treat individuals at high risk of CVDs are very important, they are resource-intensive and likely benefit few patients. They have limited impact on reducing a population's risk, are costly, require extensive health-sector involvement and resources, and are unsustainable in the long term. Capewell et al. had used the IMPACT Coronary Heart Disease Model, a validated statistical model, to determine the relative contributions of improved treatments and population-level interventions in over 15 countries.[13,14] In most HICs where significant

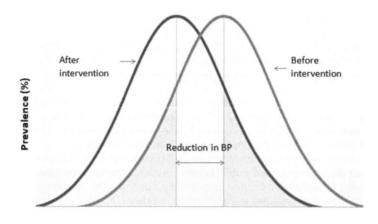

| Reduction in SBP | % Reduction in Mortality | | |
|:---:|:---:|:---:|:---:|
| (mm Hg) | Stroke | CHD | Total |
| 2 | -6 | -4 | -3 |
| 3 | -8 | -5 | -4 |
| 5 | -14 | -9 | -7 |

**Figure 9.1** Impact of modest changes in population blood pressure on CVD mortality.

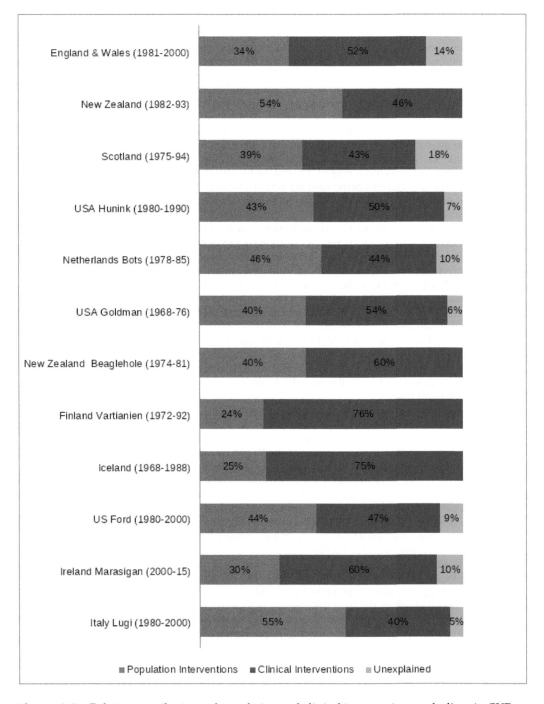

**Figure 9.2** Relative contributions of population and clinical interventions to declines in CVD mortality in high-income countries.

declines have been observed in mortality from CVDs, most of the decline has been attributable to population-wide changes in risk factors (Figure 9.2), achieved largely through lifestyle change supported by an enabling policy environment. Of note, even in the high-risk approach, extensive use of evidence-based therapies rather than tertiary care–based high-end interventions have contributed to much of the decline.[13,14]

## POLICY LESSONS FOR ADDRESSING THE INCREASING BURDEN IN LMICS

Thus, the scientific evidence base accumulated over the past half a century holds important lessons for LMICs and clearly indicates that CVD risk factors are highly amenable to preventive efforts. Promoting healthy lifestyles and behaviors through effective public health policies can reduce tobacco use, promote healthier diets, and increase physical activity at the population level and reduce the risk of premature CVDs. What is needed is a synergistic mix of both prevention at the population level and making widely available proven and affordable clinical treatments at the individual level to those requiring them equitably. Moreover, preventive efforts have been reported to be cost-effective and feasible to implement at the population level.

Despite the availability of proven and effective prevention and treatment strategies for CVDs, there is a huge "know-to-do gap", especially in most LMICs. For instance, the detection and control rates of hypertension, which is a major CVD risk factor, are abysmally low. In most LMICs, less than half of those who have hypertension are actually detected, less than half of those detected receive appropriate treatment, and less than half of those receiving treatment have their blood pressure treated to recommended targets ("the rule of halves").[15,16] In addition to poor control rates, of considerable concern is the fact that once hypertension-related CVD occurs, the use of proven, inexpensive, evidence-based secondary prevention therapies is also very low in primary and secondary care, leading to a large and escalating burden of avoidable and premature mortality. A global study indicated that up to 80% of individuals were not on proven and effective lifesaving drug treatments after a stroke or heart attack.[17] Furthermore, there were also large inequalities in access to lifesaving CVD treatments between the rich and poor nations and significant inequalities within countries.[18] This results in avoidable complications, increased healthcare costs, poor quality of life, premature disability, and death.

Given this, it is increasingly clear that LMICs, which currently bear a disproportionate disease burden, cannot adopt the resource-intensive model of healthcare to address CVDs and should therefore prioritize prevention approaches concomitantly with evidence-based clinical approaches focused on early detection and treatment, which can have substantially greater impact on improving population heart health.

The landmark UN High Level Meeting on the prevention and control of noncommunicable diseases (NCDs) in 2011 provided an impetus to concerted global efforts to reduce NCDs, including CVDs, which are a major contributor to the NCD disease burden in most countries. Subsequently, in 2013, the World Health Assembly endorsed the World Health Organization's (WHO's) Global Action Plan for the Prevention and Control of NCDs 2013–2020, which called for a 25% reduction in premature NCD mortality by 2025, with a focus on achieving nine voluntary targets for 2025 against a baseline from 2010 (Figure 9.3).[19] This Global Action Plan aims to help countries reduce the preventable and avoidable burden of morbidity, mortality, and disability due to NCDs by means of multisectoral collaboration and cooperation at national, regional, and global levels. The Sustainable Development Goals (SDGs), which were released in 2015, call for a more ambitious 30% reduction in premature NCD mortality by 2030.[20] These global targets include risk factor targets and health system targets, with most related to CVD prevention and control. These targets were chosen based on high epidemiological and public health relevance, coherence with major global NCD reduction strategies, availability of evidence-based and feasible public health interventions, evidence of achievability at the country level, existence of unambiguous data collection instruments, and potential to set a baseline and monitor changes over time.

The WHO advocates that member countries implement a complement of evidence-based interventions called the 'Best Buys', which targets all the chief CVD risks as well as management (Figure 9.4).[19,20]

Based on synthesis of available scientific evidence, the WHO has developed global strategies and technical guidance for countries to implement public health policies and health system actions. These include the Framework Convention on Tobacco Control (FCTC) and the MPOWER strategy for reducing tobacco use[21]; the Global Strategy on Diet, Physical Activity and Health to improve diets and increase activity levels[22]; the Global Strategy to Reduce the Harmful Use of Alcohol[23]; the SHAKE Package[24] and Global Sodium Benchmarks for Different Food Categories to advance salt reduction[25]; recommendations on the marketing of foods and nonalcoholic beverages to children[26]; the REPLACE action framework for elimination of trans fatty acids[27]; and the Package of Essential Noncommunicable Disease Interventions (PEN) for providing evidence-based primary care for NCDs in low-resource settings.[28]

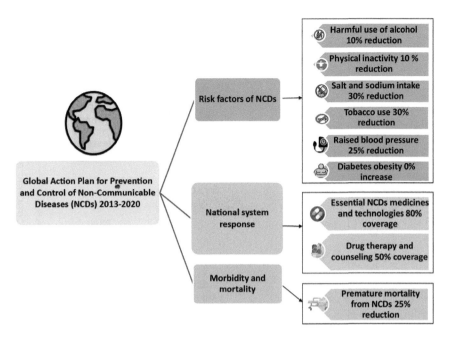

**Figure 9.3** Global NCD targets

| Population-Based Interventions Addressing NCD/CVD Risk Factors | | | Individual-Based Interventions Addressing NCDs/CVDs in Primary Care | |
|---|---|---|---|---|
| Tobacco use | Harmful use of alcohol | Unhealthy diet and physical activity | Cancer | Cardiovascular diseases and diabetes |
| • Increase in excise tax and price<br><br>• Plain packaging, health information, and graphic warnings about tobacco<br><br>• Bans on advertising, promotion, and sponsorship<br><br>• Smoke-free indoor workplaces, public places, and public transport<br><br>• Mass media use to educate the public | • Increase in excise tax<br><br>• Comprehensive restrictions and bans on alcohol marketing<br><br>• Restrictions on the availability of retailed alcohol | • Salt reduction through reformulation<br><br>• Establish supportive environments in public institutions and provide low-salt options<br><br>• Mass media campaigns<br><br>• Implementation of front-of-pack labeling<br><br>• Community-wide public education and awareness programs about physical activity | • Prevention of cervical cancer through screening (visual inspection with acetic acid [VIA]) and treatment of pre-cancerous lesions<br><br>• Vaccination against human papillomavirus | • Multidrug therapy (including glycemia control for diabetes mellitus) and counseling for individuals who have had a heart attack or stroke and to persons at high risk (>30%) of a cardiovascular event within 10 years |

**Figure 9.4** The 'best buys': An evidence-based intervention package.

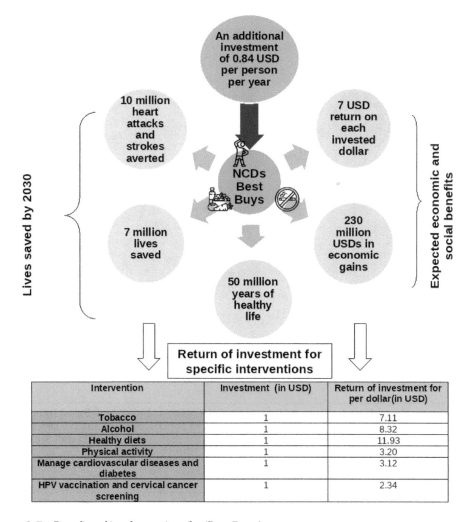

**Figure 9.5** Benefits of implementing the 'Best Buys'.

A recent analysis reports that the implementation of the 'Best Buys' by countries leveraging the aforementioned strategies and technical guidance has the potential to save 7 million lives, avert 10 million heart attacks and strokes, and result in a gain of 50 million life years and 230 million in economic and social gains (Figure 9.5).[20] This could be achieved by investing just an additional USD 84 per person per year in LMICs. The overall return on investment (ROI) was estimated to be USD 7 per dollar invested, with the ROI for healthy diets being the highest (USD 11.93 per dollar invested).[20] This makes the 'Best Buys' not only affordable for LMIC governments but has the potential to have a multiplier effect to deliver long-term social and economic benefits, as well as likely contribute to building back better from the adverse impact on the ongoing COVID-19 pandemic. Notably, some of them, such as increased taxes on tobacco and alcohol products, while reducing CVD-related health risks, will also continue to generate revenue for many years for governments.

The rising burden of CVDs, especially in LMICs, warrants concerted evidence-based public health action anchored on contextual factors. Public health policy making and implementation in LMICs should take into consideration the following tenets:

1. A life-course approach, which entails adopting a comprehensive and integrated response to addressing the continuum of risk and risk modification throughout the lifespan.

2. Building and utilizing a contextually relevant evidence base in LMICs for policy implementation.

3. Considering the financial feasibility of implementing relevant evidence-based policies.

4. Determining the social acceptance of policies that are prioritized for implementation.

5. Assessing the readiness of the health system to implement policies in the domain of CVD prevention and control.

6. Assessing likely equity issues and adopting mitigating measures to reach the most vulnerable population sub-groups.

7. Recognizing the cultural sensitivities and tailoring policy implementation to suit the context.

8. Meaningfully engaging communities, patients, and other relevant stakeholders and measuring the impact through newer approaches such as photo voice, patient voice surveys, and discrete choice experiments.

Closing the current know-to-do gaps between available scientific evidence and policy implementation is necessary to achieve the WHO and SDGs goals of reduction in NCD/CVD mortality. A recent report indicates that that no LMIC is on track achieve these goals if their 2010–2016 average rates of decline for both men and women are maintained or exceeded. Reassuringly, the report also showed that effective and integrated health systems interventions, combined with tobacco and alcohol control, could transform NCD/CVD control such that most countries could achieve the SDG target.[29]

## CONCLUSION

Evidence and experience from HICs indicate the need to prioritize risk factor modification and prevention, as well as early diagnosis and evidence-based management of established disease. The evidence also indicates that greatest benefits vis-à-vis reductions in CVD mortality and morbidity can be achieved using the previously mentioned approach, which is also the most cost-effective. Thus, in alignment with the Global Action Plan and the associated global strategies for initiating action on CVD and its determinants, national health policies and programs should prioritize a comprehensive approach comprising policy measures involving multiple stakeholders, multisectoral whole-of-society action, population-based risk factor modification, and evidence-based, cost-effective management of individuals with CVD.

## REFERENCES

1. WHO. Cardiovascular Diseases [Internet]. 2017 Available from: www.who.int/news-room/fact-sheets/detail/cardiovascular-diseases-(cvds). Assessed 29 March, 2022.
2. Roth GA, Mensah GA, Johnson CO, Addolorato G, Ammirati E, Baddour LM, Barengo NC, Beaton AZ, Benjamin EJ, Benziger CP, Bonny A, Brauer M, Brodmann M, Cahill TJ, Carapetis J, Catapano AL, Chugh SS, Cooper LT, Coresh J, Criqui M, DeCleene N, Eagle KA, Emmons-Bell S, Feigin VL, Fernández-Solà J, Fowkes G, Gakidou E, Grundy SM, He FJ, Howard G, Hu F, Inker L, Karthikeyan G, Kassebaum N, Koroshetz W, Lavie C, Lloyd-Jones D, Lu HS, Mirijello A, Temesgen AM, Mokdad A, Moran AE, Muntner P, Narula J, Neal B, Ntsekhe M, Moraes de Oliveira G, Otto C, Owolabi M, Pratt M, Rajagopalan S, Reitsma M, Ribeiro ALP, Rigotti N, Rodgers A, Sable C, Shakil S, Sliwa-Hahnle K, Stark B, Sundström J, Timpel P, Tleyjeh IM, Valgimigli M, Vos T, Whelton PK, Yacoub M, Zuhlke L, Murray C, Fuster V; GBD-NHLBI-JACC Global Burden of Cardiovascular Diseases Writing Group. Global burden of cardiovascular diseases and risk factors, 1990–2019: Update From the GBD 2019 Study. J Am Coll Cardiol 2020;76:2982–3021.
3. Mahmood SS, Levy D, Vasan RS, Wang TJ. The framingham heart study and the epidemiology of cardiovascular disease: a historical perspective. Lancet 2014;383:999–1008.
4. Mensah GA, Wei GS, Sorlie PD, Fine LJ, Rosenberg Y, Kaufmann PG, Mussolino ME, Hsu LL, Addou E, Engelgau MM, Gordon D. Decline in cardiovascular mortality: possible causes and implications. Circ Res 2017;120:366–380.
5. Kannel WB, McGee D, Gordon T. A general cardiovascular risk profile: the Framingham Study. Am J Cardiol 1976;38:46–51.
6. Wilson PW, D'Agostino RB, Levy D, Belanger AM, Silbershatz H, Kannel WB. Prediction of coronary heart disease using risk factor categories. Circulation 1998;97:1837–1847.

7. Hartley A, Marshall DC, Salciccioli JD, Sikkel MB, Maruthappu M, Shalhoub J. Trends in mortality from ischemic heart disease and cerebrovascular disease in Europe: 1980 to 2009. Circulation 2016;133:1916–1926.

8. Vartiainen E. The North Karelia Project: Cardiovascular disease prevention in Finland. Glob Cardiol Sci Pract 2018;2018:13.

9. Dowse GK, Gareeboo H, Alberti KG, Zimmet P, Tuomilehto J, Purran A, Fareed D, Chitson P, Collins VR. Changes in population cholesterol concentrations and other cardiovascular risk factor levels after five years of the non-communicable disease intervention programme in Mauritius. Mauritius non-communicable disease study group. BMJ 1995; 311:1255–1259.

10. Zatonski WA, McMichael AJ, Powles JW. Ecological study of reasons for sharp decline in mortality from ischaemic heart disease in Poland since 1991. BMJ 1998;316:1047–1051.

11. Whelton PK, He J, Appel LJ, Cutler JA, Havas S, Kotchen TA, Roccella EJ, Stout R, Vallbona C, Winston MC, Karimbakas J; National High Blood Pressure Education Program Coordinating Committee. Primary prevention of hypertension: clinical and public health advisory from the national high blood pressure education program. JAMA 2002;288:1882–1888.

12. Cook NR, Cohen J, Hebert PR, et al. Implications of small reductions in diastolic blood pressure for primary prevention. Arch Intern Med 1995;155:701–709.

13. Ford ES, Ajani UA, Croft JB, Critchley JA, Labarthe DR, Kottke TE, Giles WH, Capewell S. Explaining the decrease in U.S. deaths from coronary disease, 1980–2000. N Engl J Med 2007;356:2388–2398.

14. Ford ES, Capewell S. Proportion of the decline in cardiovascular mortality disease due to prevention versus treatment: public health versus clinical care. Annu Rev Public Health 2011;32:5–22.

15. Chow CK, Teo KK, Rangarajan S, Islam S, Gupta R, Avezum A, Bahonar A, Chifamba J, Dagenais G, Diaz R, Kazmi K, Lanas F, Wei L, Lopez-Jaramillo P, Fanghong L, Ismail NH, Puoane T, Rosengren A, Szuba A, Temizhan A, Wielgosz A, Yusuf R, Yusufali A, McKee M, Liu L, Mony P, Yusuf S; PURE (Prospective Urban Rural Epidemiology) Study investigators. Prevalence, awareness, treatment, and control of hypertension in rural and urban communities in high-, middle-, and low-income countries. JAMA 2013;310:959–968.

16. NCD Risk Factor Collaboration (NCD-RisC). Worldwide trends in hypertension prevalence and progress in treatment and control from 1990 to 2019: a pooled analysis of 1201 population-representative studies with 104 million participants. Lancet 2021;398:957–980.

17. Yusuf S, Islam S, Chow CK, Rangarajan S, Dagenais G, Diaz R, Gupta R, Kelishadi R, Iqbal R, Avezum A, Kruger A, Kutty R, Lanas F, Lisheng L, Wei L, Lopez-Jaramillo P, Oguz A, Rahman O, Swidan H, Yusoff K, Zatonski W, Rosengren A, Teo KK; Prospective Urban Rural Epidemiology (PURE) Study Investigators. Use of secondary prevention drugs for cardiovascular disease in the community in high-income, middle-income, and low-income countries (the PURE Study): a prospective epidemiological survey. Lancet 2011;378:1231–1243.

18. Murphy A, Palafox B, O'Donnell O, Stuckler D, Perel P, AlHabib KF, Avezum A, Bai X, Chifamba J, Chow CK, Corsi DJ, Dagenais GR, Dans AL, Diaz R, Erbakan AN, Ismail N, Iqbal R, Kelishadi R, Khatib R, Lanas F, Lear SA, Li W, Liu J, Lopez-Jaramillo P, Mohan V, Monsef N, Mony PK, Puoane T, Rangarajan S, Rosengren A, Schutte AE, Sintaha M, Teo KK, Wielgosz A, Yeates K, Yin L, Yusoff K, Zatońska K, Yusuf S, McKee M. Inequalities in the use of secondary prevention of cardiovascular disease by socioeconomic status: evidence from the PURE observational study. Lancet Glob Health 2018;6:e292–e301.

19. Global action plan for the prevention and control of noncommunicable diseases 2013–2020. Geneva: World Health Organization; 2013.

20. Saving lives, spending less: the case for investing in noncommunicable diseases. Geneva: World Health Organization; 2021.

21. WHO report on the global tobacco epidemic 2021: addressing new and emerging products. Geneva: World Health Organization; 2021.

22. Global strategy on diet, physical activity and health. Geneva: World Health Organization; 2004.

23. Global strategy to reduce the harmful use of alcohol. Geneva: World Health Organization; 2010.

24. World Health Organization. The SHAKE technical package for salt reduction. Geneva: World Health Organization; 2016.

25. WHO global sodium benchmarks for different food categories. Geneva: World Health Organization; 2021.
26. Set of recommendations on the marketing of foods and non-alcoholic beverages to children. Geneva: World Health Organization; 2010.
27. REPLACE trans-fat: an action package to eliminate industrially produced trans fatty acids. Geneva: World Health Organization; 2018.
28. WHO package of essential noncommunicable (PEN) disease interventions for primary health care. Geneva: World Health Organization; 2020.
29. NCD Countdown 2030 Collaborators. NCD Countdown 2030: pathways to achieving sustainable development goal target 3.4. *Lancet* 2020;396: 918–934.

# 10 Situational Analysis of Health Policies for Cardiovascular Disease Prevention and Control

*Sugitha Sureshkumar and Sailesh Mohan*

## CONTENTS

## INTRODUCTION

Cardiovascular diseases (CVDs) are a growing public health priority that needs to be urgently addressed worldwide, particularly in low- and middle-income countries (LMICs), which are disproportionately impacted. Reassuringly, there are very compelling evidence-based public health policies and clinical management strategies that, if implemented widely, can reduce or modify population risk, prevent disease progression, and improve population health outcomes (1). However, despite the availability of proven and cost-effective interventions, national health policies and policymakers in many LMICs have until recently tended to prioritize the provision of curative services over population-wide prevention efforts, which are fundamental to stemming the rising tide of CVDs.

Drawing upon the scientific evidence base formed over the past half a century and experiences from many high-income countries (HICs) which have achieved noteworthy declines in CVD-related morbidity and morbidity, the World Health Organization (WHO) constructed policies and programs for prevention and control. It has advocated that member countries implement a suite of evidence-based interventions called the "Best Buys", which target the main CVD risks. After the UN High-Level Meeting on Noncommunicable Diseases (NCDs) in 2011, the WHO called for a 25% reduction in premature mortality from NCDs, including CVDs, by 2025 through a Global Action Plan. Subsequently, the Sustainable Development Goals (SDGs) have endorsed this target and called for a 30% reduction in premature NCDs, including CVDs, by 2030 (2).

The ambitious goal of 25% by 2025 or 30% by 2030 is heavily dependent on the effective implementation of population-wide policies for risk factor reduction/modification, synergistically complemented by improving access to available proven lifesaving treatments. It is estimated that

DOI: 10.1201/b23266-19

every dollar invested in "Best Buys" will yield a return of at least seven dollars, and its global implementation will save 10 million lives by 2025 and prevent 17 million strokes and heart attacks by 2030 (3).

In this chapter, we examine the status of CVD prevention and control policies in various parts of the world and subsequently explore the recommended policy interventions (Best Buys) in terms of their implementation and ways forward for addressing the challenges and seizing opportunities. Specifically, we examine the status of policy implementation in 12 countries representing all the six WHO regions of the world. From each WHO region we selected two countries based on the CVD burden, population size, and gross domestic product (GDP), for a detailed examination to provide a broad perspective on the current situation. In addition, we also selected three large countries (India, China, and Russia) where nearly 40% of the global population resides and which together contribute to a significant proportion of global CVD burden and are facing similar health system challenges. We have used data available from the WHO Noncommunicable Diseases Progress Monitor 2020, Global Health Expenditure database 2018, Institute of Health Metrics, and the World Bank (WB).

## CURRENT STATUS OF HEALTH POLICIES FOR CVD PREVENTION AND CONTROL

The 15 countries from the six WHO-defined regions are detailed here. Twelve have been chosen to provide a contrasting picture of CVD/NCD burden and mortality in each region, while also considering the variation in population size and GDP to provide a broad perspective on the current situation. The other three have been included to present a perspective of large countries with high CVD burden. One-third of deaths globally were attributable to CVD in 2019 (18.5 million deaths). China, followed by India and Russia, were accountable for 40% of these deaths (4).

Using data from the Global Burden of Disease Study (GBD), the WB, WHO, and individual country documents, we present the CVD and NCD policies that are in place in the following WHO regions: African Region (WHO AFRO): South Africa and Uganda; Region of the Americas (WHO AMR): United States and Peru; Southeast Asia Region (WHO SEAR): Indonesia and Nepal; European Region (WHO EUR): Bulgaria and France; Eastern Mediterranean Region (WHO EMR): Morocco and Qatar; and Western Pacific Region (WHO WPR): Japan and Papua New Guinea.

Fifteen CVD Best Buys policy recommendations are advocated by the WHO (5). The last update about their implementation status in 2020 presents a mixed picture as to how various regions and countries are advancing toward the 25% by 2025 or 30% by 2030 goals.

While most countries have one CVD/NCD plan or strategy in place, Peru and Papua New Guinea have a partial national CVD/NCD plan or strategy, whereas South Africa and Uganda have no national CVD/NCD plan or strategy implemented.

### Africa Region (WHO AFRO)

Although there is still a huge burden of communicable diseases in this region, an increase in CVD has been observed over the past few decades, with considerable differences between countries (e.g., total CVD deaths in 2019 ranged from 8.5% in Niger to 48.7% in Algeria) (4). Given this, effective implementation of the Best Buys can help prevent and control CVDs as well as improve population health outcomes and quality of life.

*Uganda*

**Demographics**

Total Population: 41,488,000

GDP: 3,737,2032,558 USD[a]

**CVD Policy**

Existing NCD Action Plan: No[b]

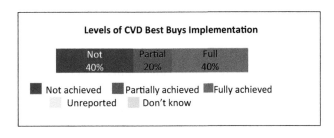

145

**CVD Profile**

Total population percentage of deaths from CVDs: 12%

Total number of CVD deaths: 28,149[c]

Total population percentage of deaths from NCDs: 33%

Total number of NCD deaths: 97,600

Probability of premature mortality from NCDs: 22%[b]

**Health Financing in USD per Person**

Current health expenditure as a % of GDP: 6.5%[d]

Total health spending: $43

Government spending: $7 (16.3%)

Development assistance: $18 (41.9%)

OOP: $17 (39.5%)

Prepaid private insurance: $1 (2.3%)[c]

In the absence of a national NCD strategy or plan, in Uganda, the Best Buys implementation level has been sub-optimal, with 40% of policies fully achieved and a further 20% partially achieved. With out-of-pocket (OOP) payments and development assistance accounting for most of the health expenditure, Uganda may benefit from implementing population-wide policies for CVD control and health system strengthening to address CVDs.

## South Africa

**Demographics**

Total population: 56,015,000

GDP: 301,924,000,000 USD[a]

**CVD Policy**

Existing NCD action plan: No[b]

**Levels of CVD Best Buys Implementation**

| Don't know | Not | Partial | Full |
|---|---|---|---|
| 7% | 33% | 33% | 27% |

**CVD Profile**

Total population percentage of deaths from CVDs: 16%

Total number of CVD deaths: 82,661[c]

Total population percentage of deaths from NCDs: 51%

Total number of NCD deaths: 269,500

Probability of premature mortality from NCDs: 26%[b]

**Health Financing in USD per Person**

Current health expenditure as a percentage of GDP: 8.2%[d]

Total health spending: $532

Development assistance: $12 (2.2%)

Government spending: $284 (53.4%)

OOP: $41 (7.7%)

Prepaid private insurance: $195 (36.7%)[c]

South Africa reports fully implementing 27% of the Best Buys, while partially implementing 33%. South Africa spends more on health than any other African country, yet the health outcomes aren't commensurate with the spending (6). There are considerable health disparities with efforts underway to address them through several initiatives such as the Health Department's expected expansion of antiretroviral treatment, which aims to reach 6.5 million people by 2022–2023, and the roll-out of the South African National Insurance Plan (7).

### Region of the Americas (WHO AMR)

The region of the Americas has a high burden of CVDs with substantial variations between countries (e.g., total deaths due to CVD ranges between 16.7% in Guatemala and 38.5% in the Dominican Republic). CVD is the leading cause of mortality in most countries. Although remarkable declines in CVD mortality have been reported from North America due to effective implementation of population-wide policies and access to better treatments, countries in Latin America and the Caribbean are experiencing health transitions with increasing CVD-associated morbidity, disability, and mortality.

## Peru

**Demographics**

Total population: 31,774,000

GDP: 202,014,000,000 USD[a]

**CVD Policy**

Existing NCD action plan: Partial[b]

**Levels of CVD Best Buys Implementation**

| Unreported | Not | Partial | Full |
|---|---|---|---|
| 7% | 20% | 27% | 46% |

**CVD Profile**

Total population percentage of deaths from CVDs: 19%

Total number of CVD deaths: 29,215[c]

Total population percentage of deaths from NCDs: 69%

Total number of NCD deaths: 119,400

Probability of premature mortality from NCDs: 13%[b]

**Health Financing in USD per Person**

Current health expenditure as a percentage of GDP: 5.2%[d]

Total health spending: $331

Development assistance: $1 (0.3%)

Government spending: $206 (62.2%)

OOP: $96 (29%)

Prepaid private insurance: $28 (8.5%)[c]

Peru has a decentralized health care system with multiple services and insurance providers. In 2014, the first National Health Strategy for Control and Prevention of Non-Communicable Diseases was published. CVDs account for almost one-fifth of total mortality, one of the lowest CVD mortality rates in the Americas (3). There are huge health inequalities and a high proportion of OOP payments. Peru reports fully implementing 46% of the Best Buys, while partially implementing 27%. Due to the emergence of strong academic institutions such as the CRONICAS, one of Latin America's leading NCD research centers, Peru has considerably improved its capacity to monitor and address CVDs through interdisciplinary research.

## USA

**Demographics**

Total population: 322,200,000

GDP: 20,936,600,000,000 USD[a]

**CVD Policy**

Existing NCD action plan: Yes[b]

**Levels of CVD Best Buys Implementation**

| Don't know | Not | Partial | Full |
|---|---|---|---|
| 7% | 33% | 27% | 33% |

**CVD Profile**

Total population percentage of deaths from CVDs: 32.5%

Total number of CVD deaths: 957,455[c]

Total population percentage of deaths from NCDs: 88%

Total number of NCD deaths: 2,474,000

Probability of premature mortality from NCDs: 15%[b]

**Health Financing in USD per Person**

Current health expenditure as a percentage of GDP: 16.8%[d]

Total health spending: $10,243

Development assistance: $0 (0%)

Government spending: $5,365 (52.4%)

OOP: $1,177 (11.5%)

Prepaid private insurance: $3,701 (36.1%)[c]

The United States has one of the highest spending on health care in the world. Despite this, there is a high burden of CVDs as well as associated mortality. The U.S. health system is heterogenous and comprises public and private, for-profit and nonprofit insurance providers, with the government funding the national health program (Medicare) for a select group of the population (seniors, those with disabilities, and veterans), as well as Medicaid and the Children's Health Insurance Program for low-income families and children (8). The high uninsured rate decreased to 8.5% of the population from 16% in 2010, the year the Affordable Care Act was implemented. With persisting health inequalities, CVDs remain a public health priority, especially among African American and minority communities. The United States reports fully implementing 33% of the Best Buys, while partially implementing 27%.

## Southeast Asian Region (WHO SEAR)

The burden of CVD is growing in this region, which is home to a quarter of the global population. Despite the continuing challenges of communicable diseases and maternal and newborn health issues, CVD mortality has been increasing across the region. Notably, CVDs affect people in this region at relatively younger ages with high levels of premature mortality and disability. There is considerable variation in the burden between countries (e.g., total deaths due to CVD ranged from 23% in Thailand to 43% in DPR Korea).

### *Nepal*

**Demographics**

Total population: 28,983,000

GDP: 33,657,175,561 USD[a]

**CVD Policy**

Existing NCD action plan: Yes[b]

**Levels of CVD Best Buys Implementation**

| Unreported 7% | Not 40% | Partial 20% | Full 33% |
|---|---|---|---|

**CVD Profile**

Total population percentage of deaths from CVDs: 24%

Total number of CVD deaths: 46,501[c]

Total population percentage of deaths from NCDs: 66%

Total number of NCD deaths: 121,100

Probability of premature mortality from NCDs: 22%[b]

**Health Financing in USD per Person**

Current health expenditure as a percentage of GDP: 5.8%[d]

Total health spending: $51

Development assistance: $4 (7.8%)

Government spending: $11 (21.6%)

OOP: $31 (60.8%)

Prepaid private insurance: $5 (9.8%)[c]

In Nepal a quarter of all deaths are attributable to CVDs. Nepal reports partially implementing 20% of the Best Buys and fully implementing 33%. It has high OOP payments and low government spending on health. Recently, it has committed to achieving universal health coverage by 2030 to improve health care access and reduce high OOP costs.

### *Indonesia*

**Demographics**

Total population: 261,100,000

GDP: 1,058,420,000,000 USD[a]

**CVD Policy**

Existing NCD action plan: Yes[b]

**Levels of CVD Best Buys Implementation**

| Not 34% | Partial 33% | Full 33% |
|---|---|---|

**CVD Profile**

Total population percentage of deaths from CVDs: 38%

Total number of CVD deaths: 651,481[c]

Total population percentage of deaths from NCDs: 73%

Total number of NCD deaths: 1,365,000

Probability of premature mortality from NCDs: 26%[b]

**Health Financing in USD per Person**

Current health expenditure as a percentage of GDP: 2.9%[d]

Total health spending: $120

Development assistance: $1 (0.8%)

Government spending: $52 (43.3%)

OOP: $46 (38.4%)

Prepaid private insurance: $21 (17.5%)[c]

Indonesia is the fourth most populous country in the world. Even though it has a robust primary health care system and has improved several population health outcomes, it has high morbidity and mortality from CVDs. Indonesia reports partially implementing 33% of the Best Buys and fully implementing 33%. Indonesia's national health scheme initiated in 2014, the Jaminan Kesehatan Nasional (JKN), is one of the biggest single-payer systems in the world. It provides coverage to 83% of its total population, but the OOP payments remain high (9).

## *India*

**Demographics**

Total population: 1,324,000,000

GDP: 2,660,024,524,867 USD[a]

**CVD Policy**

Existing NCD action plan: Yes[b]

**Levels of CVD Best Buys Implementation**

| Unreported | Partial | Full |
|------------|---------|------|
| 14% | 33% | 53% |

**CVD Profile**

Total population percentage of deaths from CVDs: 26%

Total number of CVD deaths: 2,574,410[c]

Total population percentage of deaths from NCDs: 63%

Total number of NCD deaths: 5,995,000

Probability of premature mortality from NCDs: 23%[b]

**Health Financing in USD per Person**

Current health expenditure as a percentage of GDP: 3%[d]

Total health spending: $72

Development assistance: $0.5 (0.7%)

Government spending: $19.5 (27%)

OOP: $45 (63%)

Prepaid private insurance: $7 (9.3%)[c]

With the second largest CVD burden worldwide, the globe's second most populous country, despite improvements in access to health care, faces large inequalities in health care, primarily related to socioeconomic status, geography, and gender. Its multipayer health system is tasked with the care of 16.5% of the world's CVD burden of disease and is reported to be addressing almost all CVD policy recommendations to some degree.

## European Region (WHO EUR)

This region has one of the highest burdens and mortality from CVDs globally, with more than half of all deaths attributable to CVDs (e.g., total deaths due to CVD ranged from 26% in Israel to 64% in Bulgaria). Select countries of Central and Eastern Europe have very high levels of CVD and associated mortality.

## *France*

**Demographics**

Total population: 64,721,000

GDP: 2,603,000,000,000 USD[a]

**CVD Profile**

Total population percentage of deaths from CVDs: 27.6%

Total number of CVD deaths: 116,496[c]

Total population percentage of deaths from NCDs: 88%

Total number of NCD deaths: 488,500

Probability of premature mortality from NCDs: 11%[b]

**CVD Policy**

Existing NCD action plan: Yes[b]

### Levels of CVD Best Buy Implementation

| Partial | Full |
|---------|------|
| 33% | 67% |

**Health Financing in USD per Person**

Current health expenditure as a percentage of GDP: 11.3%[d]

Total health spending: $4,531

Development assistance: $0 (0%)

Government spending: $3,490 (77%)

OOP: $428 (9.5%)

Prepaid private insurance: $613 (13.5%)[c]

France has one of the highest levels of policy implementation. It has implemented 67% of the Best Buys fully and 33% partially. It has universal health care with a statutory national health insurance system, which has high coverage. The nation spends a high amount on health and has one of the lowest CVD mortality rates among the Organisation for Economic Co-operation and Development (OECD) countries.

## *Bulgaria*

**Demographics**

Total population: 7,131,000

GDP: 69,105,101,090 USD[a]

**CVD Profile**

Total population percentage of deaths from NCDs: 95%

Total number of CVD deaths: 79,119[c]

Total population percentage of deaths from CVDs: 64%

Total number of NCD deaths: 101,300

Probability of premature mortality from NCDs: 24%[b]

**CVD Policy**

Existing NCD action plan: Yes[b]

### Levels of CVD Best Buys Implementation

| Unreported | Not | Partial | Full |
|------------|-----|---------|------|
| 13% | 7% | 27% | 53% |

**Health Financing in USD per Person**

Current health expenditure as a percentage of GDP: 7.3%[d]

Total health spending: $714

Development assistance: $1 (0.1%)

Government spending: $365 (51.2%)

OOP: $336 (47%)

Prepaid private insurance: $12 (1.7%)[c]

While having both the highest mortality and morbidity attributable to CVD in the European region and high OOP payments, Bulgaria reports implementing fully 53% of CVD Best Buys and 27% partially. The new reforms of the Bulgarian health system and the National Health Insurance Fund allowed privatization after years of centralized communist rule. These measures have brought about improvements in primary care, quality of care, public health, service structure, and financing, although a high burden of CVD persists.

## Russian Federation

**Demographics**

Total population: 144,000,000

GDP: 1,483,497,784,867 USD[a]

**CVD Policy**

Existing NCD action plan: Yes[b]

**Levels of CVD Best Buys Implementation**

| Not 14% | Partial 33% | Full 53% |
|---|---|---|

**CVD Profile**

Total population percentage of deaths from NCDs: 87%

Total number of CVD deaths: 1,004,931[c]

Total population percentage of deaths from CVDs: 56%

Total number of NCD deaths: 1,635,000

Probability of premature mortality from NCDs: 25%[b]

**Health Financing in USD per Person**

Current health expenditure as a percentage of GDP: 5.6%[d]

Total health spending: $541

Development assistance: $0.4 (0.07%)

Government spending: $316 (58%)

OOP: $213 (39.5%)

Prepaid private insurance: $13 (2.5%)[c]

Federal health programs in Russia focusing on service delivery and resource mobilization for areas, including primary care provision in rural areas, have evolved from the previous highly centralized system to reform adopting mandatory health insurance, yet significant inequalities in care persist (10). The country has the third highest CVD death rate globally. This has dropped since 2005 and has more recently plateaued in the last decade (4).

### Eastern Mediterranean Region (WHO EMR)

This region has a high burden of CVD and its risk factors, especially overweight/obesity, hypertension, physical inactivity, and smoking. The region has higher rates of physical inactivity than other WHO regions. There is wide variation in the burden, as well as mortality, from CVD (e.g., total deaths due to CVD ranged from 10% in Somalia to 25% in Syria).

## Morocco

**Demographics**

Total population: 35,277,000

GDP: 112,871,000,000 USD[a]

**CVD Policy**

Existing NCD action plan: Yes[b]

**Levels of CVD Best Buy Implementation**

| Not 20% | Partial 67% | Full 13% |
|---|---|---|

**CVD Profile**

Total population percentage of deaths from CVDs: 51%

Total number of CVD deaths: 117,033[c]

Total population percentage of deaths from NCDs: 80%

Total number of NCD deaths: 144,900

Probability of premature mortality from NCDs: 12%[b]

**Health Financing in USD per Person**

Current health expenditure as a percentage of GDP: 5.3%[d]

Total health spending: $171

Development assistance: $5 (2.9%)

Government spending: $71 (41.5%)

OOP: $90 (52.7%)

Prepaid private insurance: $5 (2.9%)[c]

In Morocco over half of all deaths occur due to CVDs. Despite this high burden, Morocco reports implementing only 13% of the Best Buys fully and 67% partially. The Moroccan basic medical scheme (AMO) and medical assistance scheme (RAMED), in place since 2005, have achieved high population-wide coverage and aim to cover the whole population by 2022. It is expected that this increased coverage can contribute to reducing the high OOP and improve CVD-related outcomes.

## Qatar

**Demographics**

Total population: 2,570,000

GDP: 146,374,000,000 USD[a]

**CVD Profile**

Total population percentage of deaths from CVDs: 25%

Total number of CVD deaths: 1,121[c]

Total population percentage of deaths from NCDs: 69%

Total number of NCD deaths: 2,700

Probability of premature mortality from NCDs: 15%[b]

**CVD Policy**

Existing NCD action plan: Yes[b]

**Levels of CVD Best Buys Implementation**

| Not | Partial | Full |
|-----|---------|------|
| 47% | 13% | 40% |

**Health Financing in USD per Person**

Current health expenditure as a percentage of GDP: 2.5%[d]

Total health spending: $1,958

Development assistance: $0 (0%)

Government spending: $1,612 (82.3%)

OOP: $159 (8.1%)

Prepaid private insurance: $187 (9.6%)[c]

Qatar reports implementing 40% of the Best Buys interventions fully and 13% partially. Government spending on health is high, and therefore OOP is quite low when compared to other countries in the region. However, non-Qatari migrant workers account for more than 80% of the population. This group has high levels of CVD and is reported to utilize the health system less than Qatari nationals, leading to health disparities.

## Western Pacific Region (WHO WPR)

Some of the Pacific Island countries and areas have a very high prevalence of overweight/obesity, with adult prevalence as high as 75%. CVD is the leading cause of death in this region, with most deaths occurring prematurely. There is considerable variation in the CVD burden and mortality between the countries (e.g., total deaths due to CVD ranges from 22% in Papua New Guinea to 43% in China).

### *Papua New Guinea*

**Demographics**

Total population: 8,085,000

GDP: 23,591,523,025 USD[a]

**CVD Profile**

Total population percentage of deaths from CVDs: 22%

Total number of CVD deaths: 15,540[c]

Total population percentage of deaths from NCDs: 56%

Total number of NCD deaths: 31,400

Probability of premature mortality from NCDs: 30%[b]

**CVD Policy**

Existing NCD action plan: Partial[b]

**Levels of CVD Best Buy Implementation**

| Not | Partial | Full |
|-----|---------|------|
| 40% | 53% | 7% |

**Health Financing in USD per Person**

Current health expenditure as a percentage of GDP: 2.4%[d]

Total health spending: $54

Development assistance: $9 (16.7%)

Government spending: $40 (74%)

OOP: $5 (9.3%)

Prepaid private insurance: $0 (0%)[c]

About one-fifth of all deaths in Papua New Guinea are due to CVDs. The probability of dying prematurely from an NCD is high, and CVD-related risks factors are also high, especially over-weight/obesity, hypertension, and smoking. Papua New Guinea reports implementing only 7% of the Best Buys fully and 53% partially.

## Japan

**Demographics**

Total population: 127,700,000

GDP: 5,064,870,000,000 USD[a]

**CVD Profile**

Total population percentage of deaths from CVDs: 27%

Total number of CVD deaths: 372,483[c]

Total population percentage of deaths from NCDs: 82%

Total number of NCD deaths: 1,080,000

Probability of premature mortality from NCDs: 8%[b]

**CVD Policy**

Existing NCD action plan: Yes[b]

**Levels of CVD Best Buys Implementation**

| Don't know 20% | Not 40% | Partial 40% |
|---|---|---|

**Health Financing in USD per Person**

Current health expenditure as a percentage of GDP: 11%[d]

Total health spending: $4,290

Development assistance: $0 (0%)

Government spending: $3,606 (84.1%)

OOP: $553 (12.9%)

Prepaid private insurance: $131 (3%)[c]

Japan has one of the highest life expectancies globally. NCDs account for 82% of total mortality, with CVDs contributing to 27% of deaths. Despite high levels of health spending and low levels of OOP, Japan reports implementing only 40% of the Best Buys partially. Health spending has increased over time as a percentage of GDP, owing mainly to population aging and increased health care costs.

## People's Republic of China

**Demographics**

Total population: 1,404,000,000

GDP: 14,722,730,697,890 USD[a]

**CVD Profile**

Total population percentage of deaths from CVDs: 43%

Total number of CVD deaths: 3,955,275[c]

Total population percentage of deaths from NCDs: 89%

Total number of NCD deaths: 9,259,000

Probability of premature mortality from NCDs: 17%[b]

**CVD Policy**

Existing NCD action plan: Yes[b]

**Levels of CVD Best Buys Implementation**

| None 33% | Partial 47% | Full 20% |
|---|---|---|

**Health Financing in USD per Person**

Current health expenditure as a percentage of GDP: 5.4%[d]

Total health spending: $521

Development assistance: $0.18 (0.03%)

Government spending: $296 (57%)

OOP: $185 (35%)

Prepaid private insurance: $40 (8%)[c]

The most populous country, China reports the highest CVD death toll globally. In 2019, close to 4 million CVD-related deaths occurred in China. The country has made considerable progress in ensuring that more than half of the Best Buys have been partially implemented. It is estimated that effective implementation of the Best Buys may avert the 23.4% of the CVD burden in China (11).

153

## Table 10.1 Aggregate CVD Best Buys for the 15 Countries Discussed in This Chapter

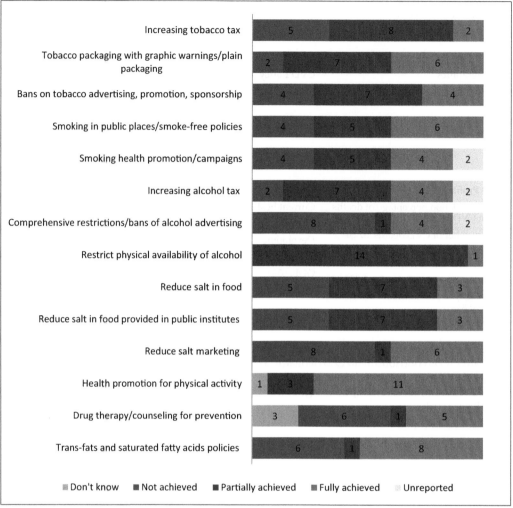

## SITUATIONAL ANALYSIS

### Barriers

CVD prevention and control attained worldwide importance and recognition as a priority health issue to be addressed at the population level only after the UN High-Level Meeting in 2011, which helped galvanize global action. The WHO's 25×25 Global Action Plan adopted in 2013 with the Best Buys as the recommended package of interventions has spurred action and development of multisectoral action plans at the country levels to advance policy implementation and strengthen health services. However, progress has been impeded by resource constraints, inefficient or low health spending, lack of multisectoral involvement and action to address the underlying root causes, and poor health system capacity (Table 10.1).

A multistakeholder approach is a cornerstone for achieving effective action on the risk factors and determinants of CVDs, including social, economic, and environmental determinants. For this to happen, countries need to have "health in all policies" and a "whole-of-society" approach with collaboration between health and nonhealth sectors at all levels of government and society so that the policies have long-term effectiveness and sustainability. Barriers to adopting such an approach can arise both from within the health sector or from other sectors, including industries linked to food, tobacco, and alcohol. Further, non–health-sector stakeholders may have competing priorities or vested interests and lack an understanding of their role in the development and implementation of CVD control policies. There can also be logistical challenges in multisectoral collaboration, resulting in a lack of stakeholder engagement or buy-in, which makes effective and sustained implementation of population-level policies for CVD control difficult.

## Challenges

The profound health transitions (epidemiological, nutritional, and demographic) propelling the rise of CVDs in most LMICs has occurred very rapidly within a compressed time frame compared to HICs. These countries face a triple burden of diseases concomitantly. Thus, until recently, low priority was accorded to addressing CVDs, as infectious disease and maternal and newborn health issues continued to pose serious challenges to governments and societies. This is compounded by low spending on health, lack of universal health coverage, high OOP expenditure, and resource-constrained health systems, especially the primary care systems with functional referral systems that are yet to reorient to also provide care for NCDs, which require continued and integrated long-term care.

Notably, there were also limited data to catalyze policy action and a lack of surveillance systems to track the changes in disease profile until very recently, when large-scale global efforts in this direction such as the GBD Study have released regular estimates of risk factors and various NCDs, including CVDs, for most countries of the world.

Lack of political commitment to implement the "Best Buys" interventions is another significant challenge. Health policymakers have largely prioritized curative services of CVD over population-wide prevention efforts, as investments in curative services bring in more political capital for policymakers and impact public support and opinion, while prevention efforts appear a less attractive option that doesn't entail high visibility, immediate benefits, or community-level recognition.

A lack of adequate investment in health and an absence of universal health coverage present another important challenge. CVD care is resource-intensive and places a disproportionate burden on individuals in the absence of universal health coverage, contributing to poor health outcomes. This is particularly evident for socioeconomically disadvantaged populations, leading to a widening of the existing health disparities.

## CONCLUSION

The benefits of CVD prevention and control are clear. The "Best Buys" offer an evidence-based package of interventions, which, if implemented effectively, can reduce the increasing burden of CVDs globally and more so in LMICs, which can ill-afford to treat their way out of the CVD epidemic. For this to be realized, it is imperative that countries prioritize both health promotion for disease prevention and clinical disease management. The root causes can be addressed effectively through multisectoral action to implement risk-reducing policies at the population level, while improving health system capacity through higher levels of investment and strengthening of the primary care systems and referral systems through universal health coverage to provide evidence-based and integrated care to those with disease, which can improve health outcomes and quality of life. This should be supplemented with improved surveillance with standardized tools to collect data for action and monitoring. Lastly, it is vital to secure, strengthen, and sustain political will and commitment for addressing CVDs.

## REFERENCES

1. Promoting Cardiovascular Health in the Developing World—A Critical Challenge to Achieve Global Health; Institute of Medicine (US) Committee on Preventing the Global Epidemic of Cardiovascular Disease: Meeting the Challenges in Developing Countries. Washington (DC). In: Kelly VFaBB, editor. National Academies Press (US); 2010. ISBN-13: 978-0-309-14774-3ISBN-10: 0-309-14774-3.
2. Joseph P. Reducing the global burden of cardiovascular disease, part 1 the epidemiology and risk factors. Circ Res 2017;121(6):677–694. doi: 101161 CIRCRESAHA117308903.
3. World Health Organization (WHO). Noncommunicable diseases progress monitor 2020. Geneva: World Health Organization; 2020.
4. Institute for Health Metrics and Evaluation (IHME). Global Burden of disease (GBD) database. Seattle, WA: IHME, University of Washington, 2021.
5. Mendis S, World Health Organization, World Heart Federation, et al. Global atlas on cardiovascular disease prevention and control. World Health Organization, 2011.

6. Kleinhert S. South Africa's health: Departing for a better future? Lancet 2009;374(9692):759–760. doi: 101016/S0140-6736(09)61306-4
7. Department of Health. National Health Act 2003, national health insurance policy- towards universal health care coverage. Government of South Africa, 2003. www.gov.za/sites/default/files/gcis_document/201707/40955gon627.pdf
8. The Commonwealth Fund December 2020. Health system overview—The United States, 2020. www.commonwealthfund.org/international-health-policy-center/countries/united-states
9. Herawati H. Research report – universal health coverage: tracking Indonesia's progress. Prakasara, 2020.
10. Popovich L. Russian federation: health system review. Health Syst Transit 2011;13(7):1–190.
11. Wei X. Implementation of a comprehensive intervention for patients at high risk of cardiovascular disease in rural China: A pragmatic cluster randomized controlled trial. PLoS ONE 2017;12(8): e0183169.
a. The World Bank. World Development Indicators (WDI) 2021. Washington: World Bank, 2021. https://databank.worldbank.org/home.aspx Accessed 27 July 2021.
b. World Health Organization (WHO). Noncommunicable Diseases Progress Monitor 2020. Geneva: World Health Organization, 2020. www.who.int/publications/i/item/9789240000490 Accessed 27 July 2021.
c. Institute for Health Metrics and Evaluation (IHME). Seattle, WA: IHME, University of Washington, 2021. www.healthdata.org Accessed 10 August 2021.
d. World Health Organization (WHO). Global Health Expenditure Database. Geneva: World Health Organization, 2018. https://apps.who.int/nha/database Accessed 09 August 2021.

# 11 Role of Surveillance Systems and Health Observatories for an Intelligent Public Health Approach to Cardiovascular Diseases

*Anand Krishnan and Lorraine Oldridge*

## CONTENTS

## INTRODUCTION

The term "surveillance" is derived from the French word meaning "to watch over" and, as applied to public health, means the close monitoring of the occurrence of selected health conditions in the population. Public health surveillance is the foundation for modern public health. The goal of surveillance is the use of data collected for the formulation of policies and programs to promote health and prevent disease and for measuring the impact of preventive efforts. It involves the systematic collection of data to ensure consistent and comparable data are collected in a regular fashion over a period. While infectious disease surveillance has focused largely on diseases as a part of its surveillance program, given the long time-lag between exposure to risk factors and the occurrence of noncommunicable diseases (NCDs), the surveillance of disease indicators is not enough to inform public health decision making adequately. Therefore, during recent years the concept of public health surveillance has evolved to encompass a much wider range of conditions or exposures known to have an impact on the occurrence of the disease of interest. Data and health intelligence have long been acknowledged as a first step in optimizing improvements in outcomes and a major driver of change in public health.

## A GENERAL FRAMEWORK FOR PUBLIC HEALTH SURVEILLANCE

Public health surveillance activities conform to the principles of a proposed general model of health surveillance (Figure 11.1) developed for a review of health surveillance functions in Canada.[1] This model clearly shows the interconnected elements that make up the complete "system" required to provide and support surveillance activities.

As the model describes, there are three layers that drive surveillance and inform the output of information, such as data collectors, surveillance experts and sponsors. These have both operational and leadership roles and are underpinned and influenced by the degree of capacity support provided. Data collectors ensure that comparable data are provided to, and available for, the surveillance experts. Surveillance experts are required to ensure that data are analyzed and interpreted so that the findings can be translated to support an informed response and improved service delivery. This also informs policy development and the role of the sponsor and should be collaborative with knowledge experts. Surveillance, along with the relevant knowledge and evidence base, informs policy decisions and ensures as far as possible that the appropriate mandate is in place, underpinned by relevant legislation and/or agreements. Sponsors are the authorities responsible for making sure that the correct systems are in place to prevent gaps and identify issues relevant to population health and well-being at an early stage.

DOI: 10.1201/b23266-20

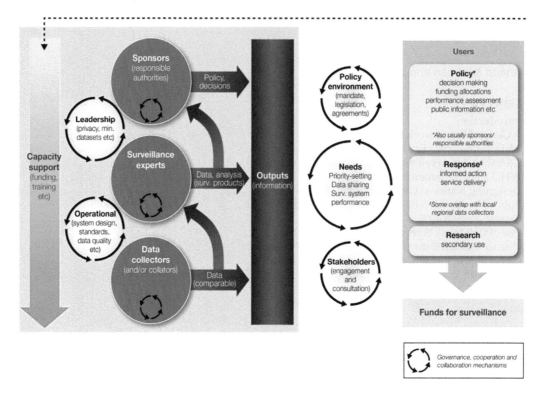

**Figure 11.1** A general model for health surveillance.[1]

## CVD SURVEILLANCE FRAMEWORK

Cardiovascular diseases (CVDs) are the leading cause of NCD mortality globally.[2] A central goal of cardiovascular surveillance would be to understand the determinants of the trends in CVD and the respective role of primary prevention versus that of the care of established disease in determining the CVD trends. A direct extension of surveillance is its application to assess the effectiveness of care and the response to interventions designed to improve the quality of care. Surveillance constitutes a comprehensive approach designed to track disease at the community level, is less costly and is more efficient than cohort studies. CVD surveillance typically tracks CVD deaths, the incidence and outcomes of some indicator conditions (say myocardial infarction or stroke), which is essential to monitor CVD trends and prevent CVD.

A CVD surveillance system would establish mechanisms (data collection tools and systems) to collect and analyze information on CVDs, prevention policies and environments affecting preventable risk factors for CVD. An indicative list of indicators, type of data and different sources for a comprehensive CVD surveillance system is shown in Table 11.1. CVD surveillance system will also make this information available to the public and health care professionals as well as to the cardiovascular health program managers to assist them in developing strategies and evaluating their effectiveness.

## GLOBAL NCD SURVEILLANCE AND MONITORING FRAMEWORK

To accelerate national efforts to address NCDs, in 2013 the World Health Assembly adopted a comprehensive global monitoring framework with 25 indicators and nine voluntary global targets for 2025, including an overarching target of reducing premature mortality from the four main NCDs (CVDs, chronic respiratory diseases, cancers, and diabetes) by 25% relative to their 2010 levels by 2025 (referred to as the 25×25 target).[3] Countries also agreed on targets for selected NCD risk factors: tobacco use, harmful alcohol use, salt intake, obesity, raised blood pressure, raised blood glucose and diabetes, and physical inactivity. Two additional targets focus on treating people at high risk of heart attack and stroke and on the availability of drugs to treat NCDs.

## Table 11.1 Possible Information Sources for Comprehensive CVD Surveillance

| Source | Information | Example of Indicators |
|---|---|---|
| Surveys | Population-based data | • Prevalence of ischemic heart disease or other CVD conditions<br>• Treatment coverage for disorders<br>• Prevalence of risk factors |
| Disease registries (hospital or population based) | Incidence and case fatality | • Incidence of different cancers<br>• Door-to-needle time for myocardial infarction<br>• Case fatality rates for specific conditions |
| Hospital data | Morbidity<br>Health service availability indicators | • Proportion of hospital user (inpatient/outpatient) by disease category<br>• Service availability indicators |
| Administrative data | Births, deaths medication use, health systems performance insurance claims, hospital audits | • Cause-specific mortality indicators<br>• Sales of different treatment modalities (medicines, stents, etc.) |
| Aggregate consumption data | Per capita consumption | • Per capita alcohol consumption or food items/groups |
| Economic data | Economic indicators | • Program budgeting<br>• Cost of care |

Three major components of NCD surveillance as proposed by the World Health Organization (WHO) are a) monitoring exposures (risk factors); b) monitoring outcomes (morbidity and disease-specific mortality); and c) assessing health system capacity and response, which also includes national capacity to prevent NCDs (in terms of policies and plans, infrastructure, human resources and access to essential health care, including medicines). Monitoring of risk factors at the population level (or in a subset of the population) has been recommended by the WHO to be the mainstay of national NCD surveillance in most countries. In this context, the WHO STEPS approach[4] to NCD risk factor surveillance is a good example of an integrated and phased approach that has been used and tested by many countries.

## WHO STEPS FRAMEWORK FOR NCD SURVEILLANCE

The WHO STEPS wise approach to Surveillance (WHO STEPS)[4] of NCDs is based on sequential levels of surveillance of different aspects of NCDs, allowing flexibility and integration at each step by maintaining standardized questionnaires and protocols to ensure comparability over time and across locations. The WHO STEPS wise approach advocates that small amounts of good-quality data are more valuable than large amounts of poor-quality data. WHO STEPS offers an entry point for low- and middle-income countries (LMICs) to get started in NCD activities. The WHO STEPS wise approach allows for the development of an increasingly comprehensive and complex surveillance system depending on local needs and resources. A strong argument can also be made for the benefits of monitoring a few modifiable NCD risk factors, since they reflect both a large part of future NCD burden as well as indicating the success of interventions considered to be beneficial to a wide range of NCDs. In the WHO STEPS approach, the recommended surveillance measures are categorized according to the degree of complexity and cost in obtaining the data. The degree of difficulty equates to whether instruments alone are used, physical measures are collected in the field or laboratory measurements requiring external expertise are required. The key feature of the WHO STEPS framework is the distinction between the different levels of risk factor assessment:

- self-report information by questionnaire (Step 1),

- objective information by physical measurements (Step 2), or

- objective information by blood samples for biochemical analyses (Step 3);

and at each of the steps, modules for each risk factor have core, expanded and optional items/questions. The key premise is that, by using the same standardized questions and protocols, all countries can use the information not only for informing within-country trends but also for between-country comparisons. The questionnaires and methods recommended must therefore be relatively simple.

## DESIGNING NATIONAL CVD SURVEILLANCE SYSTEMS

The 2017 national-level capacity assessment for NCD prevention and control by the WHO[5] also assessed the status of NCD surveillance in member countries and is shown in Table 11.2. It highlights major deficiencies in the surveillance systems in LMICs.

## PUBLIC HEALTH SURVEILLANCE DELIVERED THROUGH THE PUBLIC HEALTH OBSERVATORY MODEL

NCD surveillance systems need to be integrated into existing national health systems. This is even more important where resources are limited. Major challenges facing countries include not only weak systems for sustainable data collection and lack of availability of data but also inability to use the data to make evidence-based decision making. A model that has increasingly become recognized for its ability to support decision making is that of public health observatories (PHOs).

A PHO is a policy-oriented virtual center aimed at performing systematic, ongoing and integrated observations of population health and health systems to support effective evidence-based health policy, planning, decision making and action. A PHO serves as a platform for building better links between the available public health information and the application to public health action. The observatory is conceived as a "think-tank", an organization performing complex health situation analyses in a shorter timespan than conventional research centers and producing local epidemiological profiles and health priority assessments with greater impartiality than government agencies with a political agenda or community groups with specific interests. Some of the functions performed by PHOs are a) monitoring health and disease trends; b) identifying gaps in health information and advising ways to fill those; c) health inequality impact assessment; d) compiling and synthesizing information for public health managers; and e) forecasting to give early warning of future public health problems. One of the best examples of networked health intelligence through the PHO model globally is in England.

There has been sustained national investment in public health intelligence expertise within the national public health agency, Public Health England (PHE). Health intelligence being embedded in a national arms-length body working alongside and in collaboration with national and local government public health policy colleagues has contributed to the significant impact in public health policy development to date.

## Table 11.2 Results of WHO National-Level Capacity Assessment for NCD Surveillance in 2017

| Domain | Key Findings |
|---|---|
| NCD Surveillance Responsibility | Less than a quarter of countries (23%) reported having an office, department or administrative division within their ministry of health exclusively dedicated to NCD surveillance. Overall, high-income countries reported the highest prevalence of responsibility being shared across several divisions within the Ministry of Health, while low-income countries were most likely to report having an office/department/ administrative division within the Ministry of Health responsible for NCD surveillance but not exclusively dedicated to this. |
| Mortality Data | Ninety percent of countries reported having a system for collecting mortality data by cause of death on a routine basis, with 100% of high-income and 96% of upper-middle-income countries reporting such a registration system. |
| Disease Registries | While 84% of countries reported having a cancer registry, only half (51%) had a population-based cancer registry. While 82% of high-income countries had population-based cancer registries, availability decreased with lower-income groups. Almost half of all countries (46%) reported having a diabetes registry; however, only 16% had a population-based registry. No country in the low-income group reported having population-based diabetes registries. In comparison, at least one in five upper-middle- and high-income countries had population-based diabetes registries. |
| Risk Factor Data | Nineteen percent of countries had not conducted any recent (i.e., from 2012 onwards) national adult risk factor surveys; however, nearly half (49%) of countries had conducted recent, national adult surveys for eight or nine of the nine major NCD risk factors: In the low-income group, 42% of countries had carried out no recent adult risk factor surveys, compared with 13–16% of middle- and high-income countries. |
| Service Availability and Readiness | Approximately a quarter of countries (24%) had conducted a survey of facilities to assess service availability and readiness for NCDs, with just over two-thirds of these being national assessments. Slightly more countries in the lower-middle-income group had conducted a survey of facilities compared with other income levels. |

It could be argued that a major sea-change in the development of health intelligence in England was through the formal establishment of PHOs in 2000 following the publication of the UK government's white paper—*Saving Lives: Our Healthier Nation.*[6] This strategic publication provided the national financial and strategic support from both the chief medical officer in England as well as the Department of Health (Ministry of Health). Nine regional PHOs were consequently established to provide reliable intelligence across England (population around 56 million), synthesizing existing data, targeting specific areas for data collection and developing strong networks for access to new and innovative data.[7] The PHO teams tended to be small, though highly qualified. However, their networks allowed them to extend across a wide area, creating more than the sum of their parts in the networks they engaged in, the information they disseminated and the influence that they could have on policy. As well as "core functions", all PHOs had several national specialist areas. This enabled PHOs to develop expertise in specific areas such as cancer, CVD and inequalities (see Box 11.1 for a summary of key learning from England's national specialist CVD public health observatory—the National Cardiovascular Intelligence Network [NCVIN]).

The NCVIN in England is a partnership of leading national cardiovascular organizations (government agencies, health service national bodies, charities, research and academic organizations, professional bodies) which analyze information and data and turn it into meaningful, timely health intelligence for commissioners, policy makers, clinicians and health professionals to improve services and outcomes. PHE provides the system leadership across these national and local partners to encourage the collection, analysis and publication of comparative national statistics on diagnosis, treatment and outcomes for all types of CVD, including nondiabetic hyperglycemia, diabetes, heart disease, stroke and kidney disease. These collaborations are important in ensuring all opportunities are explored for aligning existing and new health intelligence tools and resources, thereby assisting local leaders to navigate to the material that will serve them best.

Investment has been made within PHE to sustain a team of specialist CVD analysts with comprehensive knowledge of the breadth of surveillance data. They bring significant experience and knowledge of CVD-related datasets and have built long-standing relationships with national organizations that hold specialist national audit or disease registers. Their focus is to ensure oversight of nationally available data and curate for a range of different public health and health service managers to drive outcomes in CVD. Key products and tools include disease-specific profiles that bring together summary data along with supporting a narrative for local geographies, highlighting opportunities for quality improvement. The team develops appropriate indicators for reporting at local geographies through appropriate reporting platforms and works proactively with clinical and expert colleagues to undertake headline analysis of a range of datasets, drafting initial key findings and providing analytical input to the national and thematic reports as required.

To ensure active engagement and implementation within local geographies, NCVIN leads a broad range of dissemination and engagement activity such as high-profile national events and regional workshops/masterclasses/translational support. PHE also has strong dissemination routes through a complimentary Local Knowledge and Intelligence Service (LKIS) embedded across England that supports dissemination to a wide network of National Health Service (NHS) and public health local systems. NCVIN also has a comprehensive network of stakeholders and customers with active communications through blogs, newsletters and social media activity.

PHE also facilitates access to wider specialist knowledge and expertise from its national health economics and specialist modeling unit, its comprehensive data science function, wider expertise in indicator development and data automation together with learning and development in new methodologies and techniques such as R programming, data visualization, etc.

## BOX 11.1 ESTABLISHING A SPECIALIST CVD PUBLIC HEALTH OBSERVATORY: KEY LEARNING FROM ENGLAND'S NATIONAL CARDIOVASCULAR INTELLIGENCE NETWORK

**Working as a network:** Having an effective network has a huge multiplier effect on impact. Working together reduces duplication and produces much greater clarity of the message. Information specialists can become familiar with work being carried out in other places and other countries and so the opportunities for learning and disseminating good practice become greatly enhanced.

161

Being part of a network encourages public health intelligence staff to be much more outward-facing and consequently understand the broader relevance of their analysis.

**Embedding health intelligence within broader policy:** The importance of embedding health intelligence within the broader policy context cannot be underestimated. Working closely with public health policy colleagues ensures that the health intelligence focus remains strategically relevant and impactful.

**Recognizing the local context:** Recognizing the importance of the local context and engaging through a broader network with the end users of health intelligence analysis is key. Public Health England has invested in a Local Knowledge and Intelligence Service (LKIS), which facilitates the translation of national health intelligence resources but also provides comprehensive user feedback and insight.

**Program and clinical leadership:** Appropriate program and clinical leadership to build a strong and active network is imperative. Senior leaders of the network need to take responsibility and provide leadership to drive the activity. Personal investment must be made in the relationships across the network and the added value each partner brings to the collaboration.

**Effective governance:** Effective governance structures need to be established that are embedded in the broader national strategic implementation governance structures. An influential chair provides the strategic steering, and the board provides protected time to share and agree on priorities, identify opportunities for innovation and develop the longer-term vision.

**Varied cultural and organizational approaches:** Cultures and organizational approaches can be varied, and investment must be made in developing a core purpose of the network to illustrate the benefits of being part of the partnership.

**Investment in learning and development:** Investing in learning and development across the network to ensure that health intelligence expertise and knowledge are maintained and enhanced. Success comes from a deep and comprehensive knowledge of the clinical priority as well as the intricacies of the data that support the clinical priority.

## DISEASE REGISTRIES

A disease registry is a special database that contains information about people diagnosed with a specific type of disease. Most disease registries are either hospital based or population based. A hospital-based registry contains data on all the patients with a specific type of disease diagnosed and treated at that hospital. A population-based registry (PBR) contains records for people diagnosed with a specific type of disease who reside within a defined geographic region.

Hospital-based disease registries play an important part in improving health outcomes. They also help reduce the costs of health care. Using such registries, health care providers can compare, identify and adopt best practices for patients. One way this is done is by benchmarking. Benchmarking is helpful because it highlights variation. It has long been acknowledged that some variation is inevitable in the health care and outcomes experienced by patients. Much of the variation is unwarranted—i.e. it cannot be explained based on illness, medical evidence or patient preference, but is accounted for by the willingness and ability of doctors to offer treatment. The variation that exists between demographically similar clusters/units/health facilities illustrates the local potential to improve care and outcomes for CVDs. Some of the global examples of a hospital-based registry in the area of acute cardiovascular events are CREATE (89 centers from 50 cities in India with 20,468 patients),[8] EPICOR (555 hospitals in 20 countries in Europe and Latin America covering 10 568 Acute Coronary Syndrome (ACS) survivors),[9] and PROVE in Iran.[10]

PBRs, i.e. the comprehensive collection of all disease cases that occur in a well-characterized population, are generally defined by geographic residency. PBRs are characterized by the following main features: a) the implementation in a defined population of a reasonable size, in order to provide answers to specific research questions; b) the process of case ascertainment, often integrating several data sources, including mortality and hospital admission records, which should ensure the identification of all events independently from their clinical characteristics (completeness); and c) the process of case adjudication (validation) according to diagnostic criteria. The main aims of a PBR are to provide pattern incidence and survival rates to evaluate time trends and changing pattern of the disease in order to monitor a prevention and control program.[11] The first experience of a PBR in the field of CVD was the WHO Myocardial Infarction Community Registers[12] in 1967. In the 1990s, the WHO-MONICA (WHO Multinational MONItoring of trends and determinants in Cardiovascular disease) project provided long-term CVD trends in different European populations using a common registry protocol, which yielded to comparable estimates across populations and time periods. The main results of the WHO MONICA Registry demonstrated that contributions to changing of ischemic heart disease (IHD) mortality varied, but in populations in which mortality decreased, coronary event rates contributed to two-thirds and case fatality to one-third. These trends were related to changes in known risk factors (systolic blood pressure, total cholesterol, smoking habit and body mass index) daily living habits, health care and major socioeconomic features measured at the same time in defined communities in different countries.[13] The concept of a registry in the area of CVD has now expanded to include heart failure, cardiac surgeries, congenital heart diseases and cerebrovascular diseases.

## USE OF CVD RISK SCREENING

A variety of screening tools exist to help providers estimate the risk of a first cardiovascular event in adult patients, including the Pooled Cohort Atherosclerotic Cardiovascular Disease (ASCVD) Risk Equations, Framingham Risk Score (FRS), QRISK2 and QRISK3, Assessing Cardiovascular Risk using Scottish Intercollegiate Guidelines Network (ASSIGN), Systematic Coronary Risk Evaluation (SCORE), Prospective Cardiovascular Münster (PROCAM) and UK Prospective Diabetes Study (UKPDS). A summary of some of the key tools is given in Table 11.3. It should be acknowledged that each tool is derived from a different sample and may have associated limitations. The most well established is the Framingham Score. However, its applicability in all countries is questionable. Many studies done in India have raised doubts on its applicability in the Indian context given South Asians' unique vulnerabilities. This calls for a need for nation-specific risk scores. QRISK provides an excellent example of how it can be done.[14] It is obvious that for such local risk scores to be generated, there is a need for a local cohort or a large database of patients, as in the UK NHS.

## Table 11.3 Overview of CVD Screening Tools

| Screening Tool | Summary |
| --- | --- |
| QRISK3 | The QRISK screening algorithms calculate a person's risk of developing a heart attack or stroke over the next 10 years. **QRISK3** (the most recent version of QRISK) is a prediction algorithm for cardiovascular disease (CVD) that uses traditional risk factors (age, systolic blood pressure, smoking status and ratio of total serum cholesterol to high-density lipoprotein cholesterol) together with body mass index, ethnicity, measures of deprivation, family history, chronic kidney disease, rheumatoid arthritis, atrial fibrillation, diabetes mellitus and antihypertensive treatment. (www.qrisk.org/).[15] A new version of QRISK is released every spring, usually in April. Annual updates are required because of changes in population characteristics—for example, incidence of CVD is falling; obesity is rising; smoking rates are falling; changes in requirements for how the risk prediction scores can be used, e.g. changes in age ranges; and improvements in data quality—for example, the recording of exposures and also clinical outcomes becomes more complete over time. If the algorithm is not recalculated, then its performance would gradually decay and its clinical value would diminish as a result. |
| Framingham Heart Study | A longitudinal and multigenerational study originally launched in 1948 to identify common factors/characteristics that contribute to CVD.[16] The study is based on a small US predominantly white, middle-income community. It may overestimate the risk in countries with a low CVD mortality rate and underestimate the risk in countries with a high CVD mortality rate.[17] |
| JBS3 | The Joint British Societies recommendations on the prevention of Cardiovascular Disease (JBS3) risk calculator estimates both 10-year risk and lifetime risk of CVD in all individuals except for those with existing CVD or certain high-risk diseases, i.e. diabetes age >40 years, patients with chronic kidney disease (CKD) stages 3–5, or familial hypercholesterolemia (FH). The JBS3 project and risk calculator were managed by the British Cardiovascular Society and supported by the British Heart Foundation.[18] |
| SCORE | The Systematic Coronary Risk Evaluation (SCORE) utilized pooled data of over 250,000 individuals from 12 European studies in its development. First published in 2003, the algorithm calculated the 10-year CVD death risk with separate scores for CHD and stroke fatality.[19] |

## DISEASE BURDEN ESTIMATION

Disease burden is an indicator of health outcome. Disease burden can be expressed in many ways, such as the number of cases (e.g. incidence or prevalence), deaths or disability-adjusted life years lost (DALYs) associated with a given condition. Disease burden is the impact of a health problem as measured by mortality, morbidity, economic cost or other indicators. It is often quantified in terms of quality-adjusted life years (QALYs) or DALYs. Both of these metrics quantify the number of years lost due to disability (YLDs), sometimes also known as years lost due to disease or years lived with disability/disease. These measures allow for comparison of disease burdens and are also used to forecast the possible impacts of health interventions. One DALY can be thought of as one year of healthy life lost, and the overall disease burden can be thought of as a measure of the gap between current health status and the ideal health status (where the individual lives to old age free from disease and disability). The WHO's Global Health Estimates provide the latest available data on causes of death and disability globally, by WHO region and country, by age, by sex and by income group.[20]

## CVD DISEASE BURDEN IN INDIA AND ENGLAND

In England, CVD causes one in four premature deaths,[21] it costs the NHS over £7 billion per year (approximately USD 9.2 billion)[22] and it is a major driver of health inequalities, accounting for a quarter of the life expectancy gap between rich and poor.[23] Table 11.4 provides an overview of key national indicators.

This table shows the level of refined indicators that one can answer if the country has a good surveillance and monitoring system. Unlike in England, it is not possible to provide this information for India through a surveillance system, leaving recourse to the use of review of secondary data available publicly. The India Global Burden of Disease[24] reported that in 2016:

- cardiovascular diseases contributed 28.1% (95% UI 26.5–29.1) of the total deaths and 14.1% (12.9–15.3) of the total DALYs.

- 23.8 million (95% UI 22.6–25.0) prevalent cases of IHD were estimated in India in 2016 and 6.5 million (6.3–6.8) prevalent cases of stroke,

## Table 11.4 Overview of National CVD Prevalence and Key Indicators for England

| Indicator | Year | England Average | Measure |
|---|---|---|---|
| Under 75 mortality rates from all cardiovascular diseases | 2016–2018 | 71.7 | Age-standardized rate of mortality from all cardiovascular diseases (including heart disease and stroke) in persons less than 75 years per 100,000 population. |
| Under 75 mortality rates from cardiovascular diseases considered preventable | 2016–2018 | 45.3 | Age-standardized rate of mortality that is considered preventable from all cardiovascular diseases (including heart disease) in persons less than 75 years per 100,000 population |
| Hypertension prevalence (%) | 2018–2019 | 13.96 | Crude percentage of population |
| Coronary heart disease (CHD) prevalence (%) | 2018–2019 | 3.10 | Crude percentage of population |
| Stroke and transient ischemic attack prevalence (%) | 2018–2019 | 1.77 | Crude percentage of population |
| Percutaneous coronary intervention (PCI) procedures performed in the UK | 2017–2018 | 1,548 | Per million population (102,258 in total) |
| Number of cardiac operations performed | 2017–2018 | 32,295 | Count |
| Percent directly admitted to a stroke unit within 4 hours of arrival at hospital | 2018–2019 | 58% | Percentage |
| Percentage of stroke patients who undergo a brain scan within 1 hour | 2018–2019 | 55% | Percentage |

- 53.4% (95% UI 52.6–54.6) of crude deaths due to CVD in India in 2016 were among people younger than 70 years

The Institute of Health Metrics and Evaluation (IHME) uses a square pie chart to show the relative contribution of different diseases to the total disease burden. (*http://vizhub.healthdata.org/gbd-compare [cited 8 Apr 2021]*). The depth of color indicates the change in disease over time, and CVDs appear in the top left-hand corner of the chart. If one compares these charts for India and England, India shows an increase over a time period (1990–2017), while England shows a decrease in most conditions except for atrial fibrillation. Note that these are crude figures and are not standardized for age. These diagrams also illustrate the power of visual representation of data using technology.

## CONCLUSION

In conclusion, it is acknowledged that public health surveillance is the foundation for modern public health and provides a systematic framework for improving quality of care and outcomes in CVD. Countries should consider adapting available general frameworks for the development of thematic public health surveillance systems, building on the experience from existing surveillance approaches that have already illustrated impact.

## REFERENCES

1. Public Health England. Approach to surveillance [Internet]. London: Public Health England; 2017 [cited 2021 Apr 8]. Available from: www.gov.uk/government/publications/public-health-england-approach-to-surveillance/public-health-england-approach-to-surveillance
2. www.Euro.who.int [Internet]. WHO fact-sheets cardiovascular diseases. Available from: www.who.int/news-room/fact-sheets/detail/cardiovascular-diseases-(cvds)
3. World Health Organisation. NCD global monitoring framework [Internet]. Available from: www.who.int/nmh/global_monitoring_framework/en/
4. World Health Organisation. STEP wise approach to surveillance (STEPS) [Internet] [cited 2021 Apr 8]. Available from: www.who.int/ncds/surveillance/steps/en/#:~:text=The%20 WHO%20STEPwise%20approach%20to,data%20in%20WHO%20member%20countries
5. World Health Organisation. Assessing national capacity for the prevention and control of NCDs [Internet] [cited 2021 Apr 8]. Available from: www.who.int/ncds/surveillance/ncd-capacity/en/
6. Department of Health. Saving lives: Our healthier nation [Internet]. London: Department of Health and Social Care; 1999 [cited 2021 Apr 8]. Available from: www.gov.uk/government/publications/saving-lives-our-healthier-nation
7. Hemmings J, Wilkinson J. What is a public health observatory? *Journal of Epidemiology and Community Health* 2003;57:324–326.
8. Xavier D, Prof Pais P, Devereaux PJ, Xie C, Prabhakaran D, Srinath Reddy K, et al. Treatment and outcomes of acute coronary syndromes in India (CREATE): a prospective analysis of registry data. Lancet Volume 371, ISSUE 9622, P1435–1442, April 26, 2008.
9. Annemans L, Danchin N, Van de Werf F, et al. Prehospital and in-hospital use of healthcare resources in patients surviving acute coronary syndromes: an analysis of the EPICOR registry. *Open Heart* 2016;3:e000347.
10. Givi M, Sarrafzadegan N, Garakyaraghi M, Yadegarfar G, Sadeghi M. Persian registry of cardiovascular diseasE(PROVE): Design and methodology. *ARYA Atheroscler* 2017;13(5):239–243.
11. Palmieri L, Veronesi G, Corrao G, Traversa G, Ferrario MM, Nicoletti G, Lonardo AD, Donfrancesco C, Carle F, Giampaoli S. Cardiovascular diseases monitoring: Lessons from population-based registries to address future opportunities and challenges in Europe. *Archives of Public Health* 2018;76:31.
12. World Health Organisation Regional Office for Europe. Myocardial infarction community registers. Copenhagen: WHO, 1976, Public Health in Europe. report No 5.
13. Tunstall-Pedoe H, Kuulasmaa K, Tolonen H, Davidson M. Mendis S with 64 other contributors for the WHO MONICA project. MONICA monograph and multimedia sourcebook. Geneva: WHO; 2003.
14. Hippisley-Cox J. Predicting cardiovascular risk in England and Wales: prospective derivation and validation of QRISK2. *BMJ* 2008;336:a332 doi:10.1136/bmj.39609.449676.25
15. www.qrisk.org [Internet]. Algorithm available from: https://qrisk.org/three/index.php
16. www.framinghamheartstudy.org/ [Internet]

17. Hobbs FDR, Jukema JW, Da Silva PM, McCormack T, Catapano AL. Barriers to cardiovascular disease risk scoring and primary prevention in Europe. *QJM: An International Journal of Medicine* 2010;103(10):727–739.

18. www.jbs3risk.com [Internet]. Risk calculator. Available from: www.jbs3risk.com/pages/risk_calculator.htm

19. www.escardio.org/Education/Practice-Tools/CVD-prevention-toolbox/SCORE-Risk-Charts

20. www.who.int/data/gho/data/themes/mortality-and-global-health-estimates

21. British Heart Foundation. The CVD challenge in England [Internet]. London: British Heart Foundation; 2017. Available from: www.bhf.org.uk/informationsupport/publications/healthcare-and-innovations/cvd-challenge-in-england

22. British Heart Foundation. Key Statistics Compendium 2019 [Internet]. London: British Heart Foundation; 2019. Available from: www.bhf.org.uk/what-we-do/our-research/heart-statistics/heart-statistics-publications

23. Public Health England. Public Health Matters: Using data to improve cardiovascular outcomes [Internet]. London: Public Health England; 2019. https://publichealthmatters.blog.gov.uk/2019/03/13/health-matters-using-data-to-improve-cardiovascular-outcomes/

24. www.healthdata.org/india [Internet].

# 12 Health Systems Interventions for Preventing CVD in Low- and Middle-Income Countries

*Shreya Rao, Ricardo A. Peña Silva, and Ambarish Pandey*

## CONTENTS

## INTRODUCTION

A health system is represented by a grouping of organizations, institutions and resources that have the objective of protecting and improving the health of populations (1). The health system remains the cornerstone in the prevention and treatment of cardiovascular disease (CVD). With growing disparities within and among nations, health systems serve as a crucial anchor for the continuum-of-care paradigm which remains the bulwark of CVD care. Yet despite increased awareness and surveillance of non-communicable diseases (NCDs) globally, health systems–based interventions have been challenging to enact in many low- and middle-income countries (LMICs) as a result of significant competing interests for investment, limited evidence of efficacy and cost-efficiency in LMIC settings, and the reliance of such interventions on sustained contact with healthcare organizations in order to realize benefits (2). As a consequence, in 2017, the World Health Organization (WHO) estimated that less than 50% of member countries had endorsed evidence-based guidelines and protocols for management of NCDs at a primary care level, suggestive of inadequate capacity for managing the high anticipated burden of disease (3).

In this chapter, our focus will be on summarizing the available knowledge on pragmatic health systems interventions for reducing the CVD burden in LMICs. We will provide guidance on meaningful targets for long-term surveillance, describe existing epidemiological data to guide resource allocation and discuss evidence-based interventions with particular emphasis on experiences in low-resource settings. We begin with a discussion of national-level strategies to improve healthcare access, including universal health coverage and expanded access to essential medications. We will conclude with a discussion of interventions targeted at healthcare delivery, examining opportunities for care shifting and for the use of mobile health technology in improving the reach of existing healthcare systems.

## TARGETS FOR ACHIEVING CVD REDUCTION

The CVD epidemic we experience today is tied to the social, political and economic upheaval experienced by LMICs over the past five decades and to the rise of sister epidemics of smoking, diabetes, hypertension and obesity. In probing reductions in coronary heart disease (CHD) in high-income Western countries in recent years, modeling studies have provided a blueprint for CVD reduction by means of risk factor reduction and improvement in access to common CVD therapies. The IMPACT model, a comprehensive model developed and validated to explain the decline in CVD in the United States, United Kingdom and Europe, demonstrated that across countries experiencing reductions in CHD, between 40% and 72% of the decline in CHD deaths in the 20th century were driven by reductions in blood pressure, cholesterol levels, smoking prevalence and physical inactivity, with the remaining reductions motivated by increased access to acute and secondary prevention therapies (4–7). These findings have been corroborated by large international studies, including the INTERHEART (8) and INTERSTROKE (9) studies which found that traditional risk factors alone accounted for more than 90% of the global excess risk of acute myocardial infarction (AMI), irrespective of ethnicity or region. Of these, smoking and elevated lipids emerged as the most potent drivers of risk, accounting on their own for nearly 60% of excess global

DOI: 10.1201/b23266-21

**Table 12.1 WHO "Best Buy" Interventions for Reducing the Burden of Non-communicable Diseases – Adapted from WHO, 2011 (From Burden to "Best Buys") (12).**

| Risk Factor | Interventions |
| --- | --- |
| Tobacco use | • Tax increases<br>• Smoke-free indoor workplaces and public places<br>• Health information and warnings<br>• Bans on tobacco advertising, promotion and sponsorship |
| Harmful alcohol use | • Tax increases<br>• Restricted access to retailed alcohol<br>• Bans on alcohol advertising |
| Unhealthy diet and physical inactivity | • Reduced salt intake in food<br>• Replacement of trans fat with polyunsaturated fat<br>• Public awareness through mass media on diet and physical activity |
| Cardiovascular disease (CVD) and diabetes | • Counseling and multi-drug therapy for people with a high risk of developing heart attacks and strokes<br>• Treatment of heart attacks with aspirin |
| Cancer | • Hepatitis B immunization to prevent liver cancer<br>• Screening and treatment of pre-cancerous lesions to prevent cervical cancer |

risk. The WHO's NCD "Best Buys" (10) and 2014 Global Status Report (11) highlight these findings, encouraging tobacco and alcohol reduction; increased physical activity; improved diagnosis and control of hypertension, diabetes and obesity; and improved access to essential cardiovascular medicines as intermediate targets in the effort to curb CVD morbidity and mortality (Table 12.1).

Despite this knowledge, the prevalence of smoking, hypertension, hyperlipidemia, obesity and diabetes is on the rise in LMICs. Since 1980, the number of adults globally suffering from hypertension has increased by 90%, with prevalence in high-income countries (HICs) decreasing and that in LMICs increasing dramatically (13). Diabetes prevalence meanwhile has quadrupled worldwide, with high rates of obesity and physical inactivity seen in nearly every region of the world and every income level in the same time period (10). Rates of dyslipidemia globally were unchanged, with mean decreases in HICs and gradual but consistent increases in mean cholesterol levels among most LMICs (14). And while the prevalence of smoking and consumption of alcohol and sugar-sweetened beverages (SSBs) is on the decline in HICs, consumption, affordability and availability of these products continue to increase among LMICs (15).

Compounding the increased prevalence of risk factors is the challenge of under-diagnosis and under-treatment due to individual and systems-level factors. Findings from the PURE study showed that globally less than half of participants with hypertension were aware of their diagnosis; of these, only three-quarters in low-income countries were being treated. And while nearly 10% of adults in low-income countries had known diabetes diagnoses, only about 30% in this setting were being treated with hypoglycemic agents, compared to 53% in middle-income countries and 75% in HICs (16). The study additionally demonstrates that while absolute prevalence of cardiovascular risk factors remains highest among HICs, CVD mortality paradoxically remains higher within LMICs, demonstrating the role of inadequate access to care in driving morbidity and mortality despite lower risk factor burden in LMICs.

Furthermore, health literacy of individuals plays an important role in the maintenance of cardiovascular health and should therefore be a goal of health systems. Health literacy is defined as the "degree to which individuals have the ability to obtain, process, and understand basic health information and services needed to make appropriate health decisions" (17). Several studies have revealed that inadequate health literacy is associated with low adherence to recommendations and poor outcomes in patients with hypertension, diabetes, coronary heart disease and heart failure (18–21). There is a critical need for health system–level interventions to integrate health literacy into cardiovascular care and prevention programs. Such interventions would seek to promote the quality and effectiveness of communication strategies, introducing tools such as the "AHRQ Universal Precautions Toolkit for Health Literacy" and creating novel methods to deliver patient-oriented education and promote community engagement.

Taken together, while the increasing prevalence of CVD in LMICs is largely driven by the growing burden of cardiovascular risk factors, approaches aimed to reduce CVD morbidity and

| EARLY PREVENTION | PRIMARY PREVENTION |
|---|---|
| **Reduce smoking**<br>• Taxes on tobacco products<br>• Regulation on sales and advertising<br>• Mass media campaigns to educate public on dangers<br>• Smoking cessation programming | **Improve access to essential services**<br>• Implement universal health care essential package<br>• Promote non-physician health worker interventions to improve screening and diagnosis<br>• Utilization of mHealth interventions to improve accessibility |
| **Improve dietary quality**<br>• Taxes on sugar-sweetened beverages<br>• Regulation of sodium content<br>• Trans-fatty acid bans<br>• Promote increased fruit and vegetable consumption | **Improve awareness of risk**<br>• Mass media campaigns to educate about risk factors and symptoms of ischemic heart disease and stroke<br>• Promote self-management of T2DM and hypertension |
| **Increase physical activity**<br>• Modify built environments to promote activity<br>• Community, school-based and work-place based physical activity programs<br>• Mass media campaigns to advertise benefits | **Improve diagnosis and treatment of risk factors**<br>• Promote use of polypills and fixed-dose combinations to improve adherence and risk factor control<br>• Quality guided auditing to improve adherence to guideline-directed therapies |

**Address disparities in wealth, education and health literacy**

**Figure 12.1** Early and primary prevention targets and activities for the reduction of CVD morbidity and mortality.

mortality will require a comprehensive and nuanced effort that targets traditional CVD risk factors while addressing healthcare access and social disadvantage within these settings. Figure 12.1 provides a summary of early and primary prevention targets for intervention.

### Health System Interventions for Reducing CVD

In the following sections we will explore evidence-based approaches to addressing the rising burden of CVD in LMICs. Figure 12.2 depicts a conceptual framework developed by the Institute of Medicine which will guide this discussion, with a focus on healthcare delivery interventions. The approaches described here do not represent a comprehensive or prescriptive implementation plan, but rather aim to emphasize those interventions with demonstrated impact and feasibility in LMICs.

While primordial prevention efforts, including fiscal and regulatory policies discussed in prior chapters, maintain low costs by addressing societal determinants of health, primary prevention efforts are often reliant on health systems tasked with executing more costly prevention and therapeutic strategies on the ground. Throughout the developing world today, health systems face barriers, including inadequate care coverage, healthcare workforce shortages and challenges in engaging low- and moderate-risk individuals. Universal health coverage (UHC), first described in the constitution of the WHO and later adapted as a Sustainable Development Goal, is fundamental to the delivery of effective and equitable primary care, but LMICs must contend with other crucial infrastructure shortcomings simultaneously, including critical shortages of healthcare providers, high cost and low availability of pharmaceutical therapies, inconsistent quality of care and challenges reaching patients (22–24). In the following sections, we describe efforts toward achieving UHC and expanded access to therapies in LMICs and describe evidence-based strategies for addressing workforce shortages as well as improving quality and availability of primary prevention care.

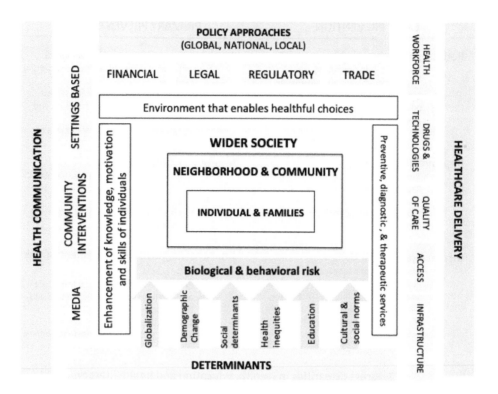

**Figure 12.2** Conceptual framework of a comprehensive strategy for addressing cardiovascular disease.

*Source*: Adapted from Institute of Medicine, Fuster and Kelly, page 187 (2).

### Universal Health Coverage

In most parts of the world today, access to CVD prevention and care is dependent on health systems, and in turn, payment structures for delivering care. In practice, UHC requires three fundamental functions: development of health programs and services to improve health, expanded access to such services and protection against financial catastrophe associated with illness (25, 26). While in HICs, discussions of UHC have come to focus on expansion of insurance coverage, LMICs must contend with discussions of both what is covered and who is covered in striving to achieve UHC (26). A 2018 study evaluating insurance coverage in LMICs highlights this distinction, demonstrating that among individuals reportedly covered by insurance in LMICs, one in seven had ineffective coverage, indicating they were unable to access basic health services like treatment of NCDs or were required to sell assets or borrow money in order to pay for essential health services (27).

Despite an increasing burden of CVD in most LMICs, cardiovascular therapies and prevention efforts continue to be excluded from most countries' UHC priorities. In a survey of LMICs, CVD was considered a top priority for coverage in only 12% of countries, with a greater proportion emphasizing antenatal and prenatal care and maternal health (28). This is due, in part, to an over-emphasis on traditional cost-effectiveness data, which may miss the true longitudinal impact of CVD on health and long-term financial risk associated with CVD. As a result, acute CVD care continues to require out-of-pocket payment in many LMICs and is associated with catastrophic health spending. One survey of patients hospitalized for acute CVD conditions found that 15-month out-of-pocket expenditures reached 40% and 45% of total household expenditures among low-income respondents in China and India, respectively. Catastrophic spending was highest among respondents in India, where insurance coverage was lowest (29).

And while CVD interventions are a necessary component of UHC, what interventions belong as part of an "essential package" vary widely and should be responsive to the needs and clinical limitations of individual countries. Table 12.2 summarizes components of a proposed essential package for early and primary prevention of CVD, developed by the Disease Control Priorities Project (DCP) (26). Of these interventions, large-scale efforts to reduce tobacco consumption and improve dietary quality are most cost-effective in most LMIC settings. The annual incremental per capita cost of implementing the essential package (including additional interventions aimed at curbing respiratory and kidney disease) is estimated by the DCP at US$21 in low-income countries and US$24 in LMICs, the majority of which would be dedicated to infrastructure building at the primary healthcare level (30).

## Table 12.2 Essential Package of Cardiovascular Interventions, Focusing on Early and Primary Prevention Interventions for Cardiovascular Disease and Heart Failure Prevention

| | All Conditions | Ischemic Heart Disease, Stroke and Peripheral Artery Disease | Heart Failure |
|---|---|---|---|
| Fiscal | 1. Tobacco taxes<br>2. Sugar-sweetened beverages tax | | |
| Intersectoral | 3. Built environment improvements to promote physical activity<br>4. School programs for nutrition and physical activity<br>5. Advertising and labeling regulation of tobacco products<br>6. Regulation of salt content in packaged foods<br>7. Trans-fat ban | | 19. Insecticide spray programs to prevent Chagas disease |
| Public health | 8. Nutritional supplementation for women of reproductive age<br>9. Mass media campaigns against unhealthy food and tobacco products | | |
| Community-based | 10. Community health workers for screening with non-lab-based risk tools, improved adherence and referral to primary health centers for ongoing management | | |
| Primary health center | 11. Screening for HTN for all adults<br>12. Targeted screening for T2DM for high-risk adults<br>13. Combination therapy for the management of multiple risk factors | 15. Management with aspirin, beta-blockers, ACEi and statins as indicated<br>16. Use of aspirin for suspected myocardial infarction | 20. Medical management with diuretics, beta-blockers, ACEi and mineralocorticoid antagonists<br>21. Treatment of acute pharyngitis to prevent rheumatic fever<br>22. Secondary prophylaxis with penicillin for rheumatic heart disease |
| First-level hospital | 14. Tobacco cessation counseling and nicotine replacement | 17. Use of unfractionated heparin, aspirin and thrombolytics in acute coronary events<br>18. Management of limb ischemia with heparin and revascularization | 23. Medical management of acute heart failure |

Source: Adapted from Prabhakaran 2017, pages 5–7 and reproduced with permission (License: Creative Commons Attribution CC BY 3.0 IGO) (30).

*Expanding Access to Essential Cardiovascular Medications*

Among individuals with diagnosed CVD, cardiovascular therapies, including anti-hypertensive agents, beta-blockers, angiotensin-converting enzyme (ACE) inhibitors, statins and anti-platelet agents have the potential to substantially reduce the risk of future events and mortality. Yet in an evaluation of access and adherence to goal-directed therapies in the PURE study, rates of the use of secondary prevention drugs in individuals with established stroke or myocardial infarction (MI) were substantially and consistently lower in LMICs when compared with HICs and in rural versus urban areas. Even for low-cost and widely available therapies such as aspirin and statins, uptake was as low as 5% and 15%, respectively, in rural low-income settings (31). A number of factors explain these findings in LMICs, including high cumulative costs of therapies, low public availability and polypharmacy (30). While compulsory licenses to manufacture and export generic alternatives have increased the affordability and accessibility of a number of essential cardiovascular agents, these drugs remain out of reach for many living in LMICs.

Two interventions designed to improve access and availability of cardiovascular therapies have the potential to change this paradigm, however. Essential Medicines Lists (EMLs), first developed by the WHO in 1977 and since adapted by a number of member countries, are one means of priority setting for drug procurement and distribution within countries. Furthermore, the introduction of polypills and fixed-dose combination therapies, at first a theoretical concept by Wald and Law in 2003, has demonstrated in clinical trials the ability to improve rates of adherence by addressing costs and reducing complexity by eliminating the need for frequent dose titrations and multi-drug regimens (32, 33).

The WHO EML has served as a guide for LMICs over the past several decades, expanding its inclusion of key cardiovascular therapies in the past 20 years, and now featuring cardiovascular therapies for lipid lowering, hypertension, heart failure, acute cardiovascular care and substance dependence (i.e. nicotine replacement therapies) (34). Medications prioritized by the WHO EML are more likely to appear among country-specific priority drug lists and become widely available. In one 2014 review, the availability of essential medicines globally was 62%, compared to 27% for non-essential medicines, with the most marked differences seen in LMICs, where availability of essential medicines was 40% compared to 7% for non-essential medicines (35). Among anti-hypertensive agents in sub-Saharan Africa, the cost of anti-hypertensive agents included in the EML were on average 41% lower than those not included, demonstrating the power of inclusion on such lists for expanding access to therapies (36).

However, access to essential medicines remains suboptimal in most LMICs, and debate about which drugs are included in EMLs, as well as incomplete translation of WHO recommendations to country-specific lists, has limited the potential impact of this intervention. A recent analysis demonstrated that of 53 countries studied, only 66% included statins on their EMLs and only two-thirds included at least one drug from four classes of essential CVD therapies, including statins and commonly used anti-hypertensive agents (37). Availability of generic drugs was higher than for brand medications across countries and was notably higher in the private compared to the public sector. Prior analyses similarly found that only one-third of low-income countries, 57% of LMICs and 50% of upper middle-income countries included aspirin, beta-blockers, statins, and ACE inhibitors among their EMLs (38). These findings highlight the need for consistency and frequent recalibration of country-specific EMLs, as well as streamlined national processes to ensure access and regulatory approval of essential medicines within countries in order to expand access to essential medicines (34, 39).

Polypills were initially proposed as alternative therapies for secondary prevention, where individual components of the combination therapy had previously demonstrated efficacy in reducing CVD outcomes but now offer a novel means for expanding access to essential cardiovascular therapies (40). The first large, randomized trial of its type, the UMPIRE trial in 2013, studied individuals with established CVD or high risk for CVD in India and Europe. The study found that combination therapy containing low-dose aspirin, statin and a combination of two anti-hypertensive agents successfully increased rates of adherence to therapy by 33%, while lowering mean systolic blood pressures and cholesterol levels at 15-month follow-up (41). Gains were greatest among communities with lower levels of baseline adherence prior to the trial. A subsequent modeling study of polypills for secondary prevention found that widespread use of polypills in LMICs had the potential to avert 40–54 major adverse cardiovascular events per 1000 patients treated, with a 3–10% reduction in DALYs attributable to CVD in 10 years. The intervention was additionally found to be cost-effective compared with usual care, amounting to 0.4–6.2% of the per capita gross domestic product (GDP) of these countries (42). Subsequent within-trial analysis among participants in India from the UMPIRE trial demonstrated consistent findings with an incremental cost-effectiveness ratio (ICER) of $75 per 10% increase in adherence (43).

A number of large clinical trials in recent years have looked to expand utilization for polypills in primary prevention as well. Most notable among these is the recently published PolyIran trial, which randomized more than 50,000 primary and secondary prevention participants to non-pharmacological interventions or combination therapy with aspirin, atorvastatin, hydrochloro-thiazide and enalapril or valsartan for five years. The once-daily pill resulted in a 35% reduction in major adverse cardiovascular events, with a nearly 60% reduction among those with highest adherence and similar adverse event rates between those on the polypill and controls. The study provides the first randomized data to support both the safety and efficacy of polypills within a primary prevention population and is the first large study to demonstrate reductions in cardiovas-cular outcomes (44). These findings support expanded use of polypills in LMICs as part of a multi-faceted approach to reducing costs and improving adherence and outcomes for both primary and secondary prevention.

### Task-Shifting Interventions

Workforce shortages, though experienced in nearly every region of the world, are exacerbated among LMICs, who bear a disproportionately high burden of disease along with disproportion-ately limited workforce resources and healthcare funding to address it (45). In 2014, the WHO reported that 95% of low-income countries and 70% of LMICs faced critical shortages of midwives, nurses and physicians. Although numbers of skilled health workers were growing in most LMICs, they are likely to be outpaced by the growth in NCD burden in these settings (46). In sub-Saharan Africa, for example, there was fewer than 1 medical doctor per 10,000 people in 2017, compared to 25–40 doctors per 10,000 individuals among Western high-income counterparts, while nurs-ing staff were outnumbered by 50 to 1 when compared with Canada and Western Europe (47). Motivating shortages are high burdens of disease leading to strain on health workers and systems, inadequate investment in healthcare and lack of economic growth, forcing systems to consider new ways to stretch existing resources to address unmet needs (45).

While retaining and recruiting skilled health workers remain important goals in LMICs, invest-ment in task shifting by redistributing non-essential functions to non-physician healthcare work-ers (NPHWs) offers the benefit of reducing burden on providers and rapidly escalating the reach of health programs in both urban and rural areas. Experience with NPHWs in addressing infectious diseases and maternal and fetal health have resulted in a cadre of community health workers (CHWs) within LMICs capable of establishing new roles.

Today, multiple large, randomized trials provide compelling evidence for the use of NPHWs and demonstrate characteristics of successful interventions (Table 12.3). In a review of nine task-shifting interventions, NPHWs, recruited from existing CHWs and newly trained with the background of a high school diploma or less, successfully performed tasks from screening and identifying high-risk individuals based on CVD algorithms to initiating therapies and providing counseling and follow up (48). Interventions across regions have capitalized on existing public health infrastructure as well as incorporation of decision-support tools to guide non-laboratory-based risk assessment and stratification by NPHWs. In one such example, recent cluster-random-ized trials in Argentina and South Asia implemented multi-component interventions, including task shifting to NPHWs and physician training, and demonstrated marked and sustained reduc-tions in blood pressure, improved blood pressure control and a trend toward mortality benefit, at a cost of less than US$11 per patient (49, 50).

Though seemingly designed to address workforce shortages only, task-shifting interventions in fact address multiple components of health system dysfunction by increasing access and affordability to therapies, increasing delivery of care and promoting guideline-driven care, while remaining flexible enough to adapt to the unique cultural context of different communities (51). In settings that identified moderate to high rates of adherence to NPHW-prescribed therapies, like South Africa, use of these interventions was actually cost-saving (30). A review of NPHW inter-ventions found that programs that emphasized a process of auditing for unique health systems challenges, accounted for regulatory limitations and gained stakeholder investment within com-munities were able to reduce implementation costs further and increase the sustainability of their interventions. Thoughtful training, periodic evaluation of training programs and the use of pilot studies prior to large-scale implementation efforts were pragmatic lessons for eventual escalating of such interventions (48).

## Table 12.3 Selected Findings of Task-Shifting Interventions Involving Non-Physician Health Workers (NPHWs)

| Country | Setting | NPHW Intervention | Outcome |
|---|---|---|---|
| **Hypertension interventions** | | | |
| India (Khetan, 2019) | Semi-urban | Home screening visits compared with usual community care | After two years, the NPHW-led group reduced SBP by 12.2 mmHg compared with 6.4 mmHg, with non-significant reductions in cigarette consumption and fasting blood glucose |
| Colombia and Malaysia (Schwalm, 2019) | Urban and rural | Screening and identification of participants with high CVD risk, initiation of medications with mobile tablet assistance | At one year, the NPHW arm achieved significant reductions in Framingham Risk Score, absolute SBP reduction of 11.45 mmHg, 0.41 mmol/L LDL reduction and significant improvement in percentage of individuals achieving BP control |
| Iran (Farzadfar, 2012) | Urban and rural | Blood pressure and BG screening, monitoring and lifestyle advice | Minor reductions in FBG and SBP for every additional NPHW available |
| India, China and Tibet (Tian, 2015) | Rural | Screening for hypertension and CVD risk, followed by lifestyle counseling (salt reduction and smoking cessation) and initiation of BP-lowering agent +/- aspirin for at-risk individuals | At one year, use of antihypertensive agents and aspirin was significantly increased in intervention arm (pre-post difference 25.5% and 17.1%, respectively) and mean SBP significantly decreased by 2.7 mmHg |
| **Physical activity and dietary education interventions** | | | |
| Ghana (Cappuccio, 2006) | Rural | Counseling on sodium restriction | SBP reduction of 2.5 mmHg in NPHW arm compared with usual care |
| Pakistan (Jafar, 2009) | Urban | Health counseling every three months by NPHW, compared to general practitioner education annually | SBP reduction of 10.8 mmHg in NPHW group versus 5.8 mmHg in usual care |
| Mexico (Denman, 2015) | Urban | 13-week educational program on physical activity | Improved dietary habits and improved physical activity levels in participants |
| India (Balagopal, 2008) | Rural | Counseling on diet, stress relief and physical activity | Reductions in fasting blood glucose levels in diabetic (25%) and non-diabetic adults |

| Country | Setting | NPHW Role/Intervention | Outcome |
|---|---|---|---|
| **Multi-component interventions** | | | |
| Argentina (He, 2017) | Urban | NPHW-led home coaching, BP monitoring, BP audit and feedback; physician intervention; and mobile health intervention | At 18 months, intervention arm achieved significant reductions in SBP and DBP, with proportion of those with controlled hypertension increasing from 17% to 73% |
| Bangladesh, Pakistan and Sri Lanka (Jafar, 2020) | Rural | NPHW-led home visits for BP monitoring and counseling; increased physician training; care-coordination | Significant reduction in SBP and DBP, improved BP control and non-significant mortality reduction (1.4%) |
| **Evaluations of NPHW and provider agreement** | | | |
| India and Pakistan (Abegunde, 2007) | Urban | Comparison of NPHW and provider advice | Over 80% agreement between NPHW and provider-issued counseling |
| India (Joshi, 2012) | Rural | Identification of high-risk individuals using algorithm; organized health promotion | Improved identification of high-risk individuals (63% compared with 51% in control) |
| Kenya (Pastakia, 2013) | Rural | Efficacy of NPHWs in detecting HTN and T2DM with home-based BP screening and random glucose testing | NPHWs had an increased odds of identifying elevated BP and blood sugar compared to experienced nurses and clinic staff |
| Bangladesh, Guatemala, South Africa, Mexico (Gaziano, 2015) | Rural and urban | NPHW screening for high CVD risk using risk-assessment tool; measured agreement compared with health professionals | 96.8% inter-operator agreement (CI 0.936–0.961) |

*Source*: (51–58).

## mHealth

The last decade has seen the rapid spread of mobile technology within LMICs, with a resulting transformative effect on communications systems and access to information. Today, more than 5 billion people have mobile devices, over half of which have Internet connectivity. Among emerging economies, between 25% and 60% of individuals report access to a smartphone, with an additional 25–45% reporting access to non-smartphone mobile devices (59). This growth provides a new platform for communicating about health, performing health-related tasks and sharing health information. A 2015 editorial anticipating the future of mHealth technology describes the possible phases this transition would require from initial applications focusing on provider-patient communication and passive tracking of health data, to the use of decision-support applications and eventually machine-learning algorithms, capable of integrating context-specific data to provide recommendations unique to patients and clinical settings (60).

We have witnessed these steps play out in recent years, with mHealth interventions being used increasingly to replace or augment traditional physician visits, to track metrics on physical activity and diet and to provide resources for clinical decision making. mHealth interventions include three main subgroups: 1) interactive voice response (IVR) interventions, which engage with patients via pre-recorded messages to provide tailored education to patients and feedback to providers; 2) short messaging service (SMS) tools that use the format to communicate health education and clinical reminders; and 3) smartphone interventions, which use web-based applications with audio and visual capacity to educate and communicate complex health data. Table 12.4 provides examples of each intervention type for performing various prevention tasks (61).

Although data from LMICs evaluating these interventions have lagged HICs, interventions using IVR and SMS messaging have demonstrated benefit in HICs and among limited trials from LMICs for motivating physical activity, guiding self-management and in providing timely feedback (61, 62). Table 12.5 presents a summary of studies of recent mHealth interventions in LMICs (63). Of these, clinical decision-support tools remain a common application of mHealth in resource-poor settings, frequently paired with scaled CHW interventions in order to increase capacity and develop standards of care. Recent large trials in LMICs have expanded the utility of mHealth in this setting, however, demonstrating applications in streamlining appointments and cardiac rehabilitation.

Among the most impactful of these examples are the mPower and SMART-CR/SP trials. The mPower study, based in rural India, demonstrated large and sustained reductions in clinical

## Table 12.4 Examples of mHealth Interventions, Stratified by Level of Intervention for Early, Primary and Secondary Prevention of CVD

| | Interactive Voice Response | SMS/Text | Smartphone |
|---|---|---|---|
| Early prevention | • Provide information about accessing resources<br>• Testimonials from others | • Messages promoting knowledge and demand for community-based programs promoting healthy lifestyle | • GPS for locating sources of healthy food, bike/walking paths and places to exercise nearby |
| Primary prevention | • Monitoring and goal setting for diet, physical activity and weight management with tailored reminders and reinforcement related to behavior goals | • Frequent reminders, encouragement and advice for how to prevent CVD | • Risk calculators and apps to track efforts toward behavior change goals<br>• Feedback on dietary choices and weight changes |
| Secondary prevention | • Monitoring of health and self-care using validated scales<br>• Tailored behavior-change messages using recorded voice to present complex messages | • SMS requests for reporting blood pressures<br>• Adherence reminders and encouragement reinforcing behavior change | • Dashboards for tracking adherence, blood pressures and other indicators of CVD risk<br>• Social media peer support<br>• Online information about self-care |

*Source*: Adapted from Piette et al. 2015, Circulation (61).

**Table 12.5 Summary of Recent Large Interventions Evaluated in LMICs for Improvement of Primary and Secondary Prevention of Cardiovascular Disease**

| Study | Setting | Country | Intervention | Outcome |
|---|---|---|---|---|
| **mPower Heart Project** (Vamadevan, 2016) | Rural | India | Mobile phone–based clinical decision support system to aid in developing personalized guideline-driven therapeutic recommendations for patients with hypertension and diabetes using input demographic and laboratory data. Implemented by nursing staff and physicians at community health centers in conjunction with lifestyle counseling. | Patients with hypertension, diabetes or both experienced significant and sustained reductions in SBP (–14.6 mmHg), DBP (–7.6 mmHg) and fasting blood glucose (–50 mg/dL) at 18 months after exposure to the intervention. |
| **mWellcare Trial** (Prabhakaran, 2019) | Rural | India | Multi-component intervention, including decision-support tool via mWellcare system, which provided guideline-based treatment recommendations, along with Short Message Service reminders and adherence reminders for patients. | Both arms led to reductions in SBP and glycated hemoglobin with no significant difference in reduction at 12 months when compared to enhanced usual care. |
| **Hope-4** (Yusuf, 2019) | Urban and rural | Colombia and Malaysia | Multi-component intervention involving use of tablet computer–based decision-support tools to guide initiation of free combination anti-hypertensive agents and statins by NPHWs, free access to therapies and support from family or assigned treatment supported to improve adherence. | Significant reductions in ASCVD risk after 12-month follow-up as well as SBP, DBP and LDL. |
| **Smart-CR/SP** (Dorje, 2019) | Single-center recruitment in Shanghai | China | Enrolled patients following admission for acute coronary syndrome requiring PCI in a smartphone WeChat-based home cardiac rehab program with access to a rehabilitation coach for six months via the platform. | Significant improvements in 6-minute walk distance, as well as improved markers of adherence to therapies, lipid profile and CVD health knowledge. |
| **CESCAS** (Gaziano, 2019) | Urban | Argentina | Integrated mHealth application for calculating ASCVD risk and scheduling physician appointments implemented by CHWs in a cluster-randomized design. | Intervention participants significantly more likely to attend initial physician visit and to complete follow-up visits. |

*Source*: (51, 63–66)

endpoints, including blood pressure and fasting glucose levels, with a simple combined intervention of CHW-led visits aided by mobile decision-support tools (67). The SMART-CR/SP study, based in China, used mHealth-based cardiac rehabilitation coaching to replace traditional brick-and-mortar rehabilitation post–acute coronary syndrome, finding that those exposed to the online program had better 6-minute walk distances, adherence to medications and knowledge of cardiovascular health, as well as reductions in systolic blood pressures and cholesterol levels by trial end (64).

Despite promising early results, future research focused on appropriate dosing of mHealth communications and alerts, appropriate boundaries around health information tracking and sharing, cost-effectiveness of mobile interventions and strategies for scaling is needed. Additionally, the limitations of maintaining quality and interoperability and managing patient privacy concerns will require thoughtful consideration as such interventions continue to evolve. Use of cartoons and simple vocabulary in the SMART-CR/SP study made that particular intervention more accessible to a broader population and highlights the importance of responsiveness to cultural norms and population literacy levels in designing intervention tools. Ultimately, current interventions remain at the early stages of realizing the potential of mHealth interventions, with the possibility of more refined tools still on the horizon.

### Quality-of-Care Interventions for Secondary Prevention

The longitudinal nature of CVD means that successful long-term cardiovascular care requires sustained access and affordability, clear and effective practice guidelines and systems for monitoring and improving upon quality of care (2). Healthcare settings play three crucial roles in the management of CVD: primary prevention by focusing on managing risk factors for CVD; secondary prevention in patients with established CVD; and early recognition, management and referral for potentially catastrophic acute presentations of CVD, including MI and stroke. Of these, secondary prevention, as highlighted in the PURE study, presents a major opportunity for improving CVD morbidity and mortality (31). Among LMICs, rates of adherence to at least three secondary prevention interventions—including aspirin, ACE inhibitors, statins, beta-blockers, cardiac rehabilitation and preventive care guidance—range from 4% in low-income countries to 21% in upper-middle-income countries. Meanwhile, acute care interventions, though part of an essential package for UHC, have historically been inconsistently executed, resulting in high case-fatality rates, particularly among lower socioeconomic groups (30).

While best practice guidelines and strategic plans for addressing CVD burden exist in 65% of LMICs, these systems are often under-utilized due to inconsistent access to medicines, facilities for performing interventions and rapid transportation and low levels of awareness among providers and the public of CVD risk factors and presentations (30). Addressing barriers to receiving care requires increasing access to primary care, developing simplified guidelines and packaging of therapies (in the form of combination pills or blister packs), systematically educating providers and developing strategies to audit and provide feedback to centers not achieving quality standards (68). In a 2016 systematic review, educational workshops for providers and patients, simplified guidelines and decision-support tools were all found to be associated with secondary prevention by risk factor management (69).

A number of studies have evaluated interventions to improve acute care at the provider level in acute coronary syndromes (ACSs) and stroke, though limited evidence is available to guide restructuring at a health-systems level. Bundled interventions such as that proposed in the Academic Model Providing Access to Healthcare (AMPATH) initiative in Kenya have offered examples of systematic reform targeted at both the population and patient-provider level. Acute care interventions included in the package include delivering timely guideline-directed therapies for ACS and stroke; incorporating thrombolytics and percutaneous coronary intervention (PCI) by means of provider, patient and community education; and simplified treatment algorithms (30, 70). Unfortunately, though these interventions achieved improvements in clinical process measures, results for clinical outcomes have traditionally been inconsistent (30, 69).

A recent large clinical trial in Hong Kong stands to change that, however. In this study, patients presenting with ACS after 2007 were managed under a newly implemented critical care pathway (CCP), including automated standard management orders, patient education and feedback for providers. Patients exposed to the CCP were more likely to receive guideline-directed therapies and exhibited improved early and long-term survival (71). A similar tool-kit intervention in Kerala did not demonstrate significant improvements in mortality, but did demonstrate improvements in performance measures seen in prior studies, including time to presentation after symptom onset (72). Though promising, further research to clarify the needed components of such multi-modality interventions and procedures for training and evaluating providers and staff will be needed in order to replicate successes on a larger scale.

## CONCLUSION

The rise of CVDs globally and the threat they pose to human life and economic growth demand a coordinated effort within countries to address risk factors for disease progression and provide policy-based solutions. Research investment in LMICs continues to grow, providing new opportunities for studying the impacts of health systems interventions in these settings and should be used to expand upon the existing evidence base. A number of policies have already demonstrated the ability to drive reductions in CVD and its risk factors in high- and low-income settings alike. Expansion of health coverage, access to therapies and a health workforce trained and equipped to address CVD have the potential to create significant reductions in CVD over the next several decades. A strategic approach with clear goals and activities for health systems and individuals such as those being promoted by the Global Hearts Initiative from the WHO have the potential for improving CVD outcomes in varied socioeconomical settings.

However, successful implementation of each of these strategies will require thoughtful analysis of local contexts, engagement of shareholders and effective utilization of existing resources. For example, the COVID-19 pandemic has led to the rapid incorporation of telemedicine services globally for the provision of both acute and chronic medical care (73). Although long theorized to have potential benefits in LMICs, the forced expansion of such services during the pandemic demonstrated in real time the many potential benefits of this approach, particularly for NCDs. Applied to a chronic disease model and paired with the systems reforms described in this chapter, telemedicine approaches have the potential to rapidly expand access to primary and tertiary services, reduce burden on the healthcare system and generate valuable patient data via real-time monitoring and feedback that may further inform disease prediction and provision of services. Several such programs have been employed and studied in HICs, while data from LMICs to inform best practices are greatly needed. Similarly, integrated service models linking CVD care to existing frameworks for HIV care delivery have been suggested as pragmatic models for achieving rapid scale-up in care (74). Early studies of these models demonstrate promise; however, implementation science research and translational research will further guide best practices for execution of such models moving forward.

## REFERENCES

1. WHO. Key Components of a Well Functioning Health System. www.who.int/healthsystems/EN_HSSkeycomponents.pdf?ua=1
2. Fuster V, Kelly B. Promoting Cardiovascular Health in the Developing World: A Critical Challenge to Achieve Global Health. Washington, DC: The National Academies Press; 2010.
3. WHO. The Global Health Observatory: Noncommunicable Diseases; 2017. https://www.who.int/data/gho/data/themes/noncommunicable-diseases
4. Ford ES, Ajani UA, Croft JB, Critchley JA, Labarthe DR, Kottke TE, et al. Explaining the decrease in U.S. deaths from coronary disease, 1980–2000. N Engl J Med. 2007;356(23):2388–2398.
5. Critchley J, Liu J, Zhao D, Wei W, Capewell S. Explaining the increase in coronary heart disease mortality in Beijing between 1984 and 1999. Circulation. 2004;110(10):1236–1244.
6. Critchley J, Capewell S, O'Flaherty M, Abu-Rmeileh N, Rastam S, Saidi O, et al. Contrasting cardiovascular mortality trends in Eastern Mediterranean populations: Contributions from risk factor changes and treatments. Int J Cardiol. 2016;208:150–161.
7. Goff DC, Jr., Khan SS, Lloyd-Jones D, Arnett DK, Carnethon MR, Labarthe DR, et al. Bending the curve in cardiovascular disease mortality: Bethesda + 40 and beyond. Circulation. 2021;143(8):837–851.
8. Yusuf S, Hawken S, Ounpuu S, Dans T, Avezum A, Lanas F, et al. Effect of potentially modifiable risk factors associated with myocardial infarction in 52 countries (the INTERHEART study): case-control study. Lancet. 2004;364(9438):937–952.
9. O'Donnell MJ, Chin SL, Rangarajan S, Xavier D, Liu L, Zhang H, et al. Global and regional effects of potentially modifiable risk factors associated with acute stroke in 32 countries (INTERSTROKE): a case-control study. Lancet. 2016;388(10046):761–775.
10. WHO. Noncommunicable Diseases Country Profiles; 2018. https://apps.who.int/iris/handle/10665/274512
11. WHO. Global Status Report on Noncommunicable Diseases; 2014. https://apps.who.int/iris/handle/10665/148114
12. WHO, WEF. From Burden to "Best Buys": The Economic Impact of Non-Communicable Diseases in Low- and Middle- Income Countries; 2011. https://ncdalliance.org/sites/default/files/resource_files/WHO%20From%20Burden%20to%20Best%20Buys.pdf
13. Collaboration NCDRF. Worldwide trends in blood pressure from 1975 to 2015: A pooled analysis of 1479 population-based measurement studies with 19.1 million participants. Lancet. 2017;389(10064):37–55.

14. Farzadfar F, Finucane MM, Danaei G, Pelizzari PM, Cowan MJ, Paciorek CJ, et al. National, regional, and global trends in serum total cholesterol since 1980: systematic analysis of health examination surveys and epidemiological studies with 321 country-years and 3.0 million participants. Lancet. 2011;377(9765):578–586.

15. Health Taxes to Save Lives: Employing Effective Excise Taxes on Tobacco, Alcohol and Sugary Beverages. The Task Force on Fiscal Policy for Health; 2019. https://tobacconomics. org/research/health-taxes-to-save-lives-employing-effective-excise-taxes-on-tobacco-alcohol-and-sugary-beverages/

16. Rosengren A, Smyth A, Rangarajan S, Ramasundarahettige C, Bangdiwala SI, AlHabib KF, et al. Socioeconomic status and risk of cardiovascular disease in 20 low-income, middle-income, and high-income countries: the Prospective Urban Rural Epidemiologic (PURE) study. Lancet Glob Health. 2019;7(6):e748–e760.

17. Health literacy: A Prescription to End Confusion. Washington DS: Institute of Medicine Committee on Health; 2004.

18. Magnani JW, Mujahid MS, Aronow HD, Cene CW, Dickson VV, Havranek E, et al. Health literacy and cardiovascular disease: fundamental relevance to primary and secondary prevention: a scientific statement from the american heart association. Circulation. 2018;138(2):e48–e74.

19. Shibuya A, Inoue R, Ohkubo T, Takeda Y, Teshima T, Imai Y, et al. The relation between health literacy, hypertension knowledge, and blood pressure among middle-aged Japanese adults. Blood Press Monit. 2011;16(5):224–230.

20. Li X, Ning N, Hao Y, Sun H, Gao L, Jiao M, et al. Health literacy in rural areas of China: hypertension knowledge survey. Int J Environ Res Public Health. 2013;10(3):1125–1138.

21. Shi D, Li J, Wang Y, Wang S, Liu K, Shi R, et al. Association between health literacy and hypertension management in a Chinese community: a retrospective cohort study. Intern Emerg Med. 2017;12(6):765–776.

22. WHO. Constitution of the World Health Organization; 2006. https://www.who.int/publications/m/item/constitution-of-the-world-health-organization

23. WHO. Health Systems Financing: The Path to Universal Coverage. Geneva, Switzerland; 2010.

24. UN. The Sustainable Development Goals Report 2019. New York: United Nations; 2019.

25. WHO. Everybody Business: Strengthening Health Systems to Improve Health Outcomes: WHO's Framework for Action. Geneva: Switzerland; 2007.

26. Watkins DA, Nugent RA. Setting priorities to address cardiovascular diseases through universal health coverage in low- and middle-income countries. Heart Asia. 2017;9(1):54–58.

27. El-Sayed AM, Vail D, Kruk ME. Ineffective insurance in lower and middle income countries is an obstacle to universal health coverage. J Glob Health. 2018;8(2):020402.

28. Gutierrez H, Shewade A, Dai M, Mendoza-Arana P, Gomez-Dantes O, Jain N, et al. Health Care Coverage Decision Making in Low- and Middle-Income Countries: Experiences from 25 Coverage Schemes. Popul Health Manag. 2015;18(4):265–271.

29. Huffman MD, Rao KD, Pichon-Riviere A, Zhao D, Harikrishnan S, Ramaiya K, et al. A cross-sectional study of the microeconomic impact of cardiovascular disease hospitalization in four low- and middle-income countries. PLoS One. 2011;6(6):e20821.

30. Prabhakaran D, Anand S, Gaziano TA, Mbany J-C, Wu Y, Nugent R. Cardiovascular, Respiratory, and Related Disorders. Disease Control Priorities (third edition), Volume 5. Washington, DC: World Bank; 2017.

31. Yusuf S, Islam S, Chow CK, Rangarajan S, Dagenais G, Diaz R, et al. Use of secondary prevention drugs for cardiovascular disease in the community in high-income, middle-income, and low-income countries (the PURE Study): a prospective epidemiological survey. The Lancet. 2011;378(9798):1231–1243.

32. Wald NJ, Law MR. A strategy to reduce cardiovascular disease by more than 80%. BMJ. 2003;326(7404):1419.

33. Lonn E, Bosch J, Teo KK, Pais P, Xavier D, Yusuf S. The polypill in the prevention of cardiovascular diseases: key concepts, current status, challenges, and future directions. Circulation. 2010;122(20):2078–2088.

34. Kishore SP, Blank E, Heller DJ, Patel A, Peters A, Price M, et al. Modernizing the world health organization list of essential medicines for preventing and controlling cardiovascular diseases. J Am Coll Cardiol. 2018;71(5):564–574.

35. Bazargani YT, Ewen M, de Boer A, Leufkens HG, Mantel-Teeuwisse AK. Essential medicines are more available than other medicines around the globe. PLoS One. 2014;9(2):e87576.
36. Twagirumukiza M, Annemans L, Kips JG, Bienvenu E, Van Bortel LM. Prices of antihypertensive medicines in sub-Saharan Africa and alignment to WHO's model list of essential medicines. Trop Med Int Health. 2010;15(3):350–361.
37. Husain MJ, Datta BK, Kostova D, Joseph KT, Asma S, Richter P, et al. Access to cardiovascular disease and hypertension medicines in developing countries: an analysis of essential medicine lists, price, availability, and affordability. J Am Heart Assoc. 2020;9(9):e015302.
38. Wirtz VJ, Kaplan WA, Kwan GF, Laing RO. Access to medications for cardiovascular diseases in low- and middle-income countries. Circulation. 2016;133(21):2076–2085.
39. McKee M, Scarlatescu O, Wood D, Eisele JL, Perel P, Yusuf S. Access to essential medicines for circulatory diseases: a call to action. Glob Heart. 2019;14(4):399–400.
40. Huffman MD, Xavier D, Perel P. Uses of polypills for cardiovascular disease and evidence to date. Lancet. 2017;389(10073):1055–1065.
41. Thom S, Poulter N, Field J, Patel A, Prabhakaran D, Stanton A, et al. Effects of a fixed-dose combination strategy on adherence and risk factors in patients with or at high risk of CVD: the UMPIRE randomized clinical trial. JAMA. 2013;310(9):918–929.
42. Lin JK, Moran AE, Bibbins-Domingo K, Falase B, Pedroza Tobias A, Mandke CN, et al. Cost-effectiveness of a fixed-dose combination pill for secondary prevention of cardiovascular disease in China, India, Mexico, Nigeria, and South Africa: a modelling study. Lancet Glob Health. 2019;7(10):e1346–e58.
43. Singh K, Crossan C, Laba TL, Roy A, Hayes A, Salam A, et al. Cost-effectiveness of a fixed dose combination (polypill) in secondary prevention of cardiovascular diseases in India: Within-trial cost-effectiveness analysis of the UMPIRE trial. Int J Cardiol. 2018;262:71–78.
44. Roshandel G, Khoshnia M, Poustchi H, Hemming K, Kamangar F, Gharavi A, et al. Effectiveness of polypill for primary and secondary prevention of cardiovascular diseases (PolyIran): a pragmatic, cluster-randomised trial. Lancet. 2019;394(10199):672–683.
45. Anyangwe SC, Mtonga C. Inequities in the global health workforce: the greatest impediment to health in sub-Saharan Africa. Int J Environ Res Public Health. 2007;4(2):93–100.
46. WHO. A Universal Truth: No Health Without a Workforce. Geneva; 2014. https://www.who.int/publications/m/item/hrh_universal_truth
47. WHO. The 2018 Update, Global Health Workforce Statistics. Geneva: World Health Organization; 2018.
48. Joshi R, Thrift AG, Smith C, Praveen D, Vedanthan R, Gyamfi J, et al. Task-shifting for cardiovascular risk factor management: lessons from the Global Alliance for Chronic Diseases. BMJ Glob Health. 2018;3(Suppl 3):e001092.
49. He J, Irazola V, Mills KT, Poggio R, Beratarrechea A, Dolan J, et al. Effect of a community health worker-led multicomponent intervention on blood pressure control in low-income patients in argentina: a randomized clinical trial. JAMA. 2017;318(11):1016–1025.
50. Jafar TH, Gandhi M, de Silva HA, Jehan I, Naheed A, Finkelstein EA, et al. A community-based intervention for managing hypertension in rural South Asia. N Engl J Med. 2020;382(8):717–726.
51. Schwalm JD, McCready T, Lopez-Jaramillo P, Yusoff K, Attaran A, Lamelas P, et al. A community-based comprehensive intervention to reduce cardiovascular risk in hypertension (HOPE 4): a cluster-randomised controlled trial. Lancet. 2019;394(10205):1231–1242.
52. Jafar TH, Hatcher J, Poulter N, Islam M, Hashmi S, Qadri Z, et al. Community-based interventions to promote blood pressure control in a developing country: a cluster randomized trial. Ann Intern Med. 2009;151(9):593–601.
53. Khetan A, Zullo M, Rani A, Gupta R, Purushothaman R, Bajaj NS, et al. Effect of a community health worker-based approach to integrated cardiovascular risk factor control in India: a cluster randomized controlled trial. Glob Heart. 2019;14(4):355–365.
54. Farzadfar F, Murray CJ, Gakidou E, Bossert T, Namdaritabar H, Alikhani S, et al. Effectiveness of diabetes and hypertension management by rural primary health-care workers (Behvarz workers) in Iran: a nationally representative observational study. Lancet. 2012;379(9810):47–54.
55. Cappuccio FP, Kerry SM, Micah FB, Plange-Rhule J, Eastwood JB. A community programme to reduce salt intake and blood pressure in Ghana [ISRCTN88789643]. BMC Public Health. 2006;6:13.

56. Denman CA, Bell ML, Cornejo E, de Zapien JG, Carvajal S, Rosales C. Changes in health behaviors and self-rated health of participants in Meta Salud: a primary prevention intervention of NCD in Mexico. Glob Heart. 2015;10(1):55–61.

57. Balagopal P, Kamalamma N, Patel TG, Misra R. A community-based diabetes prevention and management education program in a rural village in India. Diabetes Care. 2008;31(6):1097–1104.

58. Tian M, Ajay VS, Dunzhu D, Hameed SS, Li X, Liu Z, et al. A cluster-randomized, controlled trial of a simplified multifaceted management program for individuals at high cardiovascular risk (simcard trial) in rural Tibet, China, and Haryana, India. Circulation. 2015;132(9):815–824.

59. Pew Research Center. Smartphone Ownership Is Growing Rapidly Around the World, but Not Always Equally; 2019. https://www.pewresearch.org/global/2019/02/05/smartphone-ownership-is-growing-rapidly-around-the-world-but-not-always-equally/

60. Kazi DS, Prabhakaran D, Bolger AF. Rising above the rhetoric: mobile applications and the delivery of cost-effective cardiovascular care in resource-limited settings. Future Cardiol. 2015;11(1):1–4.

61. Piette JD, List J, Rana GK, Townsend W, Striplin D, Heisler M. Mobile health devices as tools for worldwide cardiovascular risk reduction and disease management. Circulation. 2015;132(21):2012–2027.

62. Kelli HM, Witbrodt B, Shah A. The future of mobile health applications and devices in cardiovascular health. Euro Med J Innov. 2017;2017:92–97.

63. Beratarrechea A, Abrahams-Gessel S, Irazola V, Gutierrez L, Moyano D, Gaziano TA. Using mh ealth tools to improve access and coverage of people with public health insurance and high cardiovascular disease risk in argentina: a pragmatic cluster randomized trial. J Am Heart Assoc. 2019;8(8):e011799.

64. Dorje T, Zhao G, Scheer A, Tsokey L, Wang J, Chen Y, et al. SMARTphone and social media-based cardiac rehabilitation and secondary prevention (SMART-CR/SP) for patients with coronary heart disease in China: a randomised controlled trial protocol. BMJ Open. 2018;8(6):e021908.

65. Ajay VS, Jindal D, Roy A, Venugopal V, Sharma R, Pawar A, et al. Development of a smartphone-enabled hypertension and diabetes mellitus management package to facilitate evidence-based care delivery in primary healthcare facilities in india: the mpower heart project. J Am Heart Associat. 2016;5(12).

66. Prabhakaran D, Jha D, Prieto-Merino D, Roy A, Singh K, Ajay VS, et al. Effectiveness of an mhealth-based electronic decision support system for integrated management of chronic conditions in primary care: the mwellcare cluster-randomized controlled trial. Circulation. 2018;139(3):380–391.

67. Ajay VS, Jindal D, Roy A, Venugopal V, Sharma R, Pawar A, et al. Development of a smartphone-enabled hypertension and diabetes mellitus management package to facilitate evidence-based care delivery in primary healthcare facilities in india: the mpower heart project. J Am Heart Assoc. 2016;5(12).

68. Perel P, Avezum A, Huffman M, Pais P, Rodgers A, Vedanthan R, et al. Reducing premature cardiovascular morbidity and mortality in people with atherosclerotic vascular disease: the world heart federation roadmap for secondary prevention of cardiovascular disease. Glob Heart. 2015;10(2):99–110.

69. Lee ES, Vedanthan R, Jeemon P, Kamano JH, Kudesia P, Rajan V, et al. Quality improvement for cardiovascular disease care in low- and middle-income countries: a systematic review. PLoS One. 2016;11(6):e0157036.

70. Tierney WM, Rotich JK, Hannan TJ, Siika AM, Biondich PG, Mamlin BW, et al. The AMPATH medical record system: creating, implementing, and sustaining an electronic medical record system to support HIV/AIDS care in western Kenya. Stud Health Technol Inform. 2007;129(Pt 1):372–376.

71. Hai JJ, Wong CK, Un KC, Wong KL, Zhang ZY, Chan PH, et al. Guideline-based critical care pathway improves long-term clinical outcomes in patients with acute coronary syndrome. Sci Rep. 2019;9(1):16814.

72. Huffman MD, Mohanan PP, Devarajan R, Baldridge AS, Kondal D, Zhao L, et al. Effect of a quality improvement intervention on clinical outcomes in patients in india with acute myocardial infarction: the ACS QUIK randomized clinical trial. JAMA. 2018;319(6):567–578.

73. Hoffer-Hawlik MA, Moran AE, Burka D, Kaur P, Cai J, Frieden TR, et al. Leveraging telemedicine for chronic disease management in low- and middle-income countries during Covid-19. Glob Heart. 2020;15(1):63.

74. Ojo T, Lester L, Iwelunmor J, Gyamfi J, Obiezu-Umeh C, Onakomaiya D, et al. Feasibility of integrated, multilevel care for cardiovascular diseases (CVD) and HIV in low- and middle-income countries (LMICs): A scoping review. PLoS One. 2019;14(2):e0212296.

75. Joshi R, Chow CK, Raju PK, Raju KR, Gottumukkala AK, Reddy KS, et al. The rural Andhra Pradesh cardiovascular prevention study (RAPCAPS): a cluster randomized trial. J Am Coll Cardiol. 2012;59(13):1188–1196.

76. Abegunde DO, Shengelia B, Luyten A, Cameron A, Celletti F, Nishtar S, et al. Can non-physician health-care workers assess and manage cardiovascular risk in primary care? Bull World Health Organ. 2007;85(6):432–440.

77. Pastakia SD, Ali SM, Kamano JH, Akwanalo CO, Ndege SK, Buckwalter VL, et al. Screening for diabetes and hypertension in a rural low income setting in western Kenya utilizing home-based and community-based strategies. Global Health. 2013;9:21.

78. Gaziano TA, Abrahams-Gessel S, Denman CA, Montano CM, Khanam M, Puoane T, et al. An assessment of community health workers' ability to screen for cardiovascular disease risk with a simple, non-invasive risk assessment instrument in Bangladesh, Guatemala, Mexico, and South Africa: an observational study. Lancet Glob Health. 2015;3(9):e556–563.

# 13 Advocacy and Health Promotion

*Radhika Shrivastav, Aastha Chugh, Prachi Kathuria, and Manjusha Chatterjee*

## CONTENTS

## INTRODUCTION

The global burden of cardiovascular diseases (CVDs) is a rising concern worldwide, with repeated calls for actions to address CVDs through effective multipronged health promotion and advocacy strategies.[1] The focus on addressing CVDs through health promotion looks beyond individual behavior and improving health at a population or community level through multistakeholder and multisectoral actions. According to the World Health Organization (WHO), health promotion is a process enabling people to control and improve their *health. Health promotion is therefore a multilevel, multisectoral and multidisciplinary activity.*[2] Health advocacy is closely linked to health promotion and has often been described as a key strategy for achieving health promotion. Health advocacy is defined as a "combination of individual and social actions designed to gain political commitment, policy support, social acceptance and systems support for a particular health goal or programme". Through health advocacy, the goal is to protect the vulnerable and support people to express their needs and make their own decisions.[3]

The United Nations Political Declaration on the Prevention and Control of NCD 2011 called for the development of multisectoral policies to create equitable health-promoting environments that enable healthy practices at the individual level. Subsequently, the 66th World Health Assembly endorsed WHO's Global Action Plan for prevention and control of noncommunicable diseases (NCDs), which was adopted by many countries as a roadmap to achieve a 25% relative reduction in premature mortality from CVDs, cancers, diabetes and chronic respiratory diseases by 2025 (25×25). The Sustainable Development Goals (SDGs) also explicitly target NCDs—to reduce NCD mortality by a third by 2030 (SDG 3.4). This increased attention towards NCDs from Millennium Developmental Goals (which had no mention of NCDs) to SDG 3.4 is a resultant of multistakeholder actions (including government, civil society organizations, academicians, etc.).[4]

However, despite less than five years to 2025 and less than ten years to 2030, most countries are substantially off-target, as commitments at the UN have not translated into adequate policy and programmatic action at the regional and national levels. According to the NCD Countdown 2030, only one in six countries globally, mostly high-income, will fulfil SDG target 3.4, while half of the countries worldwide are far off-track and will not fulfil it at the current rate of progress.[5] The COVID-19 pandemic further exacerbated existing weaknesses in the health response and highlighted the urgent need to address the challenges faced by people living with NCDs.

With the current raging COVID-19 pandemic, the prevention, control and management of CVDs through effective health promotion strategies and with meaningful involvement of people living with CVDs and NCDs more broadly has thus become increasingly pertinent. Research shows that clinical outcomes are worse in patients with COVID-19 and existing CVD risk factors (e.g. hypertension, diabetes and obesity).[6] Despite that, there exist crippling gaps in the healthcare systems to tackle NCDs in many countries. A rapid assessment survey conducted by the WHO found that healthcare services for CVDs have been partially or completed disrupted in nearly half of countries with COVID-19.[7] Therefore, multisectoral actions under the umbrella of health promotion are being taken up by key stakeholders nationally and globally to address CVDs. A whole-of-society approach that acknowledges the central role of civil society, including communities, is imperative to ensure that governments deliver a robust public health response. This chapter outlines effective strategies and key stakeholders for health promotion and advocacy for addressing CVDs. The chapter also illustrates the impact of effective health promotion activities through global and Indian examples.

## INTERLINKAGES BETWEEN EFFECTIVE STRATEGIES AND STAKEHOLDERS FOR TANGIBLE IMPACT OF HEALTH PROMOTION AND ADVOCACY

The NCD civil society movement has grown substantively over the past decade, although with slower strides in low- and middle-income countries (LMICs). Despite professional societies and disease-specific or risk factor–specific associations being active for several years, an organized effort to bring together like-minded organizations working across different NCDs has only recently gained momentum. The NCD Alliance (NCDA) was founded in 2009 by the International Diabetes Federation (IDF), World Heart Federation (WHF), the Union for International Cancer Control (UICC) and the International Union Against Tuberculosis and Lung Disease (The Union). Since its inception, it has been convening, mobilizing and strengthening NCD civil society to stimulate collaborative advocacy and accountability initiatives to bridge the gap on NCDs. NCDA has effectively campaigned at the successive United Nations High-Level Meetings (UN HLM) on NCDs and UHC in 2011, 2014, 2018 and 2019, calling for stronger government commitments and actions to meet NCD targets.

Today, NCDA brings together a network of over 320 members in 81 countries. In 2021, NCDA's global network included over 65 national and regional NCD alliances, including the Healthy India Alliance (India NCD Alliance). These NCD alliances around the globe monitor national progress on NCDs, identify gaps in efforts to meet global and national commitments, foster dialogue with governments and other key stakeholders, calling for multisectoral action, and advocate for improved NCD policies and programs, with meaningful involvement of civil society and people living with NCDs in decision-making processes.

At national levels, organizations such as Health Related Information and Dissemination Among Youth (HRIDAY) in India, have been working with multiple health and nonhealth/developmental partners to achieve the national NDC targets and SDG Goal 3.4. Multisectoral action lies at the heart of promoting meaningful engagement of young people, people living with NCDs, grassroots civil society organizations (CSOs) and marginalized communities. To achieve this, HRIDAY adopts a two-pronged approach: to empower stakeholders (with information, knowledge, resources, support, etc.) to make informed choices and decisions about their health and well-being and strengthening people's voices in shaping and implementing policies and programs. HRIDAY to strengthen several international organizations, including the WHF Roadmap for reducing premature CVD mortality in India and developing action plans for strengthening health systems for hypertension and secondary prevention, augmenting implementation of the Framework Convention on Tobacco Control (FCTC) and National Tobacco Control Programme (NTCP) in India.

### Multistakeholder and Multisectoral Action

Translating global commitments on SDGs, NCDs and universal health coverage (UHC) into national action demands leadership at the highest levels and a "whole-of-society" approach that engages all sectors. Civil society, including youth and people living with NCDs, plays a critical role in strengthening the health response by creating awareness, improving uptake of services and advocating for strong policy action and holding stakeholders to account, along with fostering behavior change through community mobilization.

Currently, countries are struggling with a dual burden of communicable diseases and NCDs, exacerbated by the onslaught of climate change and air pollution. The COVID-19 pandemic forced the focus of public health systems and health promotion campaigns to recalibrate to immediate mitigation efforts. The pandemic had widespread health impacts, revealing the vulnerability of those with underlying conditions, mostly NCDs. It also provided opportunities for public health advocates to underscore further their demands for more robust health systems and policy environments, which can keep systems and citizens more equipped to tackle future public health challenges. The need to bring multiple stakeholders together to identify and act on common priorities, collaborative opportunities and synergistic pathways to achieve inclusiveness, with an overall goal to promote UHC for all, has never been more critical.

Following are some strategies for effective multistakeholder engagement for NCD prevention and control, relevant to cardiovascular health promotion:

1. Multipartner involvement in the operationalization of **national multisectoral action plans** for the prevention and control of NCDs, to seek support and buy-in from health and nonhealth stakeholders, both government and nongovernment, beyond the Ministry of Health and health-sector players.

2. Strengthening **multistakeholder communication strategy** through digital interventions to maximize reach at various settings—schools, workplaces, health systems and hospitals—to promote NCD prevention and management messages within the COVID-19 measures at national/subnational levels.

3. Promoting **evidence-based health promotion and advocacy** to address NCD risk factors (tobacco use, alcohol use, unhealthy diets, inadequate physical activity, exposure to air pollution) with a focus on policy formulation and effective implementation.

4. Civil society **partnerships** to integrate action on NCDs within the national COVID response strategy, as per the local needs. It is recommended to develop country/region-level case studies on effective civil society partnerships for disease prevention and control through community outreach and access to populations at the grassroots level.

5. As an important component of good health and well-being, prioritizing **health promotion (by healthcare professionals, midwives and nurses)** for building COVID- and NCD-resilient communities and health systems.

6. Recognizing the role of communities, including people living with NCDs and youth, led and convened by civil society partners in decision-making processes and addressing issues around access to and availability of essential medicines, disease prevention and control and support services.

7. Strengthening the **case for increasing investment** in NCD prevention and control, guided by a national people-centered research agenda, in turn guided and facilitated by academicians.

8. Prioritizing positive mental health promotion as an essential component of advocacy efforts tailored to targeted NCDs and CVDs.

### Meaningful Youth Engagement for Health Promotion

The global youth population, currently at 1.2 billion, is projected to rise to 1.4 billion by 2050. Often neglected and ignored, youth are affected by inequality, increased disease burden, poverty, injustice, lack of education and various prevalent social concerns. Interventions, programs and policies with and in benefit of youth can improve the prevailing socioeconomic, environmental and political aspects of the NCD response. Today's youth will not only be the ones who bear the growing burden of NCDs but will also be responsible for dealing with it. The focus should be on multiple challenges posed to the physical and mental health and well-being of adolescents and youth from a broader lens of comorbidities (including both communicable and NCD conditions) and the additional threats arising due to the COVID-19 pandemic.

Meaningful youth engagement is key in achieving the SDGs and UHC. In this space, they are still not recognized as significant stakeholders, as they are perceived to be young and healthy, with little need to access healthcare services. Conversely, young people living with NCDs, including mental health conditions, have great potential in building a youth-led public narrative around NCDs by becoming spokespersons to represent youth issues within the NCD and COVID-19 landscape.

Strategies that need to be adopted by CSOs include trainings and workshops, such as 'Train the Trainers workshops' on NCD prevention and control issues for CSOs, school teachers, youth peer leaders (in and out of schools) and community leaders. The use of social media platforms like Facebook, Twitter and other innovative online activities and technology-based apps for health promotion have also been successful at the national and international level. Innovative use of technology (m-health) and health-promoting apps are some of the recent initiatives globally. For example, over the years now, HRIDAY has been able to develop a strong, global youth network, Youth for Health (Y4H), founded in 2006 with members in 35 countries across the globe, with a global membership base of 45,000. The Y4H online initiative (Facebook and Twitter) engages with youth, policy makers, celebrities and other stakeholders to take the agenda of health promotion globally. Over the years, the Y4H movement has grown exponentially, mainly owing to its virtual presence (Facebook and Twitter). Nearly 15,000 youth like the page, and it registers an outreach of half a million people every month through regular interactivity (posts, comments, opinion polls, news, etc.).

## IMPACT OF EFFECTIVE ADVOCACY AND HEALTH PROMOTION EFFORTS: THE VOICES OF PEOPLE LIVING WITH AND AFFECTED BY NCDs

An organized civil society grounded in the communities and experiences of people living with and affected by NCDs demonstrates their crucial role in NCD decision-making, raising public demand for policies, ensuring that services are designed for and reach the communities they are meant for, and holding governments accountable for their commitments.

However, effectively addressing NCDs requires understanding how these diseases and conditions affect people and the challenges and needs people face as they navigate healthcare systems and daily life. Learning from the lived experience and firsthand knowledge of NCDs is essential to strengthening policies, services, programs and social beliefs. People living with NCDs are powerful agents of change, capable of leveraging their lived experience to reach others and help break down stigma and discrimination. The views and perspectives of people living with NCDs are essential to inform laws, policies, healthcare services, advocacy and other systemic NCD decisions.

*Our Views, Our Voices* is an initiative of the NCD Alliance and people living with NCDs dedicated to promoting their meaningful involvement in the NCD response, supporting and enabling individuals to share their views to take action and drive change. The initiative was guided by the *Advocacy Agenda of People Living with NCDs*, built with the generous input of nearly 2000 people living with NCDs who took part in the consultative efforts. The Advocacy Agenda serves as a compass for action for the NCD community and calls for the involvement of people living with NCDs in government decision-making bodies and processes. It has four pillars: prevention, treatment, care and support, social justice and meaningful involvement. The case study of the Healthy India Alliance (HIA), a coalition of 18 multidisciplinary CSOs engaged in multipronged action around NCD prevention and control, focusing on engaging with non-health-sector partners and key stakeholders like people living with NCDs and youth, is given in Box 13.1.

**BOX 13.1**

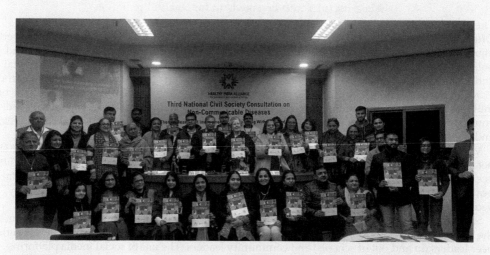

Launch of the India Advocacy Agenda of people living with NCDs, December 2019.

Since 2017, Healthy India Alliance has been closely involved with the Our Views, Our Voices initiative, leading the process of meaningfully involving people living with NCDs in the NCD response through regional and national workshops. These workshops, unique and the first of their kind, being led by HIA in India, helped build the India Advocacy Agenda of people living with NCDs. In 2020, HRIDAY also hosted the secretariat for the South-East Asia Regional NCD Alliance.

As part of the Our Views, Our Voices initiative, HIA has been prioritizing meaningful involvement of those living with NCDs to call for people-centeredness in policy formulation and program implementation.

In 2018, the UN HLM on NCDs offered a real opportunity to further the Advocacy Agenda of People Living with NCDs. As the result of concerted advocacy efforts, the contributions of people living with NCDs and civil society, as critical enablers of accelerated NCD responses, were acknowledged in the Political Declaration on NCDs adopted by the member states during the meeting.

The collective role of governments, policymakers, multilateral agencies, civil society, healthcare providers and, where and as appropriate, the private sector is imperative for creating an enabling environment to promote health and well-being and truly 'putting people first'.

### Examples of Effective Health Promotion and Advocacy Efforts
#### *Sugar Taxation in Mexico, Columbia and Chile*

A major public health concern is the rising burden of obesity in Mexico (one in three children and seven in ten adults are overweight or obese). Each year approximately 70,000 deaths are attributed to diabetes, which is the third leading cause of death in Mexico.[8,9] Various studies highlighted the role of sugar-sweetened beverages (SSBs) as a major factor contributing to the rise in overweight and obesity in the country.[10] In addition, research has also found a direct link between SSB consumption and the risk of type 2 diabetes and CVDs.[11] The concerns with SSBs entered the Mexican public agenda through mass media and CSOs.[12] As a result of intense public pressure, policy changes such as the ban on serving food that is not healthy for students at schools were adopted within the Mexican legislation. In addition, within the framework of World Health Day on April 2, 2013, the president of Mexico instructed the Ministry of Health to devise a national strategy for the prevention and control of overweight, obesity and diabetes. One of the pillars of this strategy focuses upon fiscal policies, including regulation of food and beverage advertisement, labeling and taxation.

The proposal to levy an SSB tax in Mexico is a joint effort by the government, CSOs, public-interest lobbyists, academic and medical institutions and international and multilateral institutions. This was accompanied by a major mass communication strategy carried out by CSOs. The media played an important role in publicizing the messages and awareness to key stakeholders. However, one of the greatest challenges was the response of the soft drink industry who united against the tax. One of the strategies that was used by the industry here was to present opinion makers, medical and nutritional professionals, to advance their argument against the tax in the media. Nevertheless, the Treasury Reform was approved and as a fundamental outcome of the government's work and intersectoral participation, the tax on SSBs was included within the amendments to the Special Tax on Production and Services (IEPS) Act.[13] An evaluation published in 2017 revealed that SSB purchases decreased and water purchases increased after an SSB tax was imposed in Mexico. The magnitude of these changes was greater in lower-income and urban households. While this was simulated in two other countries in Latin America (Columbia and Chile), a major constraint to implementation was the strong influence of transnational corporations (TNCs) in the policy process. A lack of transparency during agenda setting was notably enhanced by the powerful presence of TNCs.[14] As stakeholders in other countries draw up plans to combat obesity and diabetes, several lessons are to be learned from the examples of these three countries.

#### *Global Youth Meet on Health (GYM)*

HRIDAY hosted the **1st GYM in 2006**, convening youth from 32 countries from around the world, bringing together organizations from different sectors and calling for the inclusion of youth in action on key health issues. A **Y4H** movement was launched as an outcome of GYM 2006, aiming to connect youth across the world to undertake health promotion activities and advocacy at national, regional and global levels.

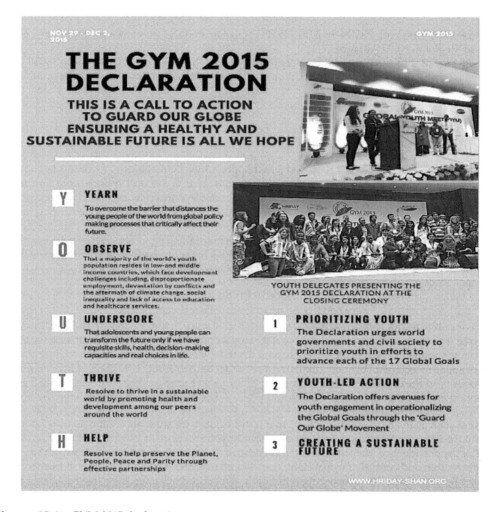

**Figure 13.1** GYM 2015 declaration.

The Y4H charter was presented in the form of an appeal with 225,000 signatures of youth and adults from across the world to the UN secretary-general Ban Ki-Moon by HRIDAY's youth advocates in 2007. The **2nd GYM** was held in 2009 as a pre-conference workshop to the 14th World Conference on Tobacco or Health (WCTOH) in Mumbai, India. Participants explored issues in tobacco control and conducted several campaigns, which led to a global movement on **No More Tobacco in the 21st Century (NMT-21C)** launched in 2013 during an International Conference on Public Health Priorities in the 21st Century: The Endgame for Tobacco. This conference was inaugurated by WHO Director-General Dr. Margaret Chan. This campaign was endorsed by several global health leaders and celebrities at the 16th WCTOH held in Abu Dhabi in 2015 (Figure 13.1). The **3rd GYM 2015** empowered youth participants with advocacy and leadership skills on all aspects of SDGs. They developed action plans for reaching the Post 2015 Sustainable Development Goals and launched the '**Guard Our Globe**' movement to call for more investment in youth for a sustainable future. Pursuing activities under Guard Our Globe leads us to the 4th GYM in 2021.

The **4th GYM (Virtual) 2021 was jointly co-organized by HRIDAY and WHO SEARO**, convened around 300 delegates, representing all six WHO regions to explore linkages between adolescent sexual and reproductive health (ASRH), communicable diseases, NCDs, environmental health and mental health within the framework of the SDGs and UHC and to mark progress following the Global Action Plan for the prevention and control of NCDs (2013–2020) (Figure 13.2). **Following earlier models, GYM 2021 culminated with the release of a GYM Youth Declaration and the**

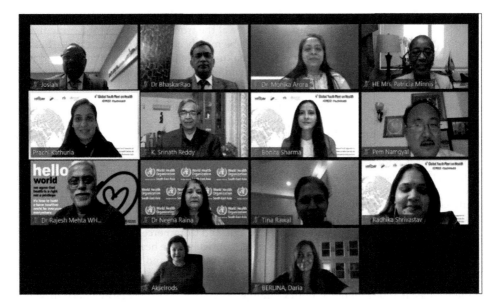

**Figure 13.2** GYM 2021 (virtual).

**adoption of concrete and time-bound youth-led GYM Regional Action Plans that are being implemented post-GYM.**

As a lead-up to GYM 2021, HRIDAY's Youth Health Ambassadors initiated online campaigns #YouthAgainstCovid19 (the youth-led online awareness campaign was launched on World Health Day, April 7, 2020) aimed at involving adolescents and young people to develop awareness materials such as posters, poems and short films outlining the risks posed due to COVID-19 and to motivate people to support the national lockdown and adopt social distancing. These efforts were streamlined with a set of pre-GYM activities aimed at building youth leadership in the COVID-19 era to address the interlinkages between communicable diseases and NCDs; specific activities included a youth-led call to action, country- and regional-level youth-led activities and calling for a comprehensive multisectoral approach in public health interventions. Skill-building workshops have been a key component of the GYM program that is based on a co-production model. These workshops are essentially framed to fabricate youth-centered and youth-led responses to address health issues of adolescents and young adults (AYAs). The workshops comprise both technical sessions and interactive discussions/activities to ensure meaningful youth involvement.

Pursuant to participation and capacity building the 4th GYM, youth public health leaders from a number of Southeast Asian countries and from several states of India planned and executed strategic campaigns focusing on key NCD-related needs and priorities within their jurisdictions. The planning and implementation of these campaigns provided these youth advocates with an opportunity to, first-hand, apply the leadership, communication and technical skills gained during GYM and pre- and post-GYM initiatives to real-life settings. A compendium of these case studies is currently being developed by HRIDAY, with support from the WHO Regional Office for South-East Asia and the WHO Country Office for India.

## CHARACTERISTICS OF SUCCESSFUL ADVOCACY AND HEALTH PROMOTION CAMPAIGNS

For an advocacy and health promotion campaign to be successful in meeting its goals and expected outcomes, it is imperative that the plan is context-specific and relevant. This implies that 'one size does not fit all' and each campaign has to be planned, implemented and evaluated considering the local social, cultural, political and economic factors. Whether the focus is upstream advocacy (e.g. with policy makers, opinion leaders, etc.) or downstream (e.g. with community groups, youth, people living with NCDs, etc.), there are certain common principles to be borne in mind, right from the conceptualization stage:

- **Community-led:** The voices of the communities affected (such as youth, people living with NCDs and other marginalized groups) should be at the front and center of the campaign planning and implementation. They should not be merely considered beneficiaries, but as key stakeholders who have a seat on the decision-making table from design, planning and implementation to evaluation. They should guide agenda-setting and strategies to engage wider stakeholders.

- **Multisectoral and multistakeholder engagement:** Given the interlinkages between determinants for CVDs and other NCDs, along with other non-NCD disease conditions and environmental factors, the solutions to a majority of issues warrant action from multiple sectors and stakeholders beyond the limited purview of the health sector. For advocacy to bring about a positive impact, addressing both government and nongovernment stakeholders is essential. For example, the Ministry of Finance would be responsible for mandating an increase in taxation on unhealthy products, such as tobacco, alcohol and processed foods; the Ministry of Education would ensure that the sale and promotion of such products are prohibited in and around educational institutions; the Ministry of Health would promulgate comprehensive legislation for the control of such products; the Ministry of Trade and Commerce would ensure that commercial interests linked to revenue generation do not outweigh the healthcare expenditure related to CVDs and NCDs (caused due to the use of these products); and the Home Ministry would ensure that all legislative provisions are enforced and violators taken to task.

- **Evidence-based and targeted at policy change:** Advocacy asks must be evidence-driven, pivoted on proven measures and strategies tested to yield impact. In the same vein, advocacy outcomes should be targeted to garner support for policy formulation and effective enforcement in the context of NCD and CVD risk factors.

- **Independent from conflict of interest:** NCDs, including CVDs, are driven by commercial interests of the unhealthy commodity industry, including companies dealing with tobacco, alcohol, food and beverages and fossil fuels. Since advocacy to curb NCD risk factors is often incongruent with the commercial interests of these industries, they apply devious strategies to thwart policy formulation and implementation, along with promoting their products to potential customers from vulnerable population sub-groups such as youth, women, etc. Therefore, advocacy campaigns and advocates themselves should be equipped to be independent of any conflict-of-interest situations and industry interference and influence, such that public health priorities outweigh commercial interests.

- **Transparency and accountability:** It is important that all advocates and stakeholders hold a degree of accountability with respect to their role in the advocacy plan. Advocates should be accountable for the cause and the stakeholders they represent. Simultaneously, they should hold other stakeholders accountable with respect to their obligation to protect the health and well-being of citizens. It is also essential for advocacy and health promotion campaigns to be transparent about their sources of funding and reasons to promote certain arguments and not others. The ultimate goal should be to uphold larger public interests as compared to vested commercial interests.

- **Robust communication strategy:** In today's virtual living, the role of effective communication through maximum utilization of digital communication channels is imperative. In the current context, advocacy campaigns need to garner visibility and traction, both in the physical/in-person mode and in the digital/virtual mode.

## CONCLUSION

Community-led, evidence-based and context-specific advocacy campaigns and health promotion initiatives are critical to bring about a positive shift in health systems, policies and other multisectoral and multistakeholder efforts. Such interventions can steer sustained behavior change and garner support for formulation, compliance and effective health-promoting policies. Globally, there are a plethora of examples where people's movements have brought about far-reaching changes in fostering and sustaining public health and well-being, minimizing preventable morbidity and mortality. The devastating COVID-19 pandemic has underscored the urgent need to support communities to take ownership of their health and partake in key decision-making processes. To build the resilience of communities and public healthcare systems to withstand present and future challenges, advocating to change the status quo is critical. Promoting cardiovascular health bodes well for overall NCD prevention and control. Comprehensive health promotion practice to denormalize CVD and NCD risk factors requires coordinated and streamlined action across multiple government and nongovernment stakeholders. Such initiatives also provide an opportunity to realize a 'whole-of-society' approach, wherein each stakeholder has a critical role to play and all actors function in partnership towards the common goals of attaining physical and mental well-being of populations and upholding the fundamental right to health.

## NOTES

1  World Health Organization. *Health Promotion* [Online]. Available from: Health promotion (who.int) [Accessed on: Jul 1 2021].

2  Carlisle S. Health promotion, advocacy and health inequalities: a conceptual framework. *Health Promot Int.* 2000 December;15(4):369–376. https://doi.org/10.1093/heapro/15.4.369

3  Scottish Health Service Advisory Group. *Advocacy: A Guide to Good Practice.* Edinburgh: Scottish Office, 1997.

4  Ralston J, Reddy KS, Fuster V, Narula J. Cardiovascular diseases on the global agenda: The United Nations high level meeting, sustainable development goals, and the way forward. *Glob Heart.* 2016 December;11(4):375–379. https://doi.org/10.1016/j.gheart.2016.10.029. PMID: 27938821.

5  NCD Countdown Collaborators. NCD Countdown 2030: efficient pathways and strategic investments to accelerate progress towards the Sustainable Development Goal target 3.4 in low-income and middle-income countries. *The Lancet.* 2022 Mar 26;399(10331):1266–1278.

6  Chung MK, Zidar DA, Bristow MR, Cameron SJ, Chan T, Harding III CV, Kwon DH, Singh T, Tilton JC, Tsai EJ, Tucker NR. COVID-19 and cardiovascular disease: from bench to bedside. *Circ Res.* 2021 April 16;128(8):1214–1236.

7  WHO. *Rapid Assessment of Service Delivery for NCDs During the COVID-19 Pandemic.* Geneva: World Health Organization, 2020.

8  Rull JA, Aguilar-Salinas CA, Rojas R, Rios-Torres JM, Gómez-Pérez FJ, Olaiz G. Epidemiology of type 2 diabetes in Mexico. *Archives of Medical Research.* 2005 May 1;36(3):188–196.

9  GBD 2013 Mortality and Causes of Death Collaborators. Global, regional, and national age-sex specific all cause and cause specific mortality for 240 causes of death 1990–2013: a systematic analysis for the Global Burden of Disease Study 2013. *Lancet,* 2014 [Epub ahead of print].

10  Mozaffarian D, Hao T, Rimm EB, Willett WC, Hu FB. Changes in diet and lifestyle and long-term weight gain in women and men. *New England Journal of Medicine.* 2011 Jun 23;364(25):2392–2404.

11  de Ruyter JC, Olthof MR, Seidell JC, Katan MB. A trial of sugar-free or sugar-sweetened beverages and body weight in children. *New England Journal of Medicine.* 2012 Oct 11;367(15):1397–1406.

12  World Health Organization. *Taxes on Sugar Sweetened Beverages as a Public Health Strategy. The Experience of Mexico.* Mexico DF, Mexico: PAHO, 2015.

13  Colchero MA, Molina M, Guerrero-López CM. After Mexico implemented a tax, purchases of sugar-sweetened beverages decreased and water increased: difference by place of residence, household composition, and income level. *The Journal of Nutrition.* 2017 Aug 1;147(8):1552–1557.

14  Carriedo A, Koon AD, Encarnación LM, Lee K, Smith R, Walls H. The political economy of sugar-sweetened beverage taxation in Latin America: lessons from Mexico, Chile and Colombia. *Globalization and Health.* 2021 Dec;17(1):1–4.

# 14 Digital Health and Cardiovascular Disease

## *Current Status and Future Directions*

*Arun Pulikkottil Jose, Devraj Jindal, and Dorairaj Prabhakaran*

## CONTENTS

## BACKGROUND

Since the late 20th century, there has been great interest in the application of digital health to improve the health and well-being of patients as well as the population. The World Health Organization, in its digital health global strategy for 2020–24, recognizes it as one of the key mechanisms to achieve the Sustainable Development Goals by 2030.[1] There has been an increasing demand on health systems in low- to middle-income countries (LMICs) to improve affordability and accessibility to healthcare. In addition to reducing costs and improving access, technological innovations can aid in improving health service provider practices, care linkages, patient lifestyle and health-seeking behavior, thus impacting patients' overall quality of life. However, the health sector has been among the last to embrace the digital revolution. The COVID-19 pandemic of 2020 brought a dramatic shift in thought, and quite suddenly, several aspects of health care seem ripe for digitization. This has led to possible scale-up in a sustainable manner through both public and private funding opportunities for many existing and new digital health innovations.

## DEFINITION AND SCOPE OF DIGITAL HEALTH

Before we dive into the impact, potential applications and way forward for "digital health", it is important to understand its definition and scope.

The definition of the term "digital health" has remained ambiguous, and its scope has expanded over time. In an attempt to define "digital health", Fatehi et al. conducted a scholarly and general electronic search and extracted 95 unique definitions from various sources.[2] On quantitatively analyzing the terms used in these definitions, they observed that emphasis remained on the health aspect rather than technology, health and well-being and rather than disease and patients and the use of the technology rather than its technical aspects.[2] They concluded that "digital health is about the proper use of technology for improving the health and wellbeing of people at individual and population levels, as well as enhancing the care of patients through intelligent processing of clinical and genetic data".[2] Some have defined digital health simply as the convergence of digital technologies with health, health care, living and society enhancing the efficiency of health care delivery.[3] Others, however, have been more specific and have ascribed it to the "application of software or hardware, often using mobile smartphone or sensor technologies to improve patient or population health and health care delivery".[4]

The broad nature of this definition also allows for the inclusion of a wide range of applications within the ambit of digital health. For example, the US Food and Drug Administration includes mobile health, wearable devices, health information technologies, personalized medicine,

DOI: 10.1201/b23266-23

telehealth and telemedicine as digital health.[5] With the ubiquitous use of smart phones over the last decade, mobile health (mHealth) has become one of the most popular and widely used among these.[2] In addition to this, there has been increasing interest and great advances made in the use of machine learning and artificial intelligence (AI) on the large volumes of digital patient data (big data) now available for disease detection, clinical practice, patient compliance, epidemiological evaluations, drug discovery and many other applications.

## DIGITAL HEALTH FOR PREVENTION AND CONTROL OF CARDIOVASCULAR DISEASE

Digital health has been used extensively to improve cardiovascular outcomes as well as for modifying risk factors for cardiovascular disease (CVD). A systematic review and meta-analysis of 51 studies that included randomized controlled trials and cohort studies showed a nearly 40% relative risk reduction in CVD outcomes with digital health interventions, with effects largely seen in heart failure patients and secondary prevention of CVD.[6] Digital health interventions in the management of CVD have been found to be cost-effective too.[7] A systematic review of 14 studies on the cost-effectiveness of digital health interventions in CVD found that 43% of the studies showed a gain in quality-adjusted life years at a lower cost, while the remaining 57% showed a gain with an additional cost but within an acceptable incremental cost-effectiveness ratio.[7]

While there are a variety of ways in which digital health innovations are used to improve cardiovascular care (Table 14.1), there are three broad areas of focus—patient self-management (lifestyle modification and medication adherence), clinical care and health system strengthening.

## DIGITAL HEALTH TOOLS FOR IMPROVING SELF-MANAGEMENT AND MONITORING IN CVD

Digital health interventions use cell phones, smart phones, personal computers and wearables paired with numerous technologies (short messaging service [SMS], internet, software applications) to deliver lifestyle modifications using a wide range of behavioral change constructs (cognition, follow-up, goal setting, record keeping, perceived benefit, persuasion, socialization, personalization, rewards and incentives, support and self-management).[8] A systematic review and meta-analysis of randomized controlled trials using digital technology for risk factor modification in CVD patients found improvements in multiple clinical and behavioral risk factors (total cholesterol, high-density lipoprotein, low-density lipoprotein [LDL], physical inactivity, unhealthy diet) and patient compliance with therapy.[8] Text messaging programs are the most widely studied so far, while the use of smart phone apps and wearables are on the rise.[9]

## Table 14.1 Digital Health Interventions for Cardiovascular Care

**Innovations for Self-Management**

Text messaging

Smart phone applications

Intelligent wearables

**Innovations for Clinical Care**

Point-of-care diagnostics

Electronic clinical decision support systems

Telemedicine

Electronic health records

Digital pharmacies

Intelligent wearables

Smart phone–paired diagnostic innovations

**Innovations for Health System Strengthening**

Telemedicine

Electronic health records

Big data analytics

Digital education

Machine learning and artificial intelligence

## Text Messaging

This is one of the earliest and most-studied digital health innovations. The non-dependence on internet connectivity, the ability to send out messages in bulk and the widespread use of cell phones made text messaging one of the most popular digital health tools in the early 2000s.[9] The two most common applications of text messaging in CVD have been in improving lifestyle and medication adherence.[9] Smoking cessation, weight management, blood pressure management, physical activity and medication adherence are the specific areas where text messaging has been found to be effective.[9] While most trials have focused on a single behavior change, TEXT ME, a text message–based parallel-group, single-blind, randomized clinical trial designed to support multiple behavioral changes and decrease overall cardiovascular risk in patients with CVD found lower total and LDL cholesterol, blood pressure (BP), body mass index (BMI) and smoking rates and higher physical activity levels and adherence to dietary guidelines in the text-messaging group.[10–13]

## Wearables or "Intelligent Wearables"

These devices are widely popular today, with numerous variants and brands available on the market. These devices capture and process patient data through a commonly used wearable (such as a wristwatch) and provide output with relevant information on a smart phone application or itself.[9,14] They have conventionally been used to improve physical activity through tracking the number of steps covered in a day, setting of daily targets and motivational messaging through sharing of achievements with peers, among others. The limited evidence available at present shows conflicting results on the ability of these devices to improve physical activity, reduce a sedentary lifestyle, lower BP or improve a blood lipid profile.[9] More studies would be required to show conclusive benefits of using intelligent wearables in improving lifestyle behavior.

## Smart Phone Applications

Smart phone applications have been used to deliver lifestyle modification interventions through prompts, self-monitoring, health education, rewards for healthy behavior and so on. The number of smart phone applications available on app stores has mushroomed over the last couple of years. While there is potential benefit from using these applications to improve lifestyle and eventually health outcomes, one should be cautious when choosing an application, as a large majority of these applications have been developed with little to no medical expertise and rarely use evidence-based guidelines.[9,15] Poor quality of data, short follow-up periods and a paucity of clinical trial data have limited our understanding of the potential benefits of this digital innovation.[9] While existing trials have seen mixed results in improving CVD risk factors and medication adherence, follow-up periods have been too short to study clinical outcomes.[9]

## DIGITAL HEALTH TOOLS FOR IMPROVING PATIENT MANAGEMENT IN CVD

### Digital Innovations for CVD Diagnosis and Management

Availability of portable point-of-care diagnostics for blood glucose, HbA1c, BP, blood lipids, electrocardiography and other basic investigations in cardiology is now on the rise. These, coupled with telehealth and e-pharmacies, have helped in delivering complete care to patients.

In addition, several digital innovations have helped transform commonly used devices such as wearables, smart phones, tablets and laptops into diagnostic aids. For example, mobile application–based ultrasound systems now enable the plugging in of a transducer into a smart phone or tablet to work as a handheld ultrasound.[16] This has immense potential, such as the detection of valvular heart disease in limited-resource settings. Similarly, inflatable BP cuffs connected to a smart phone application via Bluetooth can help in home monitoring of BP among the elderly and can help in guiding medication.[17] Wearable devices have been used to enable continuous monitoring of patients, thereby enabling diagnosis of arrhythmias and other disorders. The Apple Heart study that included over 400,000 participants showed how wearables were able to detect an irregular pulse. Of those detected with an irregular pulse, 34% had atrial fibrillation on subsequent electrocardiogram (ECG) patch readings and 84% of notifications were concordant with atrial fibrillation.[18] This site-less study is also an example of how large-scale pragmatic and cost-effective research could be carried out using data captured on existing wearables. Although there is immense potential for such digital innovations, there is a need for standardization and further evaluation to establish their true value in CVD care. While it is exciting to explore the possibility of screening and diagnosing CVD using these innovations, it is important to weigh its benefits against the psychological impact of being falsely labeled positive as well as the risk of falsely labeling an individual negative, delaying diagnosis and timely management. Investigators and regulatory authorities have to carefully determine acceptable sensitivity and specificity values for these tools before wide implementation.

## Electronic Clinical Decision Support Systems

Digital tools like electronic clinical decision support systems (CDSS), AI and machine learning (ML) integrated with electronic health records (EHR) or a health management information system (HMIS) can assist health care providers in identifying individuals at high risk for CVD; early diagnosis of CVD; delivery of evidence-based care; referral to an appropriate level of care; and follow-up to respond to changes in health status, improve treatment adherence and ensure retention. Digital tools like an EHR with in-built CDSS can also help in ensuring proper patient workflow and task-sharing with nonphysician health care providers. A systematic review of randomized controlled trials assessing the effectiveness of computerized CDSSs has shown that it improves the performance of health care providers' performance.[19]

An interesting example of the use of an electronic CDSS to improve CVD risk factors and help in task-sharing is the mPower Heart mHealth System being used In India.[20] This nurse-facilitated, smart phone–based CDSS was developed to provide evidence-based care for hypertension and diabetes in resource-poor settings.[20] Over a period of 18 months, over 21,000 patients were screened and 6,800 patients were treated using the CDSS, which was found to significantly reduce BP (systolic BP by 14 mmHg and diastolic BP by 7 mmHg) and fasting glucose level (by 50 mg/dl).[20] The impressive results from this project led to a state-wide adoption and implementation of the CDSS in 40 government health facilities of the northeastern state of Tripura, which included all different levels of health care.[21] As of now, approximately 195,000 patients have been enrolled in the NCD clinics using the CDSS, which can be utilized to further improve the algorithms using ML and AI approaches.[21]

# DIGITAL HEALTH TOOLS FOR HEALTH SYSTEM STRENGTHENING FOR CVD CARE

## Telehealth

Innovations in health technology and telehealth have immense potential in mitigating inequities in access to good-quality health care. Barriers to health access such as distance, time, indirect health care costs, unavailability of health professionals and affordability can be alleviated using telehealth. In addition to this, appropriate and adequate use of health technology can augment the patient's and the treating physician's experience, while potentially improving quality of care delivered through telehealth. The COVID-19 pandemic exposed weaknesses in health systems around the world and made health facilities largely inaccessible to patients suffering from chronic conditions. During this time telemedicine played an important role in ensuring undisrupted care for patients with CVD. A systematic review of the role telemedicine plays in CVD found that it was an effective measure to deliver timely preventive care, reduce readmission of patients with heart failure, improve quality of care and enable remote evaluation and monitoring of patients.[22] Telemedicine helped reduce specialist shortages and the need for physical interactions between patients and health personnel, which has lately been associated with high risks of infection amidst the COVID-19 pandemic.[22]

## Electronic Health Records

Another useful digital tool in the prevention and care of CVD are EHRs. While the rate of adoption and use of EHR systems have been slow, countries across the world have started to see the merit in the maintenance of EHRs for improving quality of health care, digital surveillance, big data analytics and formulation of policy decisions. Many countries have mandatorily moved to digital health records in private- as well as public-sector health facilities. An analysis of the American College of Cardiology's PINNACLE registry in India found significantly higher documentation of receipt of guideline-directed medical therapy in coronary artery disease (CAD), heart failure and atrial fibrillation in practices with EHRs as compared with sites without EHRs.[23] In addition, EHRs have been used to estimate lifetime health care costs and outcomes of patients with stable CAD, which can help inform decisions regarding commissioning, pricing and reimbursement.[24]

Although EHRs were conceived for individual-level documentation, deidentified data are now being used for digital surveillance of CVD events and risk factor burden.[25] An example of this application is the analysis by Rudy JE et al., who were able to monitor improvement in cardiovascular health metrics in the Guideline Advantage (TGA) data repository comprising EHR data of patients from eight diverse health care systems.[26] Big data derived from EHR have been used in various early and late cardiovascular research studies, including drug development, genomic approaches to drug target validation, precision medicine and many more.[27]

## Digital Education

While digital technology has been found to be extremely useful in delivering patient-level health education, it also plays a major in role capacity building of primary care physicians and training for task-shifting in allied health professionals. Digital education platforms offer a cost-effective and convenient way to impart medical education and provide recent updates to large audiences, build referral linkages and collaboration networks and decrease therapeutic inertia in CVD.[28] With the COVID-19 pandemic, almost all forms of education, including medical education, moved into a virtual format. Considering this may be a long-term adaptation, digital education should be seen as a tool for health system strengthening through skill building and task-sharing among the health care workforce.

## CURRENT BARRIERS AND THE WAY FORWARD

A recent rapid review of the role of digital health interventions in mitigating drivers of the health disparities in populations disproportionately affected by atherosclerotic-related CVD showed significantly improved health and health care delivery outcomes (access, utilization and quality) in 24 of 38 included studies.[29] Telemedicine, mobile health and CDDSs were the most commonly used digital health interventions to reduce health inequities, while hypertension control was the most frequently improved outcome.[29] However, there are inequities in access to digital health itself.

The utilization of digital health remains subpar in rural as well as urban areas across the world. Low digital literacy and language barriers play an important role in its poor acceptance. Most digital health technology and telehealth services, although available, remain inaccessible. Complex user interfaces and inattention to user experience are some of the probable reasons. Moreover, a large majority of these services are designed for an educated and English-speaking audience, leaving digital health a luxury for the rural as well as urban uneducated population. Neglecting affordability, language, digital literacy and technology barriers during design, deployment and delivery of digital health services is a key contributor to inequality.

It is important to remember that use of digital health is still a revolutionary innovation in many areas. Its deployment has to be complemented with patient motivation and education to ensure adequate utilization. A focus on optimizing the user interface and experience when designing the intervention would be critical to its acceptance and continued utilization. It has been observed that digital health tools with greater user engagement and interaction are associated with greater levels of behavior modification.[30]

Innovative models of health delivery that use a hybrid of conventional and telehealth care may help transitioning populations ease into the new digital health paradigm. An interesting example of this is the "Digisahayam project" being implemented by the Public Health Foundation of India, where a trained health care worker acts as bridge personnel connecting the patient to the telephysician using an interoperable telemedicine platform paired with multiple state-of-the-art technologies (Box 14.1).

---

### BOX 14.1

**"Digisahayam"** is an assisted telemedicine solution being implemented by the Public Health Foundation of India to ensure uninterrupted care for patients during COVID-19. Telemedicine clinics established with trained health personnel help bridge current gaps in telemedicine by acting as a link between patients and physicians, improving access to health care for the poor and vulnerable populations living in remote locations and providing uninterrupted services during the pandemic.

In this model, trained health care workers connect, convey findings, facilitate doctor-patient interactions and prevent wasteful visits. General physician, specialist and super-specialist teleconsultations are made available. The trained health care worker collects a history, performs a physical examination and carries out lab investigations before initiating a teleconsultation, thereby saving time and improving quality of care. The unique "Digisahayam" assisted telemedicine platform embeds electronic health records, point-of-care diagnostics (13 common lab tests, including ECG), an in-built clinical decision support system for noncommunicable disease (NCD) care and numerous state-of-the-art digital health technologies (digital stethoscope for remote auscultation and physician-controlled camera), thereby facilitating teleconsultations of superior quality aiming at standardizing treatment and avoiding errors in diagnosis. The Swasthya Sahayak device used in the program, also an innovation by the Public Health Foundation of India, is another example of the integration of multiple point-of-care diagnostics into a single device and a robust EHR. The tests that can be carried out by this compact device include vitals such as BP, oxygen saturation, temperature and pulse rate, as well as screening tests such as urine protein and sugar, blood glucose, hemoglobin and urine pregnancy test and tests for common diseases such as malaria, hepatitis B, typhoid, dengue, syphilis and HIV.

To date, three telemedicine centers have been established in India and have provided over 2500 free telemedicine consultations over a span of five months. The World Health Organization is currently supporting the setting up of a demonstration project site in the state of Karnataka in south India. It is aimed to enhance CVD care through digital innovations at the frontline and further adapt and expand this unique model of health care delivery to other parts of the Southeast Asian region.

Another exciting and fast-progressing area in digital health is big data. An interesting review of big data from EHRs for early and late translational cardiovascular research by Hemmingway et al. identifies challenges and opportunities, as well as some excellent exemplars of the use of big data from EHR in early and late translational research.[27] Some of the important challenges mentioned include nonstandardization of data collected, data sharing, data quality, legal and ethical frameworks for its use and building and maintaining public trust, among others.[27] Silverio et al. point out missing data, selection bias, complexity of analysis, data privacy issues and translational applicability as some of the other challenges.[31] Exciting opportunities for big data include accelerated understanding of disease causation and progression, delineating richer disease profiles, discovery of new mechanisms of disease causation and treatment, creation of machine learning models, development of quality of care and performance measures and understanding the health and disease burden of whole populations.[27]

The success of future digital health technologies will depend largely upon cooperation between multiple stakeholders. Lack of communication and trust between different players in the digital health field leads to delay in implementation and hampers the scalability of many proven health technologies. There is a need for a global digital health standardization body, a responsive and accepting regulatory body at the national level, funding and commercialization opportunities from business and philanthropic organizations and a good-quality manufacturing and maintenance infrastructure. On the health technology developer and implementation side, we need to ensure that technologies designed to meet requirements of both private and government sectors are interoperable, follow standard guidelines and most importantly ensure privacy, safety and respect of human data. Further, the recent surge in active mobile internet and social media users has created an opportunity to reach millions of people to deliver health communication messages and personalized care.

Development and implementation agencies for digital health technologies must follow a rigorous iterative process that includes identification of health care needs, formative research, development and evaluation of the digital solution by following a user-centric approach and implementation of the innovative solution. It will be important to support and encourage research in this area and standardize reporting of findings on the development, implementation and impact of digital health interventions. Careful consideration of baseline characteristics of the study population is vital to avoid overestimation as well as underestimation of the effects.

The appropriate and adequate use of digital health interventions will be essential to achieve the Sustainable Development Goals by 2030. Digital health has the ability to address multiple public health challenges, such as access, affordability, availability, quality and sustainability of health care. The applications of digital health to improve public health ranges from the use of mHealth and cellphones for mass health education to the use of big data for digital surveillance, epidemiological evaluations, health planning and public health administration. Every nation should make it an immediate priority to evaluate and effectively integrate digital health innovations in their public health system. We believe that with support from governing bodies and by taking significant steps towards building institutional and workforce capacity, a digital health ecosystem can be created that can reach hundreds of millions of people; engage and empower them in their self-care; and lead to better disease management, less disability and deaths, improved health access, reduced health inequities and lowered health care costs.

## REFERENCES

1. World Health Organization. *Draft Global Strategy on Digital Health 2020–2024.* 2020. https://www.who.int/docs/default-source/documents/gs4dhdaa2a9f352b0445bafbc79ca799dce4d.pdf
2. Fatehi F, Samadbeik M, Kazemi A. What is Digital Health? Review of Definitions. In: Alpo Värri Jdpgmhkhu-Mklbp-Hl-Mpksps, ed. *Integrated Citizen Centered Digital Health and Social Care: Studies in Health Technology and Informatics.* Vol 275. IOS Press; 2020: 67–71. http://doi.org/10.3233/SHTI200696
3. Chen CE, Harrington RA, Desai SA, Mahaffey KW, Turakhia MP. Characteristics of Digital Health Studies Registered in ClinicalTrials.gov. *JAMA Intern Med.* 2019;179(6):838–840. http://doi.org/10.1001/jamainternmed.2018.7235
4. Turakhia MP, Desai SA, Harrington RA. The Outlook of Digital Health for Cardiovascular Medicine: Challenges But also Extraordinary Opportunities. *JAMA Cardiol.* 2016;1(7):743–744. http://doi.org/10.1001/JAMACARDIO.2016.2661
5. What is Digital Health? *FDA.* www.fda.gov/medical-devices/digital-health-center-excellence/what-digital-health. Accessed August 7, 2021.
6. Widmer RJ, Collins NM, Collins CS, West CP, Lerman LO, Lerman A. Digital Health Interventions for the Prevention of Cardiovascular Disease: A Systematic Review and Meta-Analysis. *Mayo Clin Proc.* 2015;90(4):469. http://doi.org/10.1016/J.MAYOCP.2014.12.026
7. Xinchan, Ming W-K, You JH. The Cost-Effectiveness of Digital Health Interventions on the Management of Cardiovascular Diseases: Systematic Review. *J Med Internet Res.* 2019;21(6):e13166. www.jmir.org/2019/6/e13166. http://doi.org/10.2196/13166
8. Samuel A, Polson R, Skeete YD, et al. Digital Technology Interventions for Risk Factor Modification in Patients With Cardiovascular Disease: Systematic Review and Meta-analysis. *JMIR Mhealth Uhealth.* 2021;9(3):e21061 https//mhealth.jmir.org/2021/3/e21061. http://doi.org/10.2196/21061
9. Santo K, Redfern J. Digital Health Innovations to Improve Cardiovascular Disease Care. *Curr Atheroscler Rep.* 2020;22(12):1–10. http://doi.org/10.1007/S11883-020-00889-X
10. Redfern J, Thiagalingam A, Jan S, et al. Development of a Set of Mobile Phone Text Messages Designed for Prevention of Recurrent Cardiovascular Events. *Eur J Prev Cardiol.* 2014;21(4):492–499. http://doi.org/10.1177/2047487312449416
11. Chow CK, Redfern, Hillis GS, et al. Effect of Lifestyle-Focused Text Messaging on Risk Factor Modification in Patients with Coronary Heart Disease: A Randomized Clinical Trial. *JAMA.* 2015;314(12):1255–1263. http://doi.org/10.1001/JAMA.2015.10945
12. Thakkar J, Redfern J, Thiagalingam A, et al. Patterns, Predictors and Effects of Texting Intervention on Physical Activity in CHD—Insights from the TEXT ME Randomized Clinical Trial. *Eur J Prev Cardiol.* 2016;23(17):1894–1902. http://doi.org/10.1177/2047487316664190
13. Santo K, Hyun K, de Keizer L, et al. The Effects of a Lifestyle-focused Text-messaging Intervention on Adherence to Dietary Guideline Recommendations in Patients with Coronary Heart Disease: An Analysis of the TEXT ME Study. *Int J Behav Nutr Phys Act.* 2018;15(1). http://doi.org/10.1186/S12966-018-0677-1
14. Xue Y. A Review on Intelligent Wearables: Uses and Risks. *Hum Behav Emerg Technol.* 2019;1(4):287–294. http://doi.org/10.1002/HBE2.173
15. Santo K, Richtering SS, Chalmers J, Thiagalingam A, Chow CK, Redfern J. Mobile Phone Apps to Improve Medication Adherence: A Systematic Stepwise Process to Identify High-Quality Apps. *JMIR mHealth uHealth.* 2016;4(4). http://doi.org/10.2196/MHEALTH.6742

16. Chamsi-Pasha MA, Sengupta PP, Zoghbi WA. Handheld Echocardiography. *Circulation.* 2017;136(22):2178–2188. http://doi.org/10.1161/CIRCULATIONAHA.117.026622

17. Moon EW, Tan NC, Allen JC, Jafar TH. The Use of Wireless, Smartphone App—Assisted Home Blood Pressure Monitoring Among Hypertensive Patients in Singapore: Pilot Randomized Controlled Trial. *JMIR mHealth uHealth.* 2019;7(5). http://doi.org/10.2196/13153

18. Perez MV, Mahaffey KW, Hedlin H, et al. Large-Scale Assessment of a Smartwatch to Identify Atrial Fibrillation. *N Engl J Med.* 2019;381(20):1909–1917. http://doi.org/10.1056/NEJMOA1901183

19. Garg AX, Adhikari NK, McDonald H, et al. Effects of Computerized Clinical Decision Support Systems on Practitioner Performance and Patient Outcomes: A Systematic Review. *JAMA.* 2005;293(10):1223–1238. http://doi.org/10.1001/JAMA.293.10.1223

20. Ajay VS, Jindal D, Roy A, et al. Development of a Smartphone-Enabled Hypertension and Diabetes Mellitus Management Package to Facilitate Evidence-Based Care Delivery in Primary Healthcare Facilities in India: The mPower Heart Project. *J Am Heart Assoc.* 2016;5(12). http://doi.org/10.1161/JAHA.116.004343

21. Jindal D, Roy A, Ajay VS, Yadav SK, Prabhakaran D, Tandon N. Strategies for Stakeholder Engagement and Uptake of New Intervention: Experience From State-Wide Implementation of mHealth Technology for NCD Care in Tripura, India. *Glob Heart.* 2019;14(2):165–172. http://doi.org/10.1016/J.GHEART.2019.06.002

22. Battineni G, Sagaro GG, Chintalapudi N, Amenta F. The Benefits of Telemedicine in Personalized Prevention of Cardiovascular Diseases (CVD): A Systematic Review. *J Pers Med.* 2021;11(7):658. http://doi.org/10.3390/JPM11070658

23. Kalra A, Bhatt DL, Wei J, et al. Electronic Health Records and Outpatient Cardiovascular Disease Care Delivery: Insights from the American College of Cardiology's PINNACLE India Quality Improvement Program (PIQIP). *Indian Heart J.* 2018;70(5):750–752. http://doi.org/10.1016/J.IHJ.2018.03.002

24. Asaria M, Walker S, Palmer S, et al. Using Electronic Health Records to Predict Costs and Outcomes in Stable Coronary Artery Disease. *Heart.* 2016;102(10):755–762. http://doi.org/10.1136/HEARTJNL-2015-308850

25. VanWormer JJ. Methods of Using Electronic Health Records for Population-Level Surveillance of Coronary Heart Disease Risk in the Heart of New Ulm Project. *Diabetes Spectr.* 2010;23(3):161–165. http://doi.org/10.2337/DIASPECT.23.3.161

26. Rudy JE, Khan Y, Bower JK, Patel S, Foraker RE. Cardiovascular Health Trends in Electronic Health Record Data (2012–2015): A Cross-Sectional Analysis of the Guideline Advantage™. *eGEMs (Generating Evid Methods to Improv patient outcomes).* 2019;7(1):30. http://doi.org/10.5334/EGEMS.268

27. Hemingway H, Asselbergs FW, Danesh J, et al. Big Data from Electronic Health Records for Early and Late Translational Cardiovascular Research: Challenges and Potential. *Eur Heart J.* 2018;39(16):1481–1495. http://doi.org/10.1093/EURHEARTJ/EHX487

28. Lüders S, Schrader J, Schmieder RE, Smolka W, Wegscheider K, Bestehorn K. Improvement of Hypertension Management by Structured Physician Education and Feedback System: Cluster Randomized Trial. *Eur J Prev Cardiol.* 2010;17(3):271–279. http://doi.org/10.1097/HJR.0b013e328330be62

29. Thomas Craig KJ, Fusco N, Lindsley K, et al. Rapid Review: Identification of Digital Health Interventions in Atherosclerotic-related Cardiovascular Disease Populations to Address Racial, Ethnic, and Socioeconomic Health Disparities. *Cardiovasc Digit Heal J.* 2020;1(3):139–148. http://doi.org/10.1016/J.CVDHJ.2020.11.001

30. Franklin NC, Lavie CJ, Arena RA. Personal Health Technology: A New Era in Cardiovascular Disease Prevention. *Postgrad Med.* 2015;127(2):150–158. http://doi.org/10.1080/00325481.2015.1015396

31. Silverio A, Cavallo P, De Rosa R, Galasso G. Big Health Data and Cardiovascular Diseases: A Challenge for Research, an Opportunity for Clinical Care. *Front Med.* 2019:36. http://doi.org/10.3389/FMED.2019.00036

# 15 Public Health Approaches to Rheumatic Heart Disease Prevention and Management

*R. Krishna Kumar*

## CONTENTS

## BACKGROUND

Rheumatic heart disease (RHD) is essentially the result of scarring of the heart valves and their supporting tensor apparatus following an immune-inflammatory response to group A beta-hemolytic *Streptococcus* (GAS) infection.[1] While it is generally understood that these immune responses are manifest as clinically overt episodes of acute rheumatic fever (ARF), it is increasingly believed that ongoing, clinically silent smoldering inflammation of the valve may also contribute to the development of RHD.[2] This covert process is identifiable through echocardiographic screening of vulnerable populations.[3]

The prevalence of RHD and incidence of ARF have noticeably declined in many regions of the world.[4] While there are a few examples of targeted RHD control strategies that have brought about a decline in numbers in selected populations, much of the decline in RHD prevalence appears to have resulted from a general improvement in health care and human development indices.[5,6] Indeed, like many other diseases such as tuberculosis, measles, and malaria, RHD burden largely mirrors overall human development in any region. Over the years, RHD has largely been confined to the poorest and most marginalized populations of the world.[7]

With increasing health care inequity in many parts of the world, RHD has perhaps slipped out of the collective consciousness of the medical fraternity because it has largely become a disease of the voiceless. However, in absolute terms, the disease burden of RHD qualifies as an important public health priority and not just because large numbers of people are affected with considerable mortality and morbidity.[8] Additionally, most seriously affected patients are young adults who lose their most productive years of their life through disability. The most recent global burden study estimated nearly 300,000 deaths due to RHD in 2015 which was about 50% lower than the 1990 estimates.[8] There were sharp regional differences, with the highest age-standardized mortality in Oceania, South Asia, and central sub-Saharan Africa. Overall, they estimated that in 2015 there were 33.4 million cases of RHD globally. The disability-adjusted life years (DALYs) attributable to RHD was 10.5 million.[8] Established RHD often requires long-term medications, hospitalizations, surgery or catheter intervention, and loss of income that collectively contribute to an extremely high economic burden for RHD. Table 15.1 summarizes the overall burden of RHD.

The chapter will first list the unique challenges and barriers in RHD control. This will be followed by an outline of pragmatic public health approaches that integrates our current understanding of the disease epidemiology with the challenges that many regions of the world face with RHD control. The strategies include strengthening primary care to enable improved primary and secondary prophylaxis, innovative ways to improving access to tertiary care, and attention to the care continuum pathways of RHD.

DOI: 10.1201/b23266-24

## Table 15.1 Rheumatic Heart Disease in Numbers

| Region | Numbers Living with RHD | RHD Prevalence | Deaths | DALYs | Mortality Rate per 100,000 |
|---|---|---|---|---|---|
| Global | 33.4 million | | 310,000 | 9,800,000 | 2.5 |
| High-income countries | 221,000 | 3.4/100,000 | 41,000 | 540,000 | 0.77 |
| Upper-middle-income countries | | | 93,000 | 2,200,000 | 1.8 |
| Lower-middle-income countries | 33.19 million | 444/100,000 | 160,000 | 6,100,000 | 3.9 |
| Low-income countries | | | 18,000 | 900,000 | 1.9 |

DALY: Disability-adjusted life years.

Data source: Watkins D, Baker M, Kumar RK, Parks T, Epidemiology, Risk Factors, Burden and Cost of Acute Rheumatic Fever and Rheumatic Heart Disease; In *Acute Rheumatic Fever and Rheumatic Heart Disease*. Editors: Scott Dougherty, Bongani Mayosi, Jonathan Carapetis, and Nigel Wilson. Elsevier (St Louis, MO, USA) 2021, Pages 1–18.

## KEY CHALLENGES AND BARRIERS TO RHD PREVENTION AND MANAGEMENT IN POPULATIONS

A number of challenges are fairly unique to RHD, and they tend to get significantly amplified in large populations. The disease runs a long and protracted course over many years, and affected individuals need close follow-up, lifelong attention in the form of penicillin prophylaxis, heart failure medications, and one or more surgical or catheter-based interventions. Special attention is required if the affected patient becomes pregnant or develops another illness. Because of these complexities of RHD prevention and management, competing public health priorities that are easier to manage appear as better targets for allocation of limited resources.

Further, because RHD prevention requires a high level of involvement, targeted disease control strategies are very difficult to implement across large and diverse populations. This challenge is very well illustrated in a country like India (Table 15.2). Attempts to frame and implement a single policy for the entire nation are unlikely to be effective because of the way the disease is currently distributed. Sharp differences in disease prevalence exist even within small regions.[9] For example, the RHEUMATIC study demonstrated major differences in the prevalence of subclinical carditis between urban and rural populations in close geographical proximity.[10] Over the years RHD has become sequestered among the rural poor and marginalized urban populations.[10] In populations

## Table 15.2 Key Challenges and Barriers for RHD Control in India

| Broad Challenge | Details |
|---|---|
| Magnitude | The large number of people affected is well beyond the collective capacity of the health infrastructure and resources |
| Diversity | Extraordinary variability in India; a single national policy cannot shape control strategies across the country |
| Data | Little data from regions that are likely to be the worst affected because these regions have a very poor health infrastructure; data collection and implementation of RHD control strategies require a reasonably functional health infrastructure; registers are not maintained or mandated for most parts of the country |
| Awareness | Poor awareness of the magnitude of the problem and the distribution of disease among many health professionals and policy makers |
| Policy | RF-RHD are not notifiable diseases in India; there is really no clearly defined national program for RHD control. |
| Implementation | Dysfunctional health systems get in the way of implementing control; RHD registries are seldom maintained; the care continuum is largely non-existent for most regions |
| Penicillin | Erratic supply of good-quality penicillin and absence of guidelines for penicillin administration; limited governmental support to ensure widespread availability of penicillin injections |

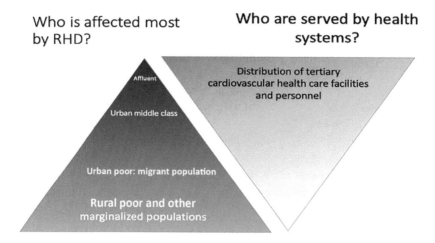

**Figure 15.1** The lopsided distribution of health care facilities and human resources for the management of rheumatic heart disease (RHD). The worst affected populations (rural poor) have the least access to facilities for the management of established RHD.

with reasonably good access to health care, such as in most urban populations, there appears to have been a sharp decline in RHD numbers.[9] Because the overwhelming majority of health care providers are living in the vicinity of these populations, there is a widespread perception that RHD burden has declined to the point that it is perhaps no longer a public health problem (Figure 15.1). There are very few among the mainstream medical professionals who perceive RHD as important enough to merit advocacy for targeted disease control. As an exemplar for a low- and middle-income country (LMIC), Table 15.2 provides key challenges and barriers for RHD control in India.

Rheumatic fever (RF) and RHD are not listed as notifiable diseases in most countries, and this contributes significantly to the paucity of data in many affected regions. Data on RHD prevalence are critically dependent on the existence of a reasonably robust health infrastructure. The unfortunate paradox is that the worst affected regions are likely to have the least developed health infrastructure. As a result, most available data on RHD are from regions with a relatively low burden. This was amply demonstrated in the Jaivigyan mission mode project that was conducted by the Indian Council of Medical Research.[11] This was one of the largest and most ambitious registry projects undertaken in RHD globally involving a population of ~10 million from various parts of India. The selected regions required a willing investigator. It was not possible to identify anyone to conduct the study from regions that were likely to be the worst affected. The data that were collected suggested a significant decline in RHD prevalence in the selected regions over the last five decades.

Another significant challenge relating to implementation of RHD prevention and management relates to the dependence on a robust primary and secondary health care infrastructure. A critical component of RHD control relates to meticulous maintenance of disease registries. It is necessary to track each patient in the registry and ensure compliance with secondary prophylaxis. Management of specific complications such as heart failure and rhythm disorders, timely referral for surgery or catheter intervention, and close follow-up after the procedures require a high level of involvement of the health care team.

RHD prevention is likely to be poorly implemented in regions with dysfunctional health systems. A vicious circle of events results from dysfunctional health systems. Deficiencies in primary health care contribute to a high disease burden and get in the way of obtaining accurate disease estimates, implementing preventive strategies, and providing effective management of affected patients.

An erratic supply of good-quality penicillin and absence of clear guidelines for penicillin administration are also proving to be massive barriers to RHD prevention. A number of countries, including India, are experiencing a serious and protracted shortfall in the supply of benzathine penicillin (BPG).[12] Additionally, there are regions where the fear of anaphylaxis has contributed to increasing reluctance to administer BPG for the prevention of RHD.[13] These two factors are serious roadblocks in the efforts to prevent RHD in many parts of the world.

The reasons behind the global shortfall of BPG are complex and relate to unique issues that affect the manufacturing process and the global supply chain. There are very few producers willing to make BPG, with only a small number of active pharmaceutical ingredient (API) manufacturers (mostly in China). Many countries have stringent regulations and compliance for medicine quality control that API manufacturers may not meet. Additionally, in some countries tight price controls restrict profit margins (e.g. in India) that deter local manufacturers. Additionally, there is a disconnect between demand and supply due to a lack of region-specific data on the prevalence of RF, RHD, and other diseases whose treatment requires penicillin.

Finally, among many health workers and patients there is a reluctance to administer or receive injections. This is due to factors such as a fear of anaphylaxis, pain, unfamiliarity with its correct use, and lack of preparedness in dealing with acute catastrophic events following injections. Deaths are reported after BPG from a number of primary health care settings. They are almost entirely limited to patients with severe heart valve disease.[13] The clinical features preceding these deaths are not well documented. Available information and anecdotes suggest that these are often not a result of anaphylaxis. This happens not necessarily with the first injection, but could occur suddenly after any injection. These deaths can potentially derail RHD prevention programs and result in local governments imposing regulations on the administration of injectable penicillin in many primary care settings.

## PUBLIC HEALTH APPROACHES TO RHD PREVENTION AND MANAGEMENT

The conventional framework for disease prevention can be applied to RHD prevention as well. This involves early, primary, and secondary prevention. Management of established heart valve disease requires tertiary care. Early prevention involves prevention of streptococcal pharyngeal and perhaps skin infection. This happens through improved living standards and access to primary health care services. An effective streptococcal vaccine would offer the ideal form of primary prevention, but in spite of several years of efforts, we do not as yet have an effective vaccine.[14] Primary prophylaxis requires timely and effective management of streptococcal pharyngitis and skin infection. While penicillin is recommended as the standard antibiotic, alternatives such as azithromycin and amoxycillin are frequently used. Secondary prophylaxis is essentially used to prevent recurrences of RF and is best achieved by three or four weekly injections of BPG. Other alternatives such as oral penicillin V or G or sulfonamides are considerably less effective.[7] Established heart valve disease requires specific treatment for the disease in addition to secondary prophylaxis. This involves heart failure management, oral anticoagulants for atrial fibrillation, catheter intervention in the form of balloon mitral valvotomy for mitral valve stenosis, and heart surgery to repair or replace damaged heart valves.[7]

It is important to acknowledge that much of the decline in RHD burden in most parts of the world has not been the result of targeted disease-specific control strategies being implemented. There are success stories of targeted RHD prevention, of course, but these are relatively few and limited to small populations with a reasonable health infrastructure. It is vital to recognize this while developing strategies for RHD control, and it is essential to never lose sight of the importance of primary health care at all times.[15] All of us need to strongly advocate for the quality of primary care services irrespective of our vocation.

However, herein lies a paradox. The extent of devastation from RHD is often best appreciated by the cardiologist. Unfortunately, most cardiologists are confined to tertiary care institutions that are typically located in urban centers that are distant and often disconnected from the community and from primary caregivers. This chasm is at the very core of the failure of advocacy for RHD control in many populations. It is essential to build robust partnerships between cardiologists committed to the prevention of RHD, primary care physicians, and public health experts to enable a strong and sustained thrust in RHD prevention. Such partnerships require an institutional framework in the public sector or one that works closely with the government and helps formulate disease control policies. Privatization of health care preferentially targets tertiary health care, and RHD care often suffers more than other chronic cardiac conditions because it is largely confined to the poorest.

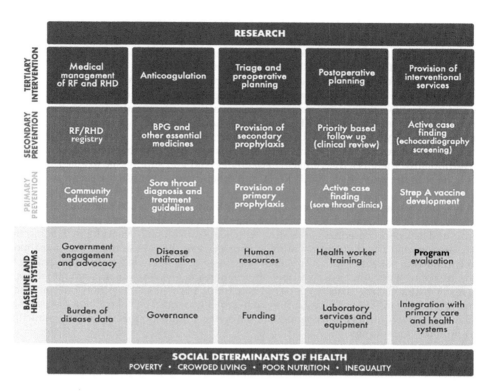

**Figure 15.2** The Tools for Implementing RHD Control Programmes (TIPS) framework for RHD control.

The Tools for Implementing RHD Control Programmes (TIPS) framework (Figure 15.2) developed by the RHD action group lays a comprehensive plan for RHD control that can be adapted and contextualized to different health care environments.[16] This is a conceptual framework of comprehensive RHD control programs that was formed by reviewing World Health Organization (WHO) recommendations and other program implementation experiences to identify common critical elements for RHD control.

## AWARENESS AND ADVOCACY

Specific advocacy strategies that could potentially work for RHD include integration of RHD control with other non-communicable diseases (NCDs). The emergence of cardiovascular disease as a major cause of death and disability in LMICs has been the focus of considerable attention in the last two decades. Management and prevention of RHD can be integrated into NCD control programs.

Awareness campaigns have to be targeted to the lay public and influential civil society members such as school teachers in high-prevalence regions and carefully integrated into RHD control programs. Table 15.3 describes an awareness and advocacy framework for RHD control.

## DISEASE REGISTRIES AND SCREENING

A uniform and simplified format for nationwide registries with integration using mHealth technologies can also allow large-scale data capture and accurately inform policy. Innovative strategies for screening, such as mandating a cardiac evaluation of children at school entry and annual check-ups, can potentially identify RHD in larger numbers. A structured cardiac evaluation integrated as a screening tool in all pregnant women could enable identification of RHD early in pregnancy and potentially avoid serious peripartum complications. The core curriculum of cardiology fellows in high-burden countries must include focused training in echocardiogram screening, preventive strategies, and management of established disease. Cardiology trainees should be encouraged to participate in public health initiatives on RHD prevention.

## Table 15.3 Awareness and Advocacy Framework for RHD Prevention

| Who? | Purpose | Specifics |
|---|---|---|
| Lay public | Improve primary prophylaxis through prompt treatment of sore throat. | Awareness campaigns for the lay public need to be thoughtfully targeted to high-prevalence regions through culturally appropriate content that has to be innovatively delivered via available media in regional languages. It greatly helps to have local champions in the form of sports persons and media celebrities endorse RHD prevention and deliver key messages. |
| School teachers | Improve primary prophylaxis; detection of RF and RHD in the community. | Targeted campaigns with specific information on RF and RHD can be delivered to school teachers to enable detection among the most vulnerable group of children between 5 and 15 years age. |
| Policy makers | Sensitize health policy makers on the disease burden, regional variations, and economic impact, as well as the opportunity to prevent RHD through public health interventions. | Resulting actions could include mandating an RF-RHD registry in high-prevalence regions; greater allocation of resources for RHD prevention and management; making RF and RHD notifiable in the worst affected regions; and ensuring adequate availability of penicillin in affected regions. |
| Medical students, primary care doctors, pediatricians, and general physicians | Improved awareness of contemporary epidemiology; sensitization on disease burden and importance of prevention | The strategies to reach out to medical professionals could include curriculum revisions for undergraduate and postgraduate education, dedicated CME programs and interactive sessions, capsules of education material that summarize recent guidelines, and dedicated sessions in major conferences. All these strategies can be implemented through close liaison with professional bodies. |
| Practitioners of alternative medicine | Making the distinction between acute rheumatic fever and arthritis from other causes. | Who needs a referral for cardiac assessment? |
| Cardiologists and cardiac surgeons | Sensitization on disease burden and affected populations and the economic challenges. Sensitization on the need to pay attention to the care continuum of RHD. | Making special efforts to ensure accurate epidemiological data are presented to challenge the perception of a sharp decline. Emphasis on the importance of liaising with primary care providers to ensure adherence to secondary prophylaxis, optimal anticoagulation, heart failure management, care during pregnancy and intercurrent illness, and timely referral for surgery or catheter interventions. |

## PREVENTION AND MANAGEMENT GUIDELINES FOR RHD

Contextualized guidelines for prevention and management of RHD need to be developed and disseminated among primary care physicians and district-level hospitals. Specifically, the importance of injectable penicillin as a cornerstone in secondary prevention needs adequate emphasis. Special efforts are needed to address and clear misconceptions and allay fears of anaphylaxis with penicillin injection. It is also necessary to ensure adequate preparedness with adverse events. Some flexibility with penicillin administration may allow for reduced fatal or near-fatal events following injections. It may perhaps be appropriate to administer oral penicillin V for patients with severe established heart valve disease. It is also necessary to consider revising the recommendations of the duration of prophylaxis. It is no longer necessary to administer penicillin for life and limit it to those under 40 years of age. The evidence base for these guidelines is not robust, but there is a growing consensus that accommodates this pragmatic approach.[7]

### Penicillin Availability

Because it is the cornerstone of RHD prevention, special efforts have to be made in conjunction with the government on procurement of the API, local formulation of injectable BPG, and distribution through effective supply chains as dictated by regional demands. The challenges on the supply side, and in particular on addressing issues with the lack of availability of the API, will need international cooperation and involvement of agencies such as the WHO. This requires sustained advocacy. There is also a need for research into better ways of administering penicillin. Preparations that can deliver penicillin over several months can greatly improve its acceptance.

## Leadership and Administration

Like many other conditions, RHD control can only be driven through a committed leadership, both nationally as well as regionally. The administrative structure of RHD control programs needs to include members from diverse backgrounds. tailored to each region depending on local challenges.

## Cost Considerations

In a recent study investigating the cost and benefit of investment in the prevention and management of RHD, it was determined that mortality can be reduced by 30% over the next decade by investing USD 100 million annually in decentralizing and integrating cardiac care at rural primary care facilities and getting those with advanced disease on the right medicines and to cardiac surgery when needed.[17] This means saving 70,000 lives. The study identifies two reasons for action: an opportunity to reduce RHD deaths by 30% through early detection, disease management, and cardiac surgery, with a very high return on investment (ROI) in the short term and an opportunity to reduce RF incidence by 30% through strep throat treatment in primary care settings, with an attractive ROI over a longer term. The results of this study help inform policy, but will need to be contextualized to each country based on specific considerations.

## International Efforts for RHD Control

The international mandate was clearly spelled out by the WHO at the 74th World Health Assembly on April 1, 2021. The key action items included assessing the magnitude and nature of the problem of RHD, providing support in developing and implementing RHD prevention, and facilitating access to existing and new medicines and technologies.[18] Table 15.4 lists the global organizations that are actively working towards RHD prevention and control. Most international organizations have alliances and connections with one another and with the WHO. Their resources and expertise are shared through collaborations within this global network.

## Table 15.4 Global Organizations that Are Actively Working Towards RHD Prevention and Control

| Name of the Organization or Agency | Scope of Action |
| --- | --- |
| World Health Organization | Lead and coordinate global efforts on prevention and control of rheumatic heart disease. To develop regional expert network on rheumatic heart disease, with the goal of supporting the development of technical guidance and accelerating in-country implementation of the regional framework. https://apps.who.int/gb/ebwha/pdf_files/WHA74/A74_40-en.pdf |
| World Heart Federation | Global advocacy efforts on RHD prevention and treatment. https://world-heart-federation.org/what-we-do/rheumatic-heart-disease/ |
| Reach | To promote the health of vulnerable populations through technical support to local, regional, and global efforts to prevent and control rheumatic fever and rheumatic heart disease. Partners with a broad range of stakeholders, including clinicians, other disease communities, academics, donors, governments, industry, and people living with RHD. www.stoprhd.org/ |
| RHD Action | RHD Action is a coalition of three global organizations: Medtronic Foundation, the World Heart Federation, and Reach, working together toward the shared goal of ending RHD. Critically reinforcing this global movement are the RHD Action Countries, a cohort of countries wherein government and partner institutions are actively engaged in achieving specific RHD targets within their geographies, while also strengthening their health systems. https://rhdaction.org/about |

| Name of the Organization or Agency | Scope of Action |
| --- | --- |
| PASCAR-ASAP Pan-African Society of Cardiology-Awareness, Surveillance, Advocacy and Prevention | The ASAP program, launched in 2006, followed a call for action from key players in Africa's health care and political realms in response to the persistent health burden attributable to RF/RHD and has agreed to a pledge of action to reduce it. The program targets efforts to raise awareness, establish surveillance systems, advocate for increased resources for treatment, and promote prevention strategies using a community-based, bottom-up approach. The ASAP program is an example of programs initiated, run, and organized by countries most affected by the disease. www.pascar.org/content/page/asap-programme |
| Global ARCH Global Alliance for Rheumatic and Congenital Hearts | The mission is to improve worldwide lifelong outcomes in childhood-onset heart disease through empowering patient and family organizations. Global ARCH brings together organizations from around the world to learn, collaborate, and speak out together about the unmet needs of those living with childhood-onset heart conditions and create a stronger voice on behalf of CHD and RHD patients and families. https://global-arch.org/ |
| Partners in Health (PIH) | A social justice organization that responds to the moral imperative to provide high-quality health care globally to those who need it most. PIH draws on the resources of the world's leading medical and academic institutions and on the lived experience of the world's poorest and sickest communities. PIH collaborates with national governments in 11 countries, across four continents, to ensure quality health care is available in some of the world's most vulnerable communities through strengthening public health systems. www.pih.org/ |

## CONCLUSIONS

Because of its overall complexity, RHD control cannot perhaps be accomplished as a vertical disease program that exists in relative isolation as a distinct entity. The care continuum of RHD is critically dependent on having a robust primary health care system. As a first step, it may be necessary to identify high-prevalence regions and target them first. Some flexibility and innovations may allow for data collection to be started simultaneously in regions presumed to have high disease burden. Sociodemographic indices are reasonable surrogates for RHD burden and may be used for the initial phases of disease control. Alterations and adjustments have to be made once data on disease burden are obtained. Echocardiographic screening of sample populations may allow for rapid estimates of the likely disease burden.

## REFERENCES

1. Tandon R, Sharma M, Chandrashekhar Y, Kotb M, Yacoub MH, Narula J. Revisiting the pathogenesis of rheumatic fever and carditis. *Nat Rev Cardiol.* 2013;10(3):171–197.
2. Carapetis JR, Beaton A, Cunningham MW, Guilherme L, Karthikeyan G, Mayosi BM, et al. Acute rheumatic fever and rheumatic heart disease. *Nat Rev Dis Primers.* 2016;2:15084.
3. Reményi B, Wilson N, Steer A, Ferreira B, Kado J, Kumar K, Lawrenson J, Maguire G, Marijon E, Mirabel M, Mocumbi AO, Mota C, Paar J, Saxena A, Scheel J, Stirling J, Viali S, Balekundri VI, Wheaton G, Zühlke L, Carapetis J. World Heart Federation criteria for echocardiographic diagnosis of rheumatic heart disease-an evidence-based guideline. *Nat Rev Cardiol.* 2012; 28:297–309.
4. Palafox B, Mocumbi AO, Kumar RK, Ali SKM, Kennedy E, Haileamlak A, Watkins D, Petricca K, Wyber R, Timeon P, Mwangi J. The WHF Roadmap for Reducing CV morbidity and mortality through prevention and control of RHD. *Glob Heart.* 2017;12(1):47–62.
5. Nordet P, Lopez R, Duenas A, Sarmiento L. Prevention and control of rheumatic fever and rheumatic heart disease: the Cuban experience (1986–1996–2002). *Cardiovasc J Afr.* 2008;19(3):135–140.
6. Bach JF, Chalons S, Forier E, Elana G, Jouanelle J, Kayemba S, et al. 10-year educational programme aimed at rheumatic fever in two French Caribbean islands. *Lancet.* 1996;347(9002):644–648.

7. Kumar RK, Antunes MJ, Beaton A, Mirabel M, Nkomo VT, Okello E, Regmi PR, Reményi B, Sliwa-Hähnle K, Zühlke LJ, Sable C. American heart association council on lifelong congenital heart disease and heart health in the young; council on cardiovascular and stroke nursing; and council on clinical cardiology. Contemporary diagnosis and management of rheumatic heart disease: implications for closing the gap: a scientific statement from the American Heart Association. *Circulation*. 2020;142(20):e337–e357.

8. Watkins DA, Johnson CO, Colquhoun SM, Karthikeyan G, Beaton A, Bukhman G, et al. Global, regional, and national burden of rheumatic heart disease, 1990–2015. *N Engl J Med*. 2017;377(8):713–722.

9. Kumar RK, Tandon R. Rheumatic fever & rheumatic heart disease: the last 50 years. *Indian J Med Res*. 2013;137:643–658.

10. Saxena A, Ramakrishnan S, Roy A, Seth S, Krishnan A, Misra P, et al. Prevalence and outcome of subclinical rheumatic heart disease in India: the RHEUMATIC (Rheumatic Heart Echo Utilisation and Monitoring Actuarial Trends in Indian Children) study. *Heart*. 2011;97(24):2018–2022.

11. India Jai Vigyan Mission Mode Project. *Community Control of Rheumatic Fever/Rheumatic Heart Disease in India Comprehensive Project Report 2001–2010*; http://ghdx.healthdata.org/record/india-jai-vigyan-mission-mode-project-community-control-rheumatic-feverrheumatic-heart. Accessed 15 May 2021.

12. Watkins D, Zuhlke L, Engel M, Daniels R, Francis V, Shaboodien G, Kango M, Abul-Fadl A, Adeoye A, Ali S, Al-Kebsi M, Bode-Thomas F, Bukhman G, Damasceno A, Goshu DY, Elghamrawy A, Gitura B, Haileamlak A, Hailu A, Hugo-Hamman C, Justus S, Karthikeyan G, Kennedy N, Lwabi P, Mamo Y, Mntla P, Sutton C, Mocumbi AO, Mondo C, Mtaja A, Musuku J, Mucumbitsi J, Murango L, Nel G, Ogendo S, Ogola E, Ojji D, Olunuga TO, Redi MM, Rusingiza KE, Sani M, Sheta S, Shongwe S, van Dam J, Gamra H, Carapetis J, Lennon D, Mayosi BM. Seven key actions to eradicate rheumatic heart disease in Africa: the Addis Ababa communiqué. *Cardiovasc J Afr*. 2016;27(3):184–187.

13. Marantelli S, Hand R, Carapetis J, Beaton A, Wyber R. Severe adverse events following benzathine penicillin G injection for rheumatic heart disease prophylaxis: cardiac compromise more likely than anaphylaxis. *Heart Asia*. 2019;11(2):e011191. doi:10.1136/heartasia-2019-011191.

14. Kumar RK, Paul M, Francis PT. Rheumatic heart disease in India, are we ready to shift from secondary prophylaxis to vaccinating high risk children. *Curr Sci*. 2009;97:397–404

15. Omurzakova NA, Yamano Y, Saatova GM, Mirzakhanova MI, Shukurova SM, Kydyralieva RB, et al. High incidence of rheumatic fever and rheumatic heart disease in the republics of Central Asia. *Int J Rheum Dis*. 2009;12(2):79–83.

16. http://rhdaction.org/sites/default/files/TIPS-HANDBOOK_World-Heart-Federation_RhEACH.pdf. Accessed 15-May-2021.

17. Coates MM, Sliwa K, Watkins DA, Zühlke L, Perel P, Berteletti F, Eiselé JL, Klassen SL, Kwan GF, Mocumbi AO, Prabhakaran D, Habtemariam MK, Bukhman G. An investment case for the prevention and management of rheumatic heart disease in the African Union 2021–30: a modelling study. *Lancet Glob Health*. 2021 May. doi:10:S2214-109X(21)00199-6.

18. https://apps.who.int/gb/ebwha/pdf_files/WHA74/A74_40-en.pdf. Accessed 30 July 2021.

# 16 Cost-Effectiveness Analysis

## *Methods, Innovations, and Applications*

*Kaitlin Harold, Shuchi Anand, and Rachel Nugent*

## CONTENTS

Cost-effectiveness analysis (CEA) is a method used to help decision-makers obtain the maximum amount of health gains per amount spent. By relating the financial and medical impacts of different health interventions, CEA is a useful tool for policymakers and decisions regarding resource allocation. At its simplest, the CEA of an intervention is the intervention's monetary cost divided by the expected health gain, compared to either a status quo or a comparable intervention. The costs are expressed in monetary terms, while the expected health gain is expressed in natural units such as lives saved. In this chapter we will introduce the basics of CEA and its applications.

## DEFINING THE PERSPECTIVE

Before detailing the different aspects of CEA, one must understand the perspective which underlies the analysis—that is, the objectives of the entity or person for whom the CEA is being conducted. Establishing the perspective not only allows the analysts to enumerate relevant costs and benefits but also allows for appropriate interpretation of the ultimate results. In other words, both the accuracy and the usefulness of a CEA are critically dependent on establishing perspective. In the current literature, the societal and the individual or the payer perspectives are adopted most commonly.

The societal perspective is for broader policy use and considers the costs incurred by society on the whole. This perspective is in contrast to the sectoral perspective or the government perspective, which is usually narrower and considers only the health care costs incurred by the government. According to the World Health Organization, the goal of the societal perspective is to "allocat[e] a fixed health budget between interventions in such a way as to maximize health in a society" and "generate the highest possible overall level of population health" (1). This requires considering different social concerns, such as prioritizing the sick and reducing inequalities in health, which would not be otherwise considered at the individual level (2, 3). It also means that the costs and benefits included in the analysis should include all paid by society, so analyses often take into account the total welfare effect of an intervention—the costs are the total welfare forgone because the resources could not be used elsewhere, and the benefits are the total welfare gain from health improvement (and include components such as increased productivity or consumption).

The payer perspective, on the other hand, is narrower than the societal perspective and more individualized. The payer perspective can be taken from the perspective of a patient, but also a provider, employer, manufacturers, and even the government if the analysis is restricted to purely government costs and benefits and does not include societal welfare or costs. This means costs, such as fees for hospitalization, physician consultations, medications, and diagnostic tests, are included where incurred and attributable to a specific payer, but also individualized welfare, such as workdays lost, suffering, and education lost may be included if the perspective includes individuals and households. For example, an insurer may want to consider the cost-effectiveness of different interventions when deciding what coverage will be included for a specific premium level.

## COSTING THE INTERVENTIONS

With these perspectives in mind, the first step of performing a CEA is cost ascertainment (4). Here it is crucial to enumerate costs of at least two states: standard care and the proposed change in care.

DOI: 10.1201/b23266-25

For example, if an assessment is being made to determine whether a health system should pay for computed tomography for kidney stone evaluation in anyone presenting with flank pain, the status quo in caring for such patients must be clearly described (e.g., at the moment such patients may get kidney ultrasounds only) and costed. The additional cost (or saving) of the alternative care—in this case, of using a computed tomography—also needs to be calculated.

There are two main categories of costs: direct and indirect costs. Direct costs are the costs of formal health care goods and services and other costs that come directly from the implementation of the intervention, such as a patient's travel time to access care. Indirect costs, on the other hand, are the estimated costs from the indirect impact of an intervention (5). Most commonly, these costs include the estimated value of income forgone due to interrupted work when obtaining the health services. Sometimes, the estimated value of informal care, or unpaid care, from family members or associates is also included. These costs, however, can be hard to factor in, as many of these resources are not equally distributed across households and cannot forcibly be distributed equally. For example, some households have higher capacity for provision of more informal care than others, making this resource hard to accurately plan for and factor into the analysis. If the scope of costs included is consistent between interventions that are being compared, the analysis nonetheless enables valid comparisons of cost and benefit, despite the imperfect nature of indirect cost estimates.

In some analyses, it is also useful to consider these costs on a time scale. Often, immediate costs are more impactful or more important to a policymaker than costs that are incurred in the future. To account for this, future costs are often discounted. As simply defined by Torgerson and Raftery, a discount rate reduces future costs, relative to current costs, since "there is an opportunity cost to spending money now and there is desire to enjoy benefits now rather than in the future" (6). The World Health Organization recommends that future costs be discounted by 3% per year and adjusted to a common year using the gross domestic product (GDP) deflator where possible (1).

## ASSESSING THE BENEFIT OF INTERVENTIONS

The next step in performing a CEA is benefit ascertainment. The benefit of the intervention is the health gain associated with it, usually measured in natural units. **This includes units such as lives saved or years of life gained**, which can greatly impact how much benefit an intervention is measured to have. For example, considering years of life gained by providing a health service, an intervention that saves an infant would provide a longer stream of health benefits than one that saves an older person. This gain is found by comparing the lifetime health experience when the status quo (or comparable) intervention against a disease is offered to the lifetime health experience with the intervention being considered, allowing the benefits of different interventions to then be compared against each other. Benefit ascertainment typically does not consider non-health benefits, but it can in certain situations. Depending on the goals of the policymaker, the reach or equity of different interventions may be factored into benefit calculations, particularly if the goal is to target a certain population group.

When measuring benefits in years of life, years are often discounted, both due to time and disease burden. To weigh more immediate health impact more than later impact, years are often discounted at a 3% rate, similar to cost. As for disease burden, analysts often want to account for the fact that different diseases and interventions will affect the quality of life differently. This is done by measuring the change from a baseline, which is often estimated from population models that can take into account the age distribution of a population and the age-specific prevalence of the disease. This change is most often measured in one of two units: disability-adjusted life years (DALY) and quality-adjusted life years (QALY). These are defined and illustrated in Box 16.1.

---

### BOX 16.1: AN ILLUSTRATION OF DALY AND QALY

Disability-adjusted life years (DALY) measure years of life lost to a disease plus years lived with a disability caused by that disease. It is calculated by summing the years of life lost (YLLs) and the years lost to disability (YLDs). A DALY is a measure of years of life lost either from a reduced life expectancy (years lost to life, or YLLs) or a reduced quality of life associated with a condition (years lost to disability, YLDs). In a cost-effectiveness analysis (CEA), one wants to calculate the benefits gained through an intervention to compare against the cost. Because DALY are years lost, CEAs that use DALY use DALY *averted* as the measure of benefit.

$$DALY = YLL + YLD$$

To calculate DALY, calculate the sum of YLL due to premature mortality and YLD. DALY are on a metric of 0 to 1: 0 is perfect health and 1 is death.

For instance, if Karpita is diagnosed with diabetes at age 55, she might be expected to live only 10 more years, whereas if she did not have diabetes she would be expected to live for 34 more years up to age 89. And if she has diabetes, she might suffer in her last 5 years from a disability caused by diabetes such as impaired eyesight and foot amputation. Hence, the DALY lost from Karpita's diabetes are 24 years of life lost plus 5 lived with disability for a total of 29 years of healthy life lost.

Quality-adjusted life years (QALY) measure years gained due to an intervention. It is calculated by finding the number of years gained by an intervention and adjusting them for the burden of the disease. Opposite to the calculation of DALY, a year in full health has a value of 1, and any years lived in less than full health are calculated by subtracting a disability weight similar to the severity weight of DALY. The World Health Organization notes that these weights do not represent the lived experience, only the state of health in relation to the societal "ideal" of good health (1).

Cost per DALY averted for use in CEA comparing an intervention (1) to its comparator (2) would then be able to be calculated with the following formula:

$$CE\,Ratio = \frac{Cost_1 - Cost_2}{DALYs\,averted_1 - DALYs\,averted_2}$$

## INNOVATIONS IN CEAS

The previously discussed methods of cost and benefit ascertainment are the basis of CEA, but the analysis has progressed over time to accommodate the complex dimensions and outcomes of health policy. For example, policymakers may want to consider protection from financial risks associated with health care expenses, as they can lead to impoverishment or unfavorable decisions to manage them. Health outcomes, such as life expectancy and access to health care, also vary largely across socioeconomic and racial groups. Public policy may aim to combat these inequalities and favor interventions that address them. Verguet, Kim, and Jamison have offered a way to integrate these factors into CEA using a methodology called extended cost-effectiveness analysis (ECEA) (7, 8). ECEAs are meant to evaluate the consequences of health policies in terms of health gains, financial risk protection benefits, the total cost of the policy to decision-makers, and distributional consequences (7).

In an ECEA, the analysis is almost the same as in a CEA, but the data considered are much more extensive. Health gains are measured through disease burden, intervention coverage, and intervention effectiveness by population subgroup. Similarly, costs may be stratified by different health groups, as different groups may have different combinations of direct health costs and indirect costs from productivity and income loss. In addition to overall cost-effectiveness for a population, interventions can be measured by their impact on one or more of the following factors: the number of catastrophic cost cases, the number of poverty cases averted, or the money-metric value of insurance provided. Catastrophic medical costs—i.e., a health event causing the affected persons to use 10% or more of their disposable household resources—may arise from paying for a health intervention and may differ for individuals along the income distribution. The number of poverty cases averted similarly compares the number of individuals no longer crossing a "poverty line" before and after the intervention. Finally, the money-metric value of insurance provided is a modeled estimate of the financial protection benefits to risk-averse individuals. The financial risk protection benefit would then be the income with uncertainty minus the income an individual is willing to have for a certain outcome due to coverage for an intervention.

ECEA is extremely useful, as it enables the design of health insurance benefits packages based on the inclusion of financial risk protection and cost and health data, taking into account both health and non-health outcomes. This allows it to be optimized to the policymakers' or users' preferences. However, to get this level of detail, ECEA can also be difficult to perform. In the article, Verguet, Kim, and Jamison (7) note that

> ECEA studies are highly context-specific and depend substantially on the local epidemiology of the setting (e.g., the endemicity and the distribution of diseases), the health system infrastructure and constraints (e.g., the presence and the distribution of health facilities), the wealth of the population (e.g., a low- vs. middle- vs. high-income country) and the underlying financial arrangements (e.g., the existence of social insurance or community-based insurance programs).
>
> (Verguet et al.)

Accounting for this across population subgroups is extremely data-intensive, and it can be difficult to get sufficient data.

## EXAMPLE OF AN APPLICATION: DISEASE CONTROL PRIORITIES' ESSENTIAL UNIVERSAL HEALTH COVERAGE PACKAGE

Disease Control Priorities (DCP3) used CEA to build its Essential Universal Health Coverage (EUHC) package (8). Since many countries may be starting with an existing small group of the population covered by a government-sponsored health plan, there exists a tension between expanding coverage or eligibility criteria to engage a larger portion of the population but also in increasing the services covered to reduce financial risk (9) (Figure 16.1).

The DCP3 EUHC package comprises 218 interventions identified as highest priority for coverage in low- and middle-income countries based on the synthesis of epidemiological and economic evidence, along with expert judgment used to extrapolate data (see www.Dcp3.org). Identifying interventions as "highest priority" was based on three dimensions: priority given to the worse off (those with significantly less lifetime health or quality because of a disease or injury, or "health-adjusted average age of death"), maximizing financial risk protection (improving the health of wage earners or addressing diseases that cause high levels of disability), and value for money, which we will focus on here (Watkins et al.).

The "value for money" dimension utilized CEA, as described earlier. It takes on a societal perspective, as the EUHC package of interventions is meant to be a set of priorities for universal health coverage policy, and the economic evidence used was from health-sector data. These data, along with price variations in technologies from subsidies in different countries and the quality

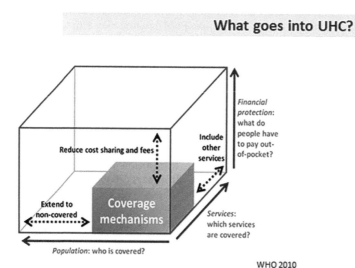

Figure 16.1 What goes into UHC? (Adapted from the World Health Organization.)

and generalizability of the data, were used to model the cost of each intervention. The benefit of each intervention was then assessed using DALY averted, as well as the epidemiological context (i.e., Is the area a high or low transmission area for the disease addressed by the intervention?). However, DALY were used only in cases where the addressed disease affected disability and premature mortality. In cases that are not easily measured in deaths, such as "met need for family planning, reductions in stillbirth rates, palliative care and relief of suffering, and remediation of intellectual losses associated with illness or poor nutritional status", a more general metric was used in place of DALY and QALY (Watkins, et al). Using these costs and benefits, the "value for money" metric was calculated for each intervention for use in the overall analysis of intervention coverage priorities.

## EXAMPLE OF AN APPLICATION: A REVIEW OF COST-EFFECTIVENESS ANALYSIS FOR HYPERTENSION MANAGEMENT

Economic evaluations are not known for their uniformity. Different studies measure outcomes differently and sometimes use different assumptions, such as the discount rate or whether to report DALY averted or QALY gained. For example, a review of studies that measure cost-effectiveness of hypertension management in low-income and middle-income countries (LMICs) described 42 studies that included cost-effectiveness (3).

In this review, the authors first narrowed their evaluation to focus on pharmacological interventions, rather than on additional potential (e.g., salt reduction, exercise promotion, or tobacco control) lifestyle modifications. Nonetheless, these studies used five different outcome measures for hypertension, included different kinds of costs, and used different thresholds for assessing whether the hypertension program was cost-effective.

There were five reported indicators of cost across all 42 studies: cost per mm Hg reduction, cost per patient with hypertension, cost per patient with controlled hypertension, cost per DALY averted, and cost per QALY gained. The cost elements across the studies varied and included costs such as that of medications, lab work, labor, equipment, transportation, and provider training for the intervention. Because of the variability in cost elements between studies, there was significant variability in cost results. However, almost all studies in all countries had a cost under $1000/patient for any intervention.

A common threshold for cost-effectiveness in LMICs is based on per capita gross domestic product (GDP). This study used the threshold of three times the annual per capita GDP, considering costs per DALY averted to be cost-effective if under this amount. The cost was considered *very* cost-effective if it did not exceed the annual per capita GDP with no multiplier. In the 42 studies, the average GDP per capita was $2188, so hypertension treatments in almost all studies were well below this threshold and therefore very cost-effective.

In spite of wide divergences in methods, the conclusions of the studies reviewed were generally aligned, showing hypertension treatment to be very cost-effective in most LMIC settings.

In summary CEAs and ECEAs attempt to rationally distribute limited resources by equipping policymakers with a systematic approach for choosing between a menu of available health care interventions. Implemented within a uniform framework across multiple sectors of health, they can be powerful tool in effective health care delivery.

## WORKS CITED

1. Edejer, T. Tan-Torres, et al. *Making Choices in Health: WHO Guide to Cost-Effectiveness Analysis*. WHO, Geneva, 2004.
2. Garrison, Louis P., et al. An overview of value, perspective, and decision context—a health economics approach: an ISPOR special task force report [2]. *Value in Health*, vol. 21, no. 2, 2018, pp. 124–130. doi:10.1016/j.jval.2017.12.006.
3. Kostova, D., Spencer, G., Moran, A.E., Cobb, L.K., Husain, M.J., Datta, B.K., Matsushita, K. and Nugent, R. The cost-effectiveness of hypertension management in low-income and middle-income countries: a review. *BMJ Global Health*, vol. 5, no. 9, 2020, p. e002213.
4. Jamison, D.T., Breman, J.G., Measham, A.R., et al., editors. *Priorities in Health*. Washington, DC: The International Bank for Reconstruction and Development/The World Bank; 2006. Chapter 3, Cost-Effectiveness Analysis.
5. Ernst, R. Indirect costs and cost-effectiveness analysis. *Value in Health*, vol. 9, no. 4, 2006, pp. 253–261. ISSN 1098–3015.
6. Torgerson, D. and Raftery, J. Discounting. *BMJ*, vol. 319, no. 7214, 1999, pp. 914–915.

7. Verguet, S., Kim, J.J. and Jamison, D.T. Extended cost-effectiveness analysis for health policy assessment: a tutorial. *Pharmaco Economics*, vol. 34, 2016, pp. 913–923.

8. Watkins, David A., et al. Chapter 3: Universal health coverage and essential packages of care. In *Disease Control Priorities. Improving Health and Reducing Poverty*, edited by Dean T. Jamison. World Bank Publications, Washington DC, 2018.

9. World Health Organization. *Health Systems Financing: the Path to Universal Coverage*. World Health Organization, 2010. https://apps.who.int/iris/bitstream/handle/10665/44371/9789241564021_eng.pdf?sequence=1&isAllowed=y

# 17 Universal Health Coverage for Better Cardiovascular Disease Outcomes in LMICs

## *Focus on Quality, Not Just Coverage*

*Giridhara R. Babu, Yamuna Ana, Min Kyung Kim, Margaret E. Kruk, and Hannah H. Leslie*

## CONTENTS

## UNIVERSAL HEALTH COVERAGE WITHIN THE SUSTAINABLE DEVELOPMENT GOALS

Universal health coverage (UHC) is the goal that all people have access to needed health services—including prevention, promotion, treatment, rehabilitation, and palliation (the whole gamut of continuum of care)—of sufficient quality to be effective, while also ensuring that the use of these services does not expose the user to financial hardship (1). The definition incorporates the different dimensions of universal health assurance: health care, which includes ensuring access to a wide range of promotive, preventive, curative, and rehabilitative health services at different levels of care; health coverage that is inclusive of all sections of the population; and health protection, which promotes and protects health through its social determinants. These services should be delivered at an affordable cost, so that people do not suffer financial hardship in the pursuit of good health. If achieved, UHC enhances population health and productivity, contributing to national and global economic and social development. UHC requires strengthening of the health system in all countries, a well-planned financial structure, pooling of funds, and investment in quality primary health care (2). The main concepts of UHC include population coverage, range of health services provided, and out-of-pocket expenditure (3). The concept of UHC began in 19th century in Europe and has been stressed by both the World Health Organization (WHO) constitution and the Alma-Ata Declaration as an important tool to achieve "Health for All" (4). Achieving UHC is among the sub-goals of the Sustainable Development Goals (SDGs) set in 2015 and endorsed by the 193 member states of the United Nations, with target indicators focusing on ensuring essential service coverage for everyone and offer financial risk protection (5, 6). Many countries have explicitly adopted UHC as a national goal and embedded this pursuit within national health policy (7). While approaches to realizing UHC vary, the core definition—and the gap between current status and true UHC—is constant across countries. We therefore consider UHC as a lens for understanding health system strengthening to address cardiovascular disease (CVD).

## THE ROLE OF UHC IN CVD PREVENTION AND TREATMENT

There is increasing recognition that access to care without the assurance of high-quality services would make UHC an empty promise (8, 9). This is particularly true for CVD, which is the single biggest contributor to amenable mortality in low- and middle-income countries (LMICs). A modeling study estimated that as of 2016, 2.4 million of the 2.8 million CVD deaths amenable to health care in LMICs (83.7%) were due to poor quality among individuals accessing health care (10). Figure 17.1 maps this mortality burden by country.

The promise of UHC for conditions like CVD is that coherent health system action with coordination across the platforms of outreach, primary, secondary, and tertiary care can bring individuals unaware of CVD risk within the ambit of health services, reduce population risk, continuously manage existing conditions, and intervene effectively in acute cases (11, 12). Effective health system action with financial protection can save at least 60 million lives and increase average life expectancy by 3.7 years by 2030 in the LMICs (13) while decreasing catastrophic health

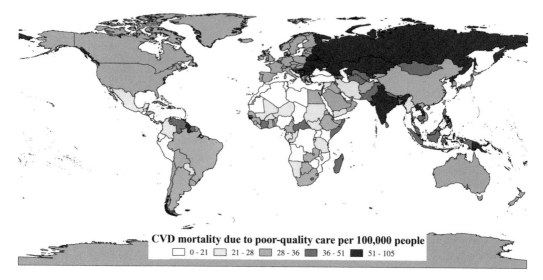

**Figure 17.1** CVD mortality due to poor-quality care, 2016.

## FOUNDATIONS

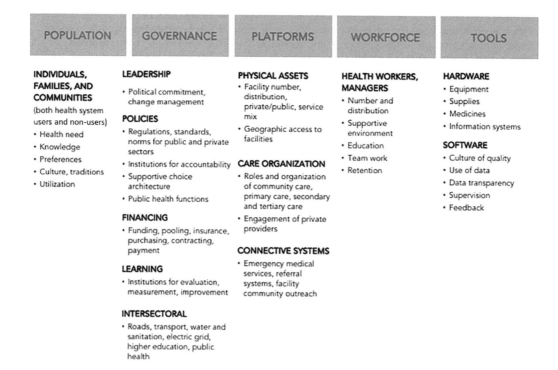

**Figure 17.2** Foundations for high-quality health systems.

expenditure (14). The national pursuit of UHC provides an opportunity to rethink health system design to optimize population health. Figure 17.2 defines the foundations required in a high-quality health system (9).

Defining these foundations enables a clear focus on the fundamentals of the health system that must be in place to effectively address CVDs. For example, platforms of care can include outreach services for screening and health promotion, primary care services for diagnosis and management of non-severe disease, and secondary care for severe disease and multimorbidity, and connective systems can ensure timely and continuous care for instances such as acute cardiac events or discharge following hospitalization. While the organization of services and delivery model will differ by context, the overarching elements of population engagement, active governance with continuous learning and evaluation, prepared workforce, and adequate tools are key foundations for a high-quality health system in all settings (9).

Health systems may be configured quite differently in different countries to build the foundations outlined earlier, including through a different mix of public and private providers and with a range of approaches to financial protection (15). Regardless of the precise configuration of care financing and delivery, higher out-of-pocket spending is closely linked with catastrophic and impoverishing health spending for families and is generally an inefficient way to finance health services, as it does not permit risk pooling (16). It is evident that, at present, achieving the goals of UHC for CVDs remains a major international challenge.

## HEALTH SYSTEM COMPETENCE FOR CVD SERVICES

For UHC to deliver widespread population health benefits, health systems must intervene effectively at multiple points along the continuum of CVD care covering both acute and chronic phases of the disease (17). This requires competent health systems, that is systems that can provide timely, integrated, and continuous care, with high-quality services delivered via multiple health system platforms, including outreach as well as primary and secondary care. Existing evidence suggests health systems are failing at multiple points along the care continuum. Table 17.1 reviews the evidence of current health system effectiveness—competent care, competent systems, user experience—across the continuum of CVD services. Competent care and systems are defined as "evidence-based, effective care: systematic assessment, correct diagnosis, appropriate treatment, counselling, and referral; capable systems: safety, prevention and detection, continuity and integration, timely action, and population health management" (9). Positive user experience includes "respect: dignity, privacy, non-discrimination, autonomy, confidentiality, and clear communication; user focus: choice of provider, short wait times, patient voice and values, affordability, and ease of use" (9).

The evidence cited in Table 17.1 indicates substantial gaps in system quality as well as inequities between and within countries. However, the current body of research is far from complete

## Table 17.1 Evidence for Health System Competence in CVD

| Level of Prevention/ Health Care | Health System Role | Evidence of Health System Quality | | |
| --- | --- | --- | --- | --- |
| | | Competent Care | Competent Systems | User Experience |
| Early prevention (avoiding risk factor development) | Outreach, continuous and effective primary care | Across 30 nationally representative surveys, one in three adults has ever been counseled on healthful eating and physical activity* | Across six Latin American and Caribbean countries, one-third to two-thirds of adults lack a regular primary care provider (18) | Primary care consultations in LMICs frequently last only 5 minutes (19) |
| Primary prevention (treating risk factors) | Continuous and effective primary care, integration of services from screening to diagnosis and management | In northern India, training of nurses in primary prevention led to shifting ~10% of participants into the low-risk category (20) | Across 30 surveys, approximately half of adults have ever had their blood pressure assessed, and under 5% report ever receiving a cholesterol test* | Patients report long wait times and overwhelmed providers in primary care settings, compounded by shortages in functioning diagnostic equipment and medications (21–23) |

*(Continued)*

## Table 17.1 (Continued)

| Level of Prevention/ Health Care | Health System Role | Evidence of Health System Quality | | |
|---|---|---|---|---|
| | | Competent Care | Competent Systems | User Experience |
| Secondary prevention (prevent progression of CVD) | Continuous and effective primary care, integration of services from screening to diagnosis and management | Only 1% of respondents across 30 surveys report regular use of aspirin or statins for CVD prevention* | Based on data on over 1.1 million individuals in 44 LMICs, one in four individuals with a known diagnosis of hypertension or elevated blood pressure at the time of assessment had never had their blood pressure checked; three-quarters of those diagnosed had received antihypertensive treatment, but only one in three treated had achieved blood pressure control (24) | Even in areas with many health facilities, patients report poor communication from providers and fragmented services (25); patients identified trust in providers and good communication as critical to medication adherence (26); households in India cite long wait times and poor quality of care as reasons for bypassing public clinics, particularly households with cardiovascular risk factors (27) |
| Acute care: myocardial infarction, angina, stroke | Timely access to emergency services, including functional transportation and 24/7 service availability, effective interventions, integration with community services and primary care for recovery and ongoing management | Across six European and central Asian countries, two in three providers misdiagnosed acute myocardial infarction in clinical vignettes Providers in India correctly diagnosed unstable angina less than 10% of the time (28, 29) | Providers in India prescribed unnecessary or harmful treatment in 55% of cases of unstable angina (29) | A study in Sri Lanka found that financial hardship following hospitalization for myocardial infarction (MI) was common and was associated with lower quality of life (30) |
| Tertiary prevention (slow or reverse disease, e.g., beta-blockers, ACE inhibitors, CABG) | Integration between specialist and primary care; continuity of management and monitoring following acute events | In hospitals in China, half of the ideal candidates for reperfusion therapy did not receive treatment, and over one in three eligible patients did not receive beta-blockers or ACE inhibitors (31) | Health system financing can incentivize unnecessary hospitalization for patients with heart failure (32) | Patients with heart failure in Uganda noted inadequate provider communication and lack of respect; their priorities of mitigating disability and economic impact of disease did not always align with health providers' focus on addressing symptoms (33) |
| Palliative care | Integration across platforms, extension to community health workers | - | Palliative care is poorly integrated within health systems in low-income countries and may be delivered primarily in vertical programs for human immunodeficiency virus (HIV) or cancer (33) | Cerebrovascular disease and non-ischemic heart disease account for 371–1280 million days of severe health-related suffering in LMICs (34) |

*Authors' analysis of STEPS and PRIMLAC data.

in describing health system quality for CVDs. The studies summarized in Table 17.1 range from quantitative analysis of over 1 million individuals to qualitative studies of small numbers of patients. Figures on testing for elevated blood pressure and cholesterol are far higher in Latin American and Caribbean countries than in sub-Saharan African and Southeast Asian countries, as is awareness of the disease among those with hypertension. Screening gaps are exacerbated in younger adults. In attention to patient experience, users experiencing challenges accessing ongoing care, receiving incomplete information about their conditions, and suffering unaddressed deficits in quality of care further undermine CVD services' continuity and effectiveness. These deficits across the continuum of care give rise to the burden of avertable mortality shown in Figure 17.1, as well as to substantial morbidity and economic harm.

## FINANCIAL PROTECTION

LMICs are witnessing a cyclical process of catastrophic out-of-pocket (OOP) expenditure on health, driving individuals into poverty and poverty worsening vulnerability to poor health and high medical expenditures (35, 36). CVD adds a burdensome financial risk in countries without UHC. Figure 17.3 shows the burden of elevated blood pressure (undiagnosed or uncontrolled hypertension) against current OOP expenditure as a percentage of health expenditure across 128 LMICs with available data, with each country scaled to size of its adult population. Much of the burden of hypertension is found in countries like India, where over half of health expenditure is borne by individuals. The weighted correlation of raised blood pressure and OOP is 43%, and Figure 17.3 makes it clear that just as there are countries with both a heavy burden of CVD risk and high reliance on individual expenditure for health services, there is substantial variability in the financing of health care at a similar prevalence of elevated blood pressure.

Major sources of financial burden include direct medical costs (consultation fees, drugs, laboratory, and hospital bed days), direct non-medical costs (transportation), and indirect costs (lost

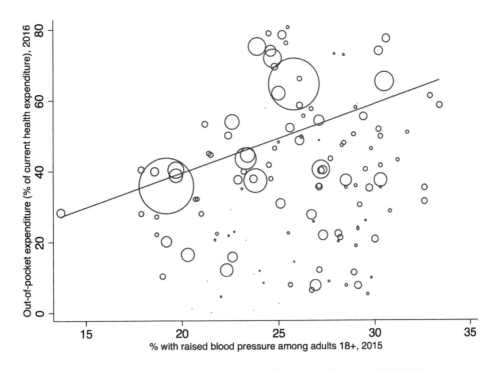

**Figure 17.3**  Burden of hypertension and out-of-pocket expenditure in 128 LMICs.

*Authors' analysis. Data*: Age-standardized prevalence of elevated blood pressure (SBP ≥ 140 or DBP ≥ 90) in adults 18 and over, World Health Organization Global Health Observatory. Out-of-pocket expenditure as percent of total health expenditure and size of adult population (proportion adults multiplied by total population size), World Bank World Development Indicators.

## PANEL 1: HOW CVDS ARE WORSENING INEQUITIES IN THE LMICS

- The total economic loss due to CVD was estimated at $3.7 trillion between 2011 and 2015, representing almost half of the non-communicable disease (NCD) economic burden and 2% of gross domestic product (GDP) across LMICs (37).

- India alone lost $237 billion over 10 years (2005–2015) due to loss of productivity and spending on health care resulting from CVDs (38).

- A systematic review of 83 studies found that the cost of treatment per episode for hypertension and CVD ranged between $500 and $1500 compared to $5000 for coronary heart disease (CHD) and stroke; the monthly cost of hypertension treatment was around $22, whereas stroke and CHD ranged between $300 and $1000 (39).

- The median out-of-pocket expenditures for CVD treatment ranged from 354 international dollars in Tanzania to 2917 international dollars in India. More than 50% of respondents in India, China, and Tanzania reported catastrophic health expenditures (40).

- A study in Ethiopia found that households in the lowest income quintile had 60 times greater odds of incurring catastrophic health expenditure for cardiovascular disease prevention and treatment services than the households in the top quintile (41).

income due to loss of productivity by patients and their attendants). In many countries, the poor fit between the configuration of primary care services for maternal and child health conditions and infectious diseases and the population need for high-quality CVD services results in extensive bypassing directly to secondary care, burdening hospitals and driving up individual costs of care (27). Chronic conditions such as CVD add higher financial costs due to the need for long-term treatment and care, loss of productivity due to long-term illness and disability, and increased costs when acute episodes occur. Households experienced catastrophic health expenditure and impoverishment, with long-term impacts to financial status due to the accumulation of debt and other risk-mitigating strategies. Panel 1 reviews evidence on the impact of CVDs on inequities within and between LMICs.

Initiatives such as the development of financial risk pooling, using generic medicines, and excluding poor patients from payments may be effective strategies for financial empowerment and reducing catastrophic and impoverishing health expenditures among cardiovascular patients. However, such interventions must be carefully planned and implemented. In India, the Rashtriya Swasthya Bima Yojana (RSBY), a publicly financed third-party payment scheme, aimed to cover more than 100 million poor. Evidence suggests that RSBY did not materially alter OOP spending either for outpatient or inpatient services. On the other hand, the likelihood of incurring any OOP spending (inpatient and outpatient) rose by 30% due to RSBY. The possible reasons for RSBY's failure include poor enrollment practices, maldistribution of roles and responsibilities, fixed package rates, and weak monitoring and supervision. There are multiple insurance schemes in LMICs, such as social health insurance, private health insurance, and community-based health insurance. Evidence from research studies to date suggests that insurance schemes appear to have improved access to hospital care but have been ineffective in preventing financial catastrophe and impoverishment (42–46). Implementing UHC could combat the shortcomings of multiple health insurance schemes.

## HEALTH SYSTEM QUALITY IN PREVENTING AND MANAGING CVD

Prevention, management, and treatment of CVD require high-quality services extending outwards into the community and integrated through primary and specialist services; similarly, a timely and competent response to acute events such as myocardial infarction and integrated, continuous response to challenges in prevention and management are required. We briefly review evidence for quality improvement organized by the framework in Figure 17.2 and the intended impact on acute versus chronic care (47, 48).

## Foundations

Relatively few studies directly address population, governance, and health platforms as foundations of the health system, reflecting the focus of quality improvement efforts on clinical services and visits (48). The largest subset of such studies considers the role of community health workers (CHWs) extending health services for CVD prevention and management into communities. Many of these studies reported that CHWs effectively screened cardiovascular risk factors in the population, suggested lifestyle modifications, and supported individuals to reduce blood pressure and glucose levels (49). While positive overall, the magnitude of impact can be small and variable across outcomes and studies (50, 51), and the effectiveness of these models in producing sustained gains remains to be established—one of the largest evaluations of a CHW-based intervention to reduce CVD risk found no appreciable impact on blood pressure over the two years of the trial (52). CHW-based extensions of health services will need to be integrated with the local health system and adapted to the context where the evidence supports their effectiveness: they may be inappropriate for settings such as urban contexts or highly privatized health care environments (53). Interventions on population health knowledge that address acute care include an integrated education program for community members and physicians on symptoms and response to acute coronary syndromes in Kerala, India, which found a decrease in time from symptoms to the health facility after the intervention (54). Observational evidence suggests that health policy reforms to ensure treatment for acute myocardial infarction (MI) decreased in-hospital mortality (55). In contrast, national or community health insurance programs have been associated with increased treatment and control of elevated blood pressure and glucose (56–58). A regional hub-and-spoke model linking hospitals performing percutaneous coronary intervention to smaller hospitals and clinics in India found no difference in timely and evidence-based reperfusion care or in-hospital mortality, but did note increased use of angiography and percutaneous coronary intervention, as well as reduced 1-year mortality post-intervention (59).

The bulk of evidence addressing quality improvement focuses on the health workforce and the tools available, with a larger body of evidence available for prevention and ongoing management than acute intervention. A substantial focus within efforts to equip the health workforce to provide services for chronic CVD is task-shifting. The use of care coordinators and non-physician health workers has been shown to reduce CVD risk scores (60) and decrease blood pressure in relatively short-term studies (61), although there is not adequate evidence to support task-sharing for lowering cholesterol (62). Failures in task shifting, such as the use of lay health workers in primary care clinics in rural South Africa (22), underscore the need for a competent health system supporting the workforce tasked with CVD care, regardless of the type of health worker.

The third area of focus in quality improvement has been the tools health workers use for CVD, particularly for detection and ongoing management. Combination pills have been associated with improved medication adherence and small improvements in disease severity (47). In addition to the relatively short assessment periods of many existing studies, a key challenge for implementing these interventions is packaging them into sustainable and scalable programs that retain efficacy, requiring integrating them within health systems not designed for CVD care. A recent study of an integrated package of interventions in 40 community health centers in India found no benefit over an enhanced version of usual care (63). Intervening on health system foundations offers the largest scope for improved health, and promising approaches have been identified, particularly for chronic care of CVD through intensified care and extension of screening services using CHWs, with less evidence to date for interventions on acute care.

## Processes

Quality improvement efforts often focus on the processes of care delivery. For example, point-of-care mobile technology interventions such as decision-support systems have demonstrated efficacy in disease management (60, 64–66), while Short Message Service reminders and mobile outreach have been successfully implemented on their own or as part of multicomponent interventions. Attempts to improve chronic CVD care have included addressing provider communication skills and care competence, with evidence of improved health behaviors and adherence (67, 68), as well as education to increase guideline implementation, with mixed results. For acute care, multiple large, randomized studies have demonstrated an impact of provider education and reminders on care competence during hospitalizations, but no effect on patient mortality or severe events (48). A challenge with these interventions to date is that the focus on the point of care and in-service interventions provides limited scope to address the underlying question of provider competence for CVD care. The current deficits in competence are likely to require broad-scale approaches such as consideration of pre-service education models to increase quality in a sustainable manner.

Considering three important dimensions is necessary while prioritizing UHC interventions, and those are the importance of money, consideration of the worse-off people, and financial risk protection. The platforms required to implement these interventions include population-based health interventions, community services, health centers, first-level hospitals, referrals, and specialized hospitals (69).

## RECOMMENDATIONS AND THE WAY FORWARD

To move from individual quality improvement efforts to high-quality health systems capable of preventing, detecting, and managing CVD requires a broad approach that tackles the foundations of the health system (9). Health system leaders need to make provision of high-quality care, with CVD services—urgently needed and potentially highly effective in reducing morbidity and mortality—as a key priority. Financing strategies and health service design must act in concert to ensure access to quality CVD services as a core function of the health system; while narrowly focused incentives may drive performance and reporting on health services, these strategies are best considered after appropriate support for the health workforce in terms of management and financing is already in place.

Prior analyses such as the Disease Control Priority Project have classified the most essential interventions for CVD by health system platform (population-based, community-based, health centers, hospitals, and referral hospitals), with the preponderance of interventions identified for CVD within the three tiers of the health system itself (70). These efforts provide guidance on potential interventions that yield high value for cost, prioritize those worst off, and enhance financial risk protection, enabling national policymakers to review the services currently covered and consider the package of service provision and financing that may best enhance population health. The successful implementation of these interventions depends upon the underlying quality of the health system; here we identify priorities for addressing the foundations for high-quality health systems.

Health service delivery must be redesigned to ensure services can be delivered with quality where the population will seek them. The innovative HWC initiative in India (Panel 2) is one approach to strengthen the role of primary care in managing CVD within the health system. Research in CVD service delivery has already identified innovative elements of the delivery redesign, such as the provision of screening and detection services using CHW and task shifting to provide routine condition management from non-physicians. Governance and redesign

---

### PANEL 2: INNOVATIONS IN SERVICE DELIVERY MODELS FOR CVD

A recent innovation with the potential to incorporate many of these advances is the health and wellness centers (HWCs) proposed in India. The HWC initiative aimed to provide universal primary health care, focusing on the principles of equity, quality, universality, and no financial hardship. The plan unveiled in 2017 was to establish 150,000 HWCs as the first point of contact for the community. Currently, the way of functioning is such that the HWCs are expected to provide primary and secondary services, reorienting service delivery to provide continuous and patient-centered care at the local level. Because India's public primary care system has historically focused on maternal and child health, developing a new tier of services may offer the opportunity to integrate CVD services, particularly screening and detection, at the primary level. If successful, this would enable a shift in care utilization for CVD services back to the primary level, reducing the system strain and individual cost incurred from the overuse of secondary care services. Progress on achieving these goals has been uneven across states in India, and questions on the capacity of HWCs to deliver on the promise of competent, first-contact care that meets population expectations remain unanswered.

must prioritize the population's expectations for care in order to deliver improved health at scale and ensure or rebuild trust in health systems. For acute care services, strengthened connections between health system levels and platforms are critical to ensure timely care in emergencies and direct integration to ongoing services thereafter. System-level interventions for strengthening acute care remain a gap in the evidence base for CVD services.

Revising and updating pre-service education will be required to ensure that the cadres tasked with delivering care, from CHWs to specialists, are equipped with the appropriate skills to do so. Team-based care and patient-centered practice are two additional elements that need to be incorporated in clinical education. Technological support for care delivery is not a substitute for underlying provider competence, but can enhance service delivery once such competence is in place.

Finally, there is latent capacity in the population to drive health system improvement, but this requires educating the community on what high-quality health systems and good-quality CVD care look like. People's input should guide efforts to govern for quality, redesign service delivery, and strengthen pre-service education.

For this to happen, tools must be developed and deployed to assess population preferences for care, and health system policymakers must enhance the capacity of the system as a learning entity, one that can monitor and learn from progress and failures. The scope for innovation must be expanded to match the scale of the challenge of CVD, and the timeframe to impact lengthened to enable fair assessment of the sustained impacts of interventions.

## REFERENCES

1. WHO. *Health Systems: Universal Health Coverage*. Available from: www.who.int/healthsystems/universal_health_coverage/en/.
2. WHO. *Universal Health Coverage (UHC)*; 2019 [cited 2021 February 8]. Available from: www.who.int/news-room/fact-sheets/detail/universal-health-coverage-(uhc).
3. Mathur M, Williams D, Reddy K, Watt R. *Universal health coverage: a unique policy opportunity for oral health*. SAGE Publications, Los Angeles, CA; 2015.
4. *The Impact of Universal Coverage Schemes in the Developing World: A Review of the Existing Evidence: World Bank* [cited 2021 February 9]. Available from: https://openknowledge.worldbank.org/handle/10986/13302.
5. Giedion U, Andrés Alfonso E, Díaz Y. The impact of universal coverage schemes in the developing world: a review of the existing evidence. UNICO Studies Series No. 25. World Bank, Washington, DC. pp. 1–139; 2013.
6. Gutierrez H, Shewade A, Dai M, Mendoza-Arana P, Gómez-Dantés O, Jain N, et al. Health care coverage decision making in low-and middle-income countries: experiences from 25 coverage schemes. *Population Health Management*. 2015;18(4):265–271.
7. Planning Commission. High-level expert group report on universal health coverage for India. Government of India. pp. 1–154; 2011.
8. Sobel HL, Huntington D, Temmerman M. Quality at the centre of universal health coverage. *Health Policy Plan*. 2016;31(4):547–549.
9. Kruk M, Gage A, Arsenault C, Jordan K, Leslie H, Roder-DeWan S, et al. High-quality health systems—time for a revolution: Report of The Lancet global health commission on high-quality health systems in the SDG era. *Lancet Global Health*. 2018;6:e1196-e252.
10. Kruk ME, Gage AD, Joseph NT, Danaei G, García-Saisó S, Salomon JA. Mortality due to low-quality health systems in the universal health coverage era: a systematic analysis of amenable deaths in 137 countries. *The Lancet*. 2018;392(10160):2203–2212.
11. Watkins DA, Nugent RA. Setting priorities to address cardiovascular diseases through universal health coverage in low- and middle-income countries. *Heart Asia*. 2017;9(1):54–58.
12. Aminde LN, Takah NF, Zapata-Diomedi B, Veerman JL. Primary and secondary prevention interventions for cardiovascular disease in low-income and middle-income countries: a systematic review of economic evaluations. *Cost Effectiveness and Resource Allocation*. 2018;16(1):22.
13. World Health Organization. Primary health care on the road to Universal Health Coverage 2019 monitoring report: conference edition. WHO Report; 2019. Available from: https://apps.who.int/iris/bitstream/handle/10665/344057/9789240004276-eng.pdf?sequence=2.

14. Huffman MD, Rao KD, Pichon-Riviere A, Zhao D, Harikrishnan S, Ramaiya K, et al. A cross-sectional study of the microeconomic impact of cardiovascular disease hospitalization in four low- and middle-income countries. PLoS ONE. 2011;6(6).

15. Mackintosh M, Channon A, Karan A, Selvaraj S, Cavagnero E, Zhao H. What is the private sector? Understanding private provision in the health systems of low-income and middle-income countries. Lancet. 2016;388(10044):596–605.

16. Brearley L, Marten R, O'Connell T. *Universal health coverage: a commitment to closing the gap.* London: Rockefeller Foundation, Save the Children, UNICEF, World Health Organization, 2013.

17. Chow CK, Gupta R. Blood pressure control: a challenge to global health systems. *The Lancet.* 2019;394(10199):613–615.

18. Macinko J, Guanais FC, Mullachery P, Jimenez G. Gaps in primary care and health system performance in six latin American and Caribbean countries. *Health Affairs (Project Hope).* 2016;35(8):1513–1521.

19. Irving G, Neves AL, Dambha-Miller H, Oishi A, Tagashira H, Verho A, et al. International variations in primary care physician consultation time: a systematic review of 67 countries. *BMJ Open.* 2017;7(10).

20. Thakur J, Vijayvergiya R, Ghai S. Task shifting of cardiovascular risk assessment and communication by nurses for primary and secondary prevention of cardiovascular diseases in a tertiary health care setting of Northern India. *BMC Health Services Research.* 2020;20(1):10.

21. Legido-Quigley H, Naheed A, de Silva HA, Jehan I, Haldane V, Cobb B, et al. Patients' experiences on accessing health care services for management of hypertension in rural Bangladesh, Pakistan and Sri Lanka: a qualitative study. *PLoS ONE.* 2019;14(1):e0211100.

22. Goudge J, Chirwa T, Eldridge S, Gómez-Olivé FXF, Kabudula C, Limbani F, et al. Can lay health workers support the management of hypertension? Findings of a cluster randomised trial in South Africa. *BMJ Global Health.* 2018;3(1).

23. Moucheraud C. Service readiness for noncommunicable diseases was low in five countries in 2013–15. *Health Affairs.* 2018;37(8):1321–1330.

24. Geldsetzer P, Manne-Goehler J, Marcus M-E, Ebert C, Zhumadilov Z, Wesseh CS, et al. The state of hypertension care in 44 low-income and middle-income countries: a cross-sectional study of nationally representative individual-level data from 1·1 million adults. *The Lancet.* 2019;394(10199):652–662.

25. Bhojani U, Mishra A, Amruthavalli S, Devadasan N, Kolsteren P, De Henauw S, et al. Constraints faced by urban poor in managing diabetes care: patients' perspectives from South India. *Global Health Action.* 2013;6:22258.

26. Legido-Quigley H, Camacho Lopez PA, Balabanova D, Perel P, Lopez-Jaramillo P, Nieuwlaat R, et al. Patients' knowledge, attitudes, behaviour and health care experiences on the prevention, detection, management and control of hypertension in Colombia: a qualitative study. *PLoS ONE.* 2015;10(4):e0122112.

27. Kujawski SA, Leslie HH, Prabhakaran D, Singh K, Kruk ME. Reasons for low utilisation of public facilities among households with hypertension: analysis of a population-based survey in India. *BMJ Global Health.* 2018;3(6):e001002.

28. Peabody JW, DeMaria L, Smith O, Hoth A, Dragoti E, Luck J. Large-scale evaluation of quality of care in 6 countries of Eastern Europe and Central Asia using clinical performance and value vignettes. *Global Health, Science and Practice.* 2017;5(3):412–429.

29. Das J, Holla A, Das V, Mohanan M, Tabak D, Chan B. In urban and rural India, a standardized patient study showed low levels of provider training and huge quality gaps. *Health Affairs (Project Hope).* 2012;31(12):2774–2784.

30. Mahesh PKB, Gunathunga MW, Jayasinghe S, Arnold SM, Mallawarachchi DSV, Perera SK, et al. Financial burden of survivors of medically-managed myocardial infarction and its association with selected social determinants and quality of life in a lower middle income country. *BMC Cardiovascular Disorders.* 2017;17(1):251.

31. Li J, Li X, Wang Q, Hu S, Wang Y, Masoudi FA, et al. ST-segment elevation myocardial infarction in China from 2001 to 2011 (the China PEACE-Retrospective Acute Myocardial Infarction Study): a retrospective analysis of hospital data. *Lancet.* 2015;385(9966):441–451.

32. Ahmedov M, Green J, Azimov R, Avezova G, Inakov S, Mamatkulov B. Addressing the challenges of improving primary care quality in Uzbekistan: a qualitative study of chronic heart failure management. *Health Policy Plan.* 2013;28(5):458–466.

33. Namukwaya E, Grant L, Downing J, Leng M, Murray SA. Improving care for people with heart failure in Uganda: serial in-depth interviews with patients' and their health care professionals. *BMC Research Notes*. 2017;10(1):184.

34. Knaul FM, Farmer PE, Krakauer EL, De Lima L, Bhadelia A, Jiang Kwete X, et al. Alleviating the access abyss in palliative care and pain relief-an imperative of universal health coverage: the Lancet commission report. *Lancet*. 2018;391(10128):1391–1454.

35. WHO. *Health financing: financial protection*. Available from: www.who.int/health_financing/topics/financial-protection/en/.

36. Saksena P, Hsu J, Evans DB. Financial risk protection and universal health coverage: evidence and measurement challenges. *PLoS Medicine*. 2014;11(9).

37. Bloom DE, Chisholm D, Jané-Llopis E, Prettner K, Stein A, Feigl A. *From burden to "best buys": Reducing the economic impact of non-communicable diseases*. World Health Org, Geneva, Switzerland; 2011.

38. Mendis S, Puska P, Norrving B, Organization WH. *Global atlas on cardiovascular disease prevention and control*. World Health Organization, Geneva; 2011.

39. Gheorghe A, Griffiths U, Murphy A, Legido-Quigley H, Lamptey P, Perel P. The economic burden of cardiovascular disease and hypertension in low-and middle-income countries: a systematic review. *BMC Public Health*. 2018;18(1):1–11.

40. Huffman MD, Rao KD, Pichon-Riviere A, Zhao D, Harikrishnan S, Ramaiya K, et al. A cross-sectional study of the microeconomic impact of cardiovascular disease hospitalization in four low-and middle-income countries. *PLoS ONE*. 2011;6(6):e20821.

41. Tolla MT, Norheim OF, Verguet S, Bekele A, Amenu K, Abdisa SG, et al. Out-of-pocket expenditures for prevention and treatment of cardiovascular disease in general and specialised cardiac hospitals in Addis Ababa, Ethiopia: a cross-sectional cohort study. *BMJ Global Health*. 2017;2(2):e000280.

42. Rezapour A, Arabloo J, Movahed MS, Faradonbeh SB, Alipour S, Alipour V. Catastrophic health expenditure and impoverishment among households with cardiovascular patients in Tehran, 2017. *Shiraz E-Medical Journal*. 2019;21(1):1–7. https://brieflands.com/articles/semj-89088.pdf

43. Karan A, Yip W, Mahal A. Extending health insurance to the poor in India: an impact evaluation of Rashtriya Swasthya Bima Yojana on out of pocket spending for healthcare. *Social Science & Medicine*. 2017;181:83–92.

44. Khetrapal S, Acharya A. Expanding healthcare coverage: an experience from Rashtriya Swasthya Bima Yojna. *The Indian Journal of Medical Research*. 2019;149(3):369.

45. van Hees SG, O'Fallon T, Hofker M, Dekker M, Polack S, Banks LM, et al. Leaving no one behind? Social inclusion of health insurance in low-and middle-income countries: a systematic review. *International Journal for Equity in Health*. 2019;18(1):134.

46. Devadasan N, Seshadri T, Trivedi M, Criel B. Promoting universal financial protection: evidence from the Rashtriya Swasthya Bima Yojana (RSBY) in Gujarat, India. *Health Research Policy and Systems*. 2013;11(1):29.

47. Lee ES, Vedanthan R, Jeemon P, Kamano JH, Kudesia P, Rajan V, et al. Quality improvement for cardiovascular disease care in low- and middle-income countries: a systematic review. *PLoS ONE*. 2016;11(6):e0157036.

48. Lee ES, Vedanthan R, Jeemon P, Kamano JH, Kudesia P, Rajan V, et al. Quality improvement in cardiovascular disease care. In: Prabhakaran D, Anand S, Gaziano TA, Mbanya J-C, Wu Y, Nugent R, editors. *Cardiovascular, respiratory, and related disorders*. 3rd ed. Washington, DC: The International Bank for Reconstruction and Development/The World Bank; 2017.

49. Khetan AK, Purushothaman R, Chami T, Hejjaji V, Mohan SKM, Josephson RA, et al. The effectiveness of community health workers for CVD prevention in LMIC. *Global Heart*. 2017;12(3):233–243. e6.

50. Poggio R, Melendi SE, Beratarrechea A, Gibbons L, Mills KT, Chen C-S, et al. Cluster randomized trial for hypertension control: effect on lifestyles and body weight. *American Journal of Preventive Medicine*. 2019;57(4):438–446.

51. Neupane D, McLachlan CS, Mishra SR, Olsen MH, Perry HB, Karki A, et al. Effectiveness of a lifestyle intervention led by female community health volunteers versus usual care in blood pressure reduction (COBIN): an open-label, cluster-randomised trial. *The Lancet Global Health*. 2018;6(1):e66–e73.

52. Peiris D, Praveen D, Mogulluru K, Ameer MA, Raghu A, Li Q, et al. SMARThealth India: a stepped-wedge, cluster randomised controlled trial of a community health worker

managed mobile health intervention for people assessed at high cardiovascular disease risk in rural India. *PLoS ONE.* 2019;14(3):e0213708.

53. Anand S, Bradshaw C, Prabhakaran D. Prevention and management of CVD in LMICs: why do ethnicity, culture, and context matter? *BMC Medicine.* 2020;18(1):7.

54. Prabhakaran D, Jeemon P, Mohanan PP, Govindan U, Geevar Z, Chaturvedi V, et al. Management of acute coronary syndromes in secondary care settings in Kerala: impact of a quality improvement programme. *The National Medical Journal of India.* 2008;21(3):107–111.

55. Nazzal NC, Campos TP, Corbalán HR, Lanas ZF, Bartolucci JJ, Sanhueza CP, et al. [The impact of Chilean health reform in the management and mortality of ST elevation myocardial infarction (STEMI) in Chilean hospitals]. *Revista médica de Chile.* 2008;136(10):1231–1239.

56. Sosa-Rubí SG, Galárraga O, López-Ridaura R. Diabetes treatment and control: the effect of public health insurance for the poor in Mexico. *Bulletin of the World Health Organization.* 2009;87(7):512–519.

57. Hendriks ME, Wit FWNM, Akande TM, Kramer B, Osagbemi GK, Tanović Z, et al. Effect of health insurance and facility quality improvement on blood pressure in adults with hypertension in Nigeria: a population-based study. *JAMA Internal Medicine.* 2014;174(4):555–563.

58. Bleich SN, Cutler DM, Adams AS, Lozano R, Murray CJ. Impact of insurance and supply of health professionals on coverage of treatment for hypertension in Mexico: population based study. *BMJ (Clinical Research ed).* 2007;335(7625):875.

59. Alexander T, Mullasari AS, Joseph G, Kannan K, Veerasekar G, Victor SM, et al. A System of care for patients with ST-segment elevation myocardial infarction in India: The Tamil Nadu—ST-segment elevation myocardial infarction program. *JAMA Cardiol.* 2017;2(5):498–505.

60. Schwalm J-D, McCready T, Lopez-Jaramillo P, Yusoff K, Attaran A, Lamelas P, et al. A community-based comprehensive intervention to reduce cardiovascular risk in hypertension (HOPE 4): a cluster-randomised controlled trial. *The Lancet.* 2019;394(10205):1231–1242. https://www.sciencedirect.com/science/article/abs/pii/S014067361931949X

61. Anand TN, Joseph LM, Geetha AV, Prabhakaran D, Jeemon P. Task sharing with non-physician health-care workers for management of blood pressure in low-income and middle-income countries: a systematic review and meta-analysis. *The Lancet Global Health.* 2019;7(6):e761–e771.

62. Anand TN, Joseph LM, Geetha AV, Chowdhury J, Prabhakaran D, Jeemon P. Task-sharing interventions for cardiovascular risk reduction and lipid outcomes in low- and middle-income countries: a systematic review and meta-analysis. *Journal of Clinical Lipidology.* 2018;12(3):626–642.

63. Dorairaj P, Dilip J, David P-M, Ambuj R, Singh K, Vamadevan SA, et al. Effectiveness of an mHealth-based electronic decision support system for integrated management of chronic conditions in primary care. *Circulation.* 2019;139(3):380–391.

64. Anchala R, Kaptoge S, Pant H, Di Angelantonio E, Franco OH, Prabhakaran D. Evaluation of effectiveness and cost-effectiveness of a clinical decision support system in managing hypertension in resource constrained primary health care settings: results from a cluster randomized trial. *Journal of the American Heart Association.* 2015;4(1):e001213.

65. Ali MK, Singh K, Kondal D, Devarajan R, Patel SA, Shivashankar R, et al. Effectiveness of a multi-component quality improvement strategy to improve diabetes care goals: the CARRS randomized controlled trial. *Annals of Internal Medicine.* 2016;165(6):399–408.

66. Chan BTB, Rauscher C, Issina AM, Kozhageldiyeva LH, Kuzembaeva DD, Davis CL, et al. A programme to improve quality of care for patients with chronic diseases, Kazakhstan. *Bulletin of the World Health Organization.* 2020;98(3):161–169.

67. Tavakoly Sany SB, Behzhad F, Ferns G, Peyman N. Communication skills training for physicians improves health literacy and medical outcomes among patients with hypertension: a randomized controlled trial. *BMC Health Services Research.* 2020;20(1):60.

68. Aung MN, Yuasa M, Moolphate S, Lorga T, Yokokawa H, Fukuda H, et al. Effectiveness of a new multi-component smoking cessation service package for patients with hypertension and diabetes in northern Thailand: a randomized controlled trial (ESCAPE study). *Substance Abuse Treatment, Prevention, and Policy.* 2019;14(1):10.

69. Watkins DA, Jamison DT, Mills A, Atun R, Danforth K, Glassman A, et al. Universal health coverage and essential packages of care. In: Jamison DT, Gelband H, Horton S, et al., editors. *Disease Control Priorities: Improving Health and Reducing Poverty*. 3rd ed. Washington, DC: The International Bank for Reconstruction and Development/The World Bank; 2017. Chapter 3. Available from: https://www.ncbi.nlm.nih.gov/books/NBK525285/.

70. Watkins DA, Jamison DT, Mills A, Atun R, Danforth K, Glassman A, et al. Universal health coverage and essential packages of care. In: Jamison DT, Gelband H, Horton S, Jha P, Laxminarayan R, Mock CN, et al., editors. *Disease control priorities: improving health and reducing poverty*. Volume 9. 3rd ed. Washington, DC: The World Bank; 2017.

# 18 Monitoring and Evaluation of Cardiovascular Disease Prevention Programs

*Rajmohan Panda and Abdul Ghaffar*

## CONTENTS

## BACKGROUND

The health system infrastructure in low- and middle-income countries (LMICs) is insufficient to support chronic disease prevention, treatment, and management (1). The scale-up of resources and initiatives for better health is unprecedented both in terms of the potential resources available and in terms of the number of initiatives involved. There is growing recognition that harmonized monitoring, evaluation, and review are required to demonstrate results, secure future funding, and enhance the evidence base for interventions. Strategic planning and program implementation should be based on strong monitoring, evaluation and review of progress and performance as the basis for information, results, and accountability (2).

Monitoring and evaluation (M&E) represent two elements of the enterprise of assessing the merit or worth of an organization or program, encompassing assessment of both performance and impact for a broad range of different audiences and purposes. The World Bank (2007) defines monitoring as "a continuing function that aims primarily to provide an ongoing intervention with early indications of progress, or lack thereof, in the achievement of results"; it defines evaluation as "the systematic and objective assessment of an on-going or completed project, program, or policy, and its design, implementation and results" (3).

The following aspects are important to consider when developing an M&E system for a cardiovascular disease (CVD) program in LMICs:

I. Principles of measurements

II. Setting up a goal and objectives

III. Designing a conceptual framework

IV. Developing and using a logic model

V. Selecting measurable program indicators

VI. Measurements for impact

### Principles of Measurements in M&E

The measurement system consists of several elements or blocks. It involves assigning numbers to characteristics of objects or events in such a way that the numbers reflect reality (4). M&E of a

DOI: 10.1201/b23266-27

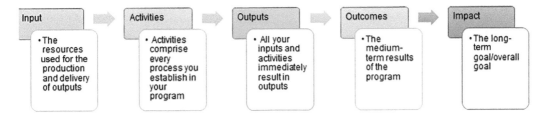

**Figure 18.1** Principles of measures in an M&E program.

program requires identification of indicators that measure inputs, process, outputs, and outcomes (5).

Measurement serves a number of critical roles in the effort to address any health problem and decision making. It helps to assess the processes, outcomes, and impact of the implemented interventions (Figure 18.1). Ultimately, measurement strategies have the potential to lead to changes in health outcomes by changing the decisions and behavior of policy makers, providers, and individuals. A number of underlying principles drive measurement as a fundamental part of efforts to decrease CVD (1):

■ First, in order to be effective, measurement needs to be relevant to the context in which it is implemented. Context includes local elements of economics, financing, existing policies, existing capacity, population demographics, and social and cultural factors.

■ Second, measurement is most effective when it is transparent and when there are feedback mechanisms to ensure that the resulting data are widely available and widely used.

■ Third, measurement is needed at all levels, from individuals to providers to policy makers.

■ According to the fourth principle, measurement needs to focus on the intermediate outcome of behavior change, for it is changes in the behavior of those at risk, of care providers, and of policy makers that will lead to lessening of the CVD burden.

### Setting Up a Goal and Objectives for the Program

A goal is a broad statement about a long-term expectation of who gets affected and what will change as a desired result of the program (6). Each goal has a set of related, more specific objectives that, if met, will collectively permit program staff to reach the stated goal (see Table 18.1). While designing a goal, but especially objectives, an organization should always keep the SMART criteria in mind. SMART equates to Specific (includes the "who", "what", and "where"), Measurable ("how much" change is expected), Achievable, Relevant (relates directly to program goals), and Time bound ("when" the objective will be achieved) (7). To set a desirable goal, one may follow the five principles called clarity, challenge, complexity, commitment, and feedback. The extent to which these principles exist within the goal is directly related to the achievement of the goal.

### Designing a Conceptual Framework

Frameworks are key elements of M&E plans that depict the components of a project and the sequence of steps needed to achieve the desired outcomes. They help increase understanding of the program's goals and objectives, define the relationships between factors key to implementation, and delineate the internal and external elements that could affect its success or failure. They

### Table 18.1 Sample CVD Prevention Program Goals Based on a Prioritized Need

| | |
|---|---|
| Long-term goal | Decrease in prevalence of CVDs |
| Medium-term goal | Ten percent reduction in premature CVD mortality in populations covered under the CVD prevention program |
| Short-term goal | Improved CVD risk factor management (hypertension control, cholesterol management, diabetes management, appropriate referrals) |

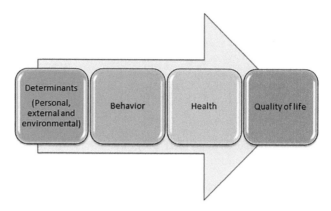

**Figure 18.2**  A conceptual framework showing relationships among behavior, health problems, quality of life, and determinants.

are crucial for understanding and analyzing how a program is supposed to work. There is no one perfect framework, and no single framework is appropriate for all situations because of the design and context of each program/project (8).

The conceptual framework is an integrated way of examining a problem under consideration for developing a health program; it is the explanation of how the health problem would be explored (9). It describes the relationship between the main aspects of the program, through which a logical structure is arranged, which aids to provide a visual display of how ideas in a program relate to one another (10).

In Figure 18.2, the conceptual framework establishes the hypothesis that causal relationships exist between the individual and social environmental factors that predispose, facilitate, and reinforce hypertension-related behaviors (exercise, nutrition, medication therapy adherence). In turn, such behaviors have a causal relationship with the development and progression of cardiovascular risk factors and, consequently, with how severe hypertension is clinically expressed.

### Developing and Using a Logic Model

Logic models are tools for planning, describing, managing, communicating, and evaluating a program or intervention. They graphically represent the relationships between a program's activities and its intended effects, state the assumptions that underlie expectations that a program will work, and frame the context in which the program operates. Logic models are not static documents. In fact, they should be revised periodically to reflect new evidence; lessons learned; and changes in context, resources, activities, or expectations (11).

A logic model can also be visually represented in a variety of ways, including as a flow chart, a map, or a table. The basic components of a good logic model are (11):

- Displayed on one page.

- Visually engaging.

- Audience specific.

- Appropriate in its level of detail.

- Useful in clarifying program activities and expected outcomes.

- Easy to relate to.

- Reflective of the context in which the program operates.

A basic logic model (Figure 18.3) typically has two "sides"—process and outcome. The process section describes the program's inputs (resources), activities, and outputs (direct products). The outcome section describes the intended effects of the program, which can be short term, intermediate, and/or long term. Assumptions under which the program or intervention operates and the contextual factors can also be included in a logic model. They are often noted in a box below or on the left side of the logic model diagram. Figure 18.3 illustrates the components of a logic model.

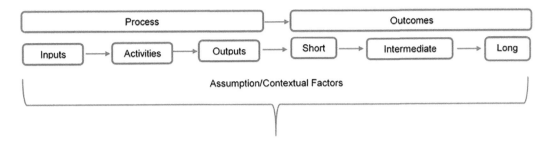

**Figure 18.3** Layout of a general logic model.

Assumptions are the beliefs we have about the program or intervention and the resources involved. Assumptions include the way we think the program will work—the "theory" we have used to develop the program or intervention. Assumptions are based on research, best practices, past experience, and common sense. The decisions we make about implementing a program or intervention are often based on our assumptions (11).

Contextual factors describe the environment in which the program exists and external factors that interact with and influence the program or intervention. These factors may influence implementation, participation, and the achievement of outcomes. Contextual factors are the conditions over which we have little or no control that affect success (11).

For example, controlling high blood pressure in an individual will reduce their risk for heart disease and stroke; when we apply this theory to a population, there are a number of confounding factors (11):

- Risk factors for high blood pressure such as obesity and diabetes are increasing in prevalence. This is likely to cause an increase in the prevalence of high blood pressure and the number of heart disease or stroke patients.

- We assume in this model that once control of high blood pressure has been achieved, it will be maintained. This might not be the case.

- We assume that once the chronic care model (CCM) is implemented and clinic-based changes occur, the changes are maintained.

This is depicted in the following logic framework (Figure 18.4).

The main activities in the framework focus on capacity building for health care providers, community screening and referral of chronic patients to clinics, and referral of patients back to frontline health workers for monitoring in the community. The outputs required to attain the desired outcomes are trained health care providers, counseled community members, screened community members, and referred patients. The outcome measures for these interventions would be improved quality of CCM management, increased access to high blood pressure screening, increased knowledge about risk factors for NCDs, and access to treatment and preventions strategies in the communities. The intermediate expected outcomes as a result of the impact of the interventions will likely be a decrease in risk behavior and an increase in access to non-communicable disease (NCD) treatment. Decreased NCD risk factors, increased NCD incidences because of access to treatment, and decreased NCD morbidity and mortality will be the impact of the interventions.

## THEORIES OF CHANGE

A theory of change is used to provide a rationale for the expected links between program resources, activities, and outcomes. They describe the set of assumptions that explain both the steps that lead to long-term objectives and the connections between program activities and outcomes that occur at each step of the way (11).

Health promotion and prevention activities are based on numerous theories of change—a reasonable explanation of why and how a certain set of activities leads to certain outcomes. Theories of change allow us to hypothesize that a program's intermediate and long-term outcomes are a result of short-term outcomes, which are a result of the activities implemented.

For example, implementing the CCM in a health care system would include use of electronic medical records that remind physicians of services needed to increase the number of patients who

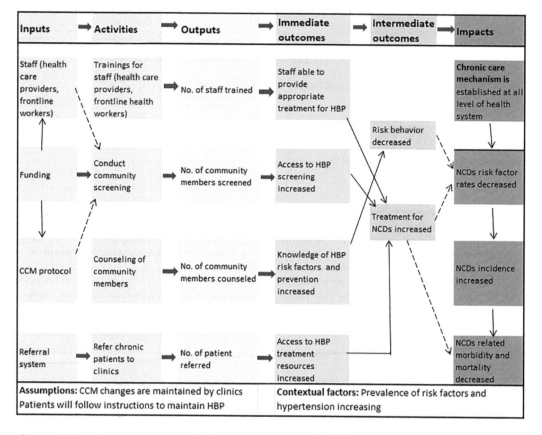

**Figure 18.4** A logic framework for the chronic care model (CCM).

have their high blood pressure under control. This, in turn, leads to changes in patient behavior that result in better management of their high blood pressure (11).

### Selecting Measurable Program Indicators

Indicators are the foundation of a monitoring system (12). Once the conceptual framework (log frame) is finalized, the next step in completing the M&E framework is selecting indicators. Indicators provide critical information on performance, achievement, and accountability, which are the cornerstone of effective M&E (13).

The key challenge with indicators is to ensure their quality and integrity. Indicators should generate data that are needed and useful. They should be technically sound. They should be easy to understand, practical, and feasible. In addition, they should have a proven record of measuring performance (13).

The question of which indicators to use and how to prioritize them must be agreed upon by the relevant stakeholders in the international community. A number of key categories of metrics are crucial to measuring CVD and its breadth of determinants and would need to be considered. These include:

- Demographics; risk and risk mitigation, including behaviors (e.g., smoking rates, physical activity, diet and nutrition).

- Biomedical measures (e.g., weight and height, blood pressure, cholesterol).

- Disease outcomes (e.g., cardiovascular events).

- Cause-specific mortality.

- Health provider and quality improvement measures.

- Health systems performance.

- Economic measures.

- Intersectoral policy measures (e.g., cigarette costs and sales data, agricultural trends, urbanization).

- Measures of global action.

Some of these measures need to be disease specific, while others need to be harmonized and coordinated with measurement strategies for related chronic diseases and for other areas of health and development.

## LEVELS OF MONITORING AND INDICATORS IN A CVD PROGRAM (14)

The CVD monitoring system consists of three types of monitoring that work together to provide the CVD management indicators.

### Health Facility Level

At the health facility level, individual patient monitoring involves monitoring of the health status and the management of a single patient over time, using an individual CVD patient treatment card (e.g., six-monthly control of blood pressure among people treated for hypertension). A facility-based register combines the details of all patients in the facility. Subsets of data from the CVD patient treatment card are extracted and used for program monitoring. The elements of the CVD patient treatment card can also be used to monitor services such as quality of care for hypertension and diabetes, including adherence to medication, follow-up examinations, and end organ damage, depending on the local context.

### Subnational Level

At a subnational level, aggregated data from health facilities can help to assess the outcomes within the program and also monitor availability of medicines. Some elements of quality of care can be assessed at the subnational level using the checklists, for example, control of blood pressure among people with hypertension within the program and availability of core CVD/diabetes drugs for people getting treated.

### Population-Level Monitoring

Population-level monitoring involves surveys in the population at the national or subnational level. Surveys use standardized tools and can provide an estimate of the prevalence of the condition and related parameters, such as the proportion of people receiving medication and the proportion with blood pressure at target, etc. Population-based indicators are a reflection of all interventions and programs in the catchment area. Over time, they can provide trends and will serve as an overall indicator of the effectiveness and coverage of the program.

## ASSESSMENT OF RISK FACTORS FOR CVD PROGRAMS

Risk assessment is central to primary prevention of CVD; a great advance in the prevention of CVD has resulted from the identification of measurable factors that predict the development of CVD. These factors are termed risk factors. This is explained in detail in Chapter 5. Several risk factors are direct causes of CVD; these are termed *major risk factors* and include tobacco smoking, high blood pressure, high serum low-density lipoprotein (LDL) cholesterol, and elevated glucose. A low level of high-density lipoprotein (HDL) cholesterol is also considered a major risk factor because it independently predicts the incidence of CVD (15).

Many prospective epidemiological studies provide estimates of the relative contributions of each major risk factor to CVD risk. Prediction equations have been developed from these estimates and can be used to estimate risk for individuals. Risk estimate based on risk equations is termed total CVD risk (15).

Total CVD risk depends on the individual's particular risk factor profile, sex, and age; it will be higher for older men with several risk factors than for younger women with few risk factors. The total risk of developing CVD is determined by the combined effect of cardiovascular risk factors, which commonly coexist and act multiplicatively. An individual with several mildly raised risk factors may be at a higher total risk of CVD than someone with just one elevated risk factor (16).

## BOX 18.1: EVALUATION FRAMEWORKS

The RE-AIM (Reach, Effectiveness, Adoption, Implementation, and Maintenance) model is intended to guide planning and evaluation of evidence-based interventions that address the different levels of the socioecological model, such as those that target individual health behavior change by increasing intrapersonal, organizational, and community resource support. It has been used to evaluate programmatic and policy interventions addressing a wide range of health conditions (e.g., diabetes, obesity, and hypertension) and health behaviors (e.g., physical activity, dietary behaviors, and smoking) (20).

The PRECEDE-PROCEED model is a cost-benefit evaluation framework that can help health program planners, policy makers, and other evaluators analyze situations and design health programs efficiently. PRECEDE stands for Predisposing, Reinforcing, and Enabling Constructs in Educational Diagnosis and Evaluation. While, PROCEED stands for Policy, Regulatory, and Organizational Constructs in Educational and Environmental Development (21).

## Measurements for Impact

Impact measurement is a concept that can be used for many purposes, at different stages of development initiatives or programs (17). It requires a well-defined theory of change–driven cycle of impact creation (18).

Measurement of a policy or program impact is a genuine desire of all interested parties, but because of complexity, it is also contested by researchers, policy makers, practitioners, and politicians. Moreover, a number of underlying principles drive impact measurement. Health indicators can show the results of health interventions as part of a program, and the monitoring of specific indicators can detect the impact of health policies, programs, services, and actions (1).

The impact of a policy or program can be measured across the domains of process, content, and outcome by understanding the approaches for enhancement of policy adoption, by identifying the elements that result in effectiveness of the policy, and by documenting the potential effects of policy or program implementation. The impact can be measured through various ways and has to include the evaluation design (whether the evaluation was quantitative, qualitative, or a mixed method); the dependent variable; and whether metrics were at an upstream, midstream, or downstream level. It is also important to examine how the measurement properties of the metrics were reported, whether there was specific attention to health disparities, and the presence or absence of economic data (1).

The emerging field of evidence-based public health encompasses individual, group, and policy-level interventions intended to have population-based impact. The social ecological framework suggests that multilevel interventions, especially those that are policy based and focus on "upstream determinants" of health, should be highly effective. Numerous planning and evaluation models have been used to conceptualize and evaluate the impact of public health interventions, including health impact assessment, PRECEDE-PROCEED, and RE-AIM (see Box 18.1). However, the vast majority of empirical applications of these models have been applied to behavior change interventions at the individual and organizational levels (19).

A major consideration in developing better measurements for evidence on policy related to CVD is the complexity of the determinants of CVD. Because of this complexity, policies in multiple sectors have the potential to affect CVD. Therefore, to comprehensively measure policy effects on CVD, there needs to be shared understanding of target outcomes, as well as comparable indicators and integrated measurement approaches to determine the health impact on chronic diseases of policies in areas such as agriculture, urban planning, and development initiatives from donors and governments (1).

## CASE STUDY 1: MILLION HEARTS CVD MODEL

The Million Hearts CVD Risk Reduction Model, run by the Centers for Medicare & Medicaid Services (CMS), seeks to improve cardiovascular care by providing incentives and supports for health care practitioners to engage in patient CVD risk calculation and population-level CVD risk management (22). CMS-enrolled organizations throughout the United States randomly assign half to the intervention and half to a control group. This study is an evaluation of the model and will assess the model impacts on patient outcomes, changes in CVD care processes, and implementation challenges and successes (23).

The evaluation team developed a logic model to guide all aspects of the evaluation. The evaluation team used a logic model to identify (a) specific incentives and supports that should be assessed in the implementation analysis, both the extent to which these supports were used and provider perceptions of them, and (b) core elements of the intervention.

The logic model was also used to identify the short-term and long-term outcomes to conduct impact evaluation. This includes the primary long-term outcomes (for example, incidence of first-time heart attacks and strokes) but also short-term or intermediate outcomes such as increased provider initiation or intensification of statins or other medications.

Once the evaluation team had collected evidence for both implementation effectiveness and outcomes, the team used the logic model to help structure an analysis of what might have driven observed impacts.

## CASE STUDY 2: THE PRECEDE MODEL

The PRECEDE model allows a portrayal of the health problem in which one desires to intervene, which is the first of the six steps of the program-planning framework (intervention mapping): evaluation of needs (diagnostic step). Based on the situational diagnosis, the following steps take place: proposing the matrix of change objectives, selecting the most appropriate theory-based methods and practical strategies, and creating a program to evaluate the results of their actions. The more specific each step of the planning process is, the greater the chances are that the program will be effective in attaining the expected results.

The model was used to guide research and the clinical practice of nurses in the clinical follow-up of patients with CVDs (24).

## CASE STUDY 3: M&E FRAMEWORK FOR HYPERTENSION CONTROL PROGRAMS (25)

The program describes the M&E framework for hypertension control programs, a collaboration between the Pan American Health Organization (PAHO) and the World Hypertension League (WHL). It provides a foundation that allows countries, based on their own resources and priorities, to select indicators for their monitoring and evaluation efforts and strongly recommends the use of the five core indicators of the Global HEARTS CVD management technical package and one additional PAHO-WHL core indicator. The framework is designed to be used at different intervention levels: national, regional, and even at the community or clinic/facility level. The intention is for hypertension programs to select quantitative indicators based on the current surveillance mechanisms that are available and what is feasible and to use the framework process indicators as a guide to program management. Programs may wish to increase or refine the number of indicators they use over time.

## CONCLUSION

A challenge that most LMICs face today is the non-availability of data for M&E of CVD programs comprehensively. There are other issues that relate to monitoring of population-based data. The monitoring process has to be in real time, has to be time efficient, has to achieve good coverage of the population, and has to help establish denominators of those that have CVD disease as well measure multiple risk factors.

The development of an M&E framework includes an understanding of utility as per a hierarchy of indicators, i.e., type of indicators required at various levels of the health system for effective M&E of the program. At higher levels of the health system (state, national), information on outcome and impact of program is most important, while at lower levels (block, district), the input, process, and output indicators, along with the data elements, are required for program management.

Implementing a system for an efficient M&E system of CVD prevention is a continuously evolving project and requires dedicated resources. Integrating the CVD M&E system into a larger NCD framework will make it more acceptable and usable. LMICs need to allocate resources for the creation of such large M&E resource pools.

There is a need for developing capacity for operational research within health ministries and state health departments. M&E experts from medical colleges and schools of public health should be empaneled for technical advice and meaningful, good-quality, publishable research.

## REFERENCES

1. Fuster V, Burke Kelly B, editors. *Promoting cardiovascular health in the developing world: a critical challenge to achieve global health.* Washington, DC: National Academies Press; 2010.
2. World Health Organization. A country-led platform for information and accountability. *A country-led platform for information and accountability* [Internet]. 2011 Nov [cited 2021 Mar 10]. Available from: www.who.int/healthinfo/country_monitoring_evaluation/1085_IER_131011_web.pdf?ua=1
3. Curry DW. Perspectives on monitoring and evaluation. *American Journal of Evaluation.* 2018;40(1):147–150.
4. Greatorex M. Types of measure. *Wiley Encyclopedia of Management.* 2015;9:1–1.
5. Krishnan A, Ritvik, Thakur J, Gupta V, Nongkynrih B. How to effectively monitor and evaluate NCD programmes in India. *Indian Journal of Community Medicine.* 2011;36(5):57.
6. Mckenzie JF, Neiger BL, Thackeray R. *Planning, implementing, and evaluating health promotion programs.* Hoboken: Pearson Higher Education; 2017.
7. Centers for Disease Control. *Framework for program evaluation—CDC* [Internet]. 2019 [cited 2021 Mar 10]. Available from: www.cdc.gov/eval/framework/index.htm
8. Boerma JT, Weir SS. Integrating demographic and epidemiological approaches to research on HIV/AIDS: the proximate-determinants framework. *The Journal of Infectious Diseases* [Internet]. 2005;191(s1):S61–S67. Available from: https://academic.oup.com/jid/article/191/Supplement_1/S61/934944
9. Liehr P, Smith MJ. Middle range theory: Spinning research and practice to create knowledge for the new millennium. *Advances in Nursing Science.* 1999;21(4):81–91.
10. Grant C, Osanloo A. Understanding, selecting, and integrating a theoretical framework in dissertation research: creating the blueprint for your "house". *Administrative Issues Journal Education Practice and Research.* 2014;4(2).
11. Centre for Disease Control. *CDC division for heart disease and stroke prevention state heart disease and stroke prevention program evaluation evaluation guide guide developing and using a logic model department of health and human services centers for disease control and prevention national center for chronic disease prevention and health promotion* [Internet]. [cited 2021 Mar 10]. Available from: www.cdc.gov/dhdsp/docs/logic_model.pdf
12. World Health Organization. *Systems for monitoring* [Internet]. 2018 [cited 2021 Mar 10]. Available from: https://apps.who.int/iris/bitstream/handle/10665/260423/WHO-NMH-NVI-18.5-eng.pdf?sequence=1
13. UNAID Monitoring and Evaluation Division. *An introduction to indicators UNAIDS monitoring and evaluation fundamentals* [Internet]. [cited 2021 Mar 10]. Available from: www.unaids.org/sites/default/files/sub_landing/files/8_2-Intro-to-IndicatorsFMEF.pdf
14. World Health Organization. *Healthy-lifestyle counselling* [Internet]. 2018 [cited 2021 Mar 10]. Available from: https://apps.who.int/iris/bitstream/handle/10665/260422/WHO-NMH-NVI-18.1-eng.pdf?sequence=1&isAllowed=y
15. Smith SC, Jackson R, Pearson TA, Fuster V, Yusuf S, Faergeman O, et al. Principles for national and regional guidelines on cardiovascular disease prevention: a scientific statement from the World Heart and Stroke Forum. *Circulation* [Internet]. 2004;109(25):3112–21 [cited 2020 Dec 8]. Available from: https://pubmed.ncbi.nlm.nih.gov/15226228/
16. World Health Organization. *Prevention of cardiovascular disease guidelines for assessment and management of cardiovascular risk* [Internet]. 2007 [cited 2021 Mar 10]. Available from: https://apps.who.int/iris/bitstream/handle/10665/43685/9789241547178_eng.pdf?sequence=1&isAllowed=y
17. YouMatter. *Impact measurement: what it is and how to measure it?* [Internet]. Youmatter. Available from: https://youmatter.world/en/definition/impact-measurement/
18. Sopact. *Impact measurement—how to measure social impact—sopact* [Internet]. www.sopact.com. Available from: www.sopact.com/social-impact-measurement
19. Jilcott S, Ammerman A, Sommers J, Glasgow RE. Applying the RE-AIM framework to assess the public health impact of policy change. *Annals of Behavioral Medicine.* 2007;34(2):105–114.
20. King DK, Glasgow RE, Leeman-Castillo B. Reaiming RE-AIM: using the model to plan, implement, and evaluate the effects of environmental change approaches to enhancing population health. *American Journal of Public Health* [Internet]. 2010;100(11):2076–2084. Available from: www.ncbi.nlm.nih.gov/pmc/articles/PMC2951937/

21. Phillips JL, Rolley JX, Davidson PM. Developing targeted health service interventions using the Precede-proceed model: two Australian Case Studies. *Nursing Research and Practice* [Internet]. 2012;2012(8):1–8. Available from: https://pdfs.semanticscholar.org/87e0/de2a55ee1e8a5bb1aa4bbe5574f9893ebab0.pdf?_ga=2.216158422.1115552367.1573495507-2071411289.1573495507

22. Conwell L, Barterian L, Rose A, Peterson G, Kranker K, Blue L, et al. *Evaluation of the million hearts ® cardiovascular disease risk reduction model: first annual report* [Internet]. 2019. Available from: https://downloads.cms.gov/files/cmmi/mhcvdrrm-firstann-evalrpt.pdf

23. *Evaluation of the million hearts CVD risk reduction model—Full text view—ClinicalTrials.gov* [Internet]. clinicaltrials.gov. 2019 [cited 2021 Mar 10]. Available from: www.clinicaltrials.gov/ct2/show/NCT04047147

24. Gallani MCBJ, Cornélio ME, Agondi R de F, Rodrigues RCM. Conceptual framework for research and clinical practice concerning cardiovascular health-related behaviors. *Revista Latino-Americana de Enfermagem*. 2013;21(Spe):207–215.

25. Campbell NRC, Ordunez P, DiPette DJ, Giraldo GP, Angell SY, Jaffe MG, et al. Monitoring and evaluation framework for hypertension programs. A collaboration between the Pan American Health Organization and World Hypertension League. *The Journal of Clinical Hypertension*. 2018;20(6):984–990.

# Index

Note: Numbers in **bold** indicate a table. Numbers in *italics* indicate a figure.

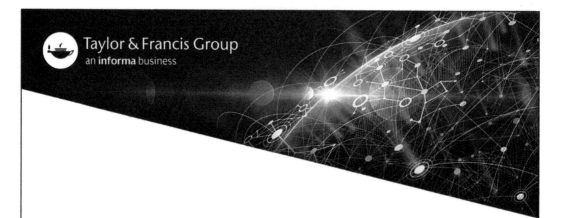

# Taylor & Francis eBooks

## www.taylorfrancis.com

A single destination for eBooks from Taylor & Francis with increased functionality and an improved user experience to meet the needs of our customers.

90,000+ eBooks of award-winning academic content in Humanities, Social Science, Science, Technology, Engineering, and Medical written by a global network of editors and authors.

## TAYLOR & FRANCIS EBOOKS OFFERS:

A streamlined experience for our library customers

A single point of discovery for all of our eBook content

Improved search and discovery of content at both book and chapter level

## REQUEST A FREE TRIAL
### support@taylorfrancis.com

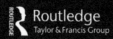

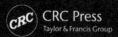